ZONE FOOD BLOCKS

The Quick & Easy, Mix & Match Counter for Staying in the Zone

Barry Sears, Ph.D.

With virtually every food item, prepared meal, and even fast-food take-out items conveniently converted to Zone Food Blocks, staying in the Zone is now easier than ever—at home, at work, and on the go.

Dr. Sears developed the Zone Food Block concept as a quick and convenient way of making Zone meals and snacks. Now, with this completely updated book, virtually every food item, prepared meal, and even fast-food take-out items have been converted to Zone Food Blocks. Simply mix and match the Blocks and making Zone meals becomes incredibly simple.

Dr. Barry Sears is the author of the *New York Times* bestsellers *The Zone* and *Mastering the Zone*. A widely-published scientist and researcher, he lives in Swampscott, Massachusetts with his wife, Lynn, and two daughters, Kelly and Kristin.

ZONE FOOD BLOCKS

ZONE FOOD BLOCKS

The Quick & Easy, Mix & Match Counter for Staying in the Zone

Barry Sears, Ph.D.

ReganBooks
An Imprint of HarperCollinsPublishers

HarperCollins books may be purchased for educational, business, or sales promotional use. For information please write: Special Markets Department, HarperCollins Publishers, Inc., 10 East 53rd Street, New York, NY 10022.

FIRST EDITION

Designed by Anne DeLozier

ISBN 0–06–039242–8

97 98 99 00 01 10 9 8 7 6 5 4 3 2 1

CONTENTS

THIS BOOK is not intended to replace medical advice or be a substitute for a physician. If you are sick or suspect you are sick, you should see a physician. If you are taking a prescription medication, you should never change diet (for better or worse) without consulting your physician, because any dietary change will affect the metabolism of that prescription drug.

Prevention will always be the best medicine. However, prevention can only be undertaken by the individual, and that includes eating correctly. This is the foundation of a healthy lifestyle. You have to eat, so you might as well eat wisely.

Although this book is about food, the author and publisher expressly disclaim responsibility for any adverse effects arising from the use of nutritional supplements to your diet without appropriate medical supervision.

ACKNOWLEDGMENTS

There are a number of people who have made this comprehensive book possible. First and foremost are my wife, Lynn Sears, and my brother, Doug Sears, who have both spent years with me in developing the concept of the Zone and the use of Zone Food Blocks. A special thanks goes to Todd Silverstein for his critical comments and expert editing of this manuscript. I am also very appreciative to Sandy Lampere for her long and often tedious hours of data entry.

But the person most responsible for this book is my publisher, Judith Regan, without whose faith and belief in the Zone, this and all of the preceding Zone books may never have been written.

PART I

Introduction

WHAT IS THE ZONE?

What is the Zone? You have probably heard many things about it. Let me first say what the Zone is not. It is not a high-protein diet, and it is not a high-fat diet, and it is not a high-carbohydrate diet. It is, however, about moderation and balance. Specifically, it's about hormonal balance—keeping hormonal responses (and in particular, the hormone insulin) generated by the food you eat within a zone: not too high, not too low. If insulin levels are too high, you can never access stored body fat for energy. If insulin levels are too low, your cells will starve to death. In essence, when you follow the Zone Diet you are treating food as if it were a drug, giving food the same respect that you would give any prescription drug. This is a revolutionary concept, and this is why the Zone is controversial. When viewed through this prism, food can be your greatest ally or your worst enemy; you just have to know how to play by the hormonal rules that haven't changed in 40 million years and are unlikely to change tomorrow.

WHY IS THE ZONE IMPORTANT TO YOU?

You need the Zone, because your life depends on it. The Zone is about hormonal thinking and how the food you eat controls very powerful hormones that are often hundreds of times more powerful than most prescription drugs. Hormones, which are the chemical messengers of your body, direct every one of your body's vital systems as they can help your body move toward illness and disease or redirect your body towards health. When they are functioning at their best, they can help your body achieve a state of wellness and optimal performance. This is what the Zone Diet is all about. Once you begin to think about food hormonally, you soon realize just how powerful a drug food actually is. This doesn't mean that food has to taste like a drug, but it does mean that it's important to realize that food can have adverse hormonal side effects, such as the overproduction of insulin.

Hormonal thinking is very different than caloric thinking. Caloric thinking can be summarized by this philosophy: "if no fat touches my lips, then no fat reaches my hips." This type of thinking has been the nutritional mantra in America for the past 15 years. During this time, fat has been made to be the villain of our society. Yet in that same 15-year period we have actually been eating less fat than ever before and, in the process, have become the fattest people on the face of the earth (1). What went wrong? Maybe fat is not the demon we have been told. This is why more and more scientists are voicing their doubts in prestigious journals like the *New England Journal of Medicine* in 1997:

> "Replacement of fat by carbohydrate has not been shown to reduce the risk of coronary disease. . . ." (2)

> "Beneficial effects of high-carbohydrate diets on the risk of cancer or body weight have also not been substantiated. . . ." (2)

Or other medical researchers who have stated:

> "The more insulin-resistant the individual, the greater the likelihood that low-fat, high-carbohydrate diets will increase the risk factors for ischemic heart disease." (3)

How could this be if we have been told that eating a high-carbohydrate diet is the key to better health? In essence, these respected scientists are saying the emperor (i.e., the low-fat diet, high-carbohydrate diet) has no clothes. Americans have been sold a pig in a poke for the last 15 years with the expectation that low-fat, high-carbohydrate diets would be the panacea for our health and wellness. The hormonal thinking behind the Zone explains why this hasn't happened. In fact, the general state of health in America is worse now than it was 15 years ago. Fortunately, there is a solution to this health crisis because it can be reversed with the Zone Diet.

ZONE BENEFITS

If dietary fat alone doesn't make you fat (besides not causing heart disease and cancer), then what does? The answer is excess levels of the hormone insulin. The power of the Zone is that this hormone can be controlled by the diet. The Zone is about keeping insulin in a range or zone—not too high, not too low. Not only can keeping insulin in a tight zone prevent you from gaining weight and help you to lose it, but also maintaining insulin in this same zone produces the following benefits:

- Thinking better
- Performing better
- Looking better
- Living better (and longer)

Who doesn't want to experience these benefits? Let's take them one by one.

Thinking Better

Maintaining peak mental acuity is simply a consequence of maintaining stable blood sugar levels. Blood sugar is the metabolic fuel your brain uses to maintain your mental activity. If blood sugar levels drop, then brain function (and your thinking ability) becomes compromised since your brain is running on empty. This is known as low blood sugar. As an example, think about how you feel three hours after eating a big pasta meal. You can barely keep your eyes open, and you find yourself in a dense mental fog. That's an example of low blood sugar. Should your blood sugar levels drop even lower, the brain will actually shut down and go into a coma. This commonly occurs with diabetics who inject too much insulin. Before that drastic step happens, most people will reach for some high-carbohydrate snack that will temporarily increase blood sugar levels, but this simply starts this vicious cycle over again.

What controls your blood sugar levels? It is the amount of insulin in the bloodstream. Insulin is a storage hormone. It tells your body to drive incoming macronutrients (protein, carbohydrate, and fat) into their respective sites for storage so that they can be used at some time in the future. Too much insulin, and you drive down the levels of blood sugar by sending it to the liver and muscles for storage. This is great for those organs, but not too good for the brain. When blood sugar levels drop, clear and concise thought becomes more difficult. I don't care how many Ph.D.'s you have, once low blood sugar sets in, your mental capacity drops like a stone. On the other hand, if you can maintain insulin in the Zone, then you stabilize blood sugar levels, giving you peak mental acuity for four to six hours after your last Zone meal. That's the good news. The bad news is that in order to maintain your insulin levels in that Zone, you must eat another Zone meal every four to six hours. In essence you are treating food as if it were a drug.

Performing Better

The average American male or female carries more than 100,000 stored calories as fat on their body. This is a remarkable amount of energy. In fact it is equivalent to eating 1,700 pancakes for breakfast. The problem is how to access this stored energy for your daily activities. The answer is to lower elevated insulin levels to get into the Zone. Once your insulin levels are in the Zone, it's as if you have a "hormonal ATM" card that allows you to tap into those 1,700 "fat pancakes" throughout the day. On the other hand, if you have high levels of insulin, there is no way you can ever access those "fat pancakes" for energy because elevated insulin blocks the enzyme that is required for their release. And here is another bit of bad news about excess insulin. If you are exercising or doing any physical activity, realize that high levels of insulin decrease oxygen transfer to your muscle cells, thereby building up lactic acid which causes muscle fatigue. So if you want to perform better throughout the day, keep your insulin levels in the Zone.

Looking Better

The loss of excess body fat should be considered a pleasant side effect of being in the Zone. The only way you can lose this extra fat is to lower insulin. Remember insulin is a storage hormone that tells your body to hang onto all the calories it has stored. And these include fat calories stored in your adipose tissue. So in fact, it's not a matter of losing weight but losing excess body fat while retaining your lean body mass. Keep in mind it's your percent body fat that indicates how good you are going to look in a swimsuit. The reason Olympic swimmers look so good in swimsuits is that they have a low percent body fat coupled with good muscle mass. They actually weigh a lot more than a marathon runner but have a lower percent body fat. So if you want to look better, then you have to keep insulin in the Zone.

Living Better (and Longer)

Excess insulin is like a loose hormonal cannon on the deck of a ship because elevated insulin is the primary risk factor associated with heart disease, which remains the number one killer of both males and females in America. Excess insulin also decreases the efficiency of your immune system by increasing the levels of certain hormones (i.e., eicosanoids) that depress the immune system. So, if you want to live better and longer, then it's simply a matter of keeping insulin in the Zone. On the other hand, if you don't have any desire to live better or live longer, then stop reading this book now.

WHAT ARE ZONE FOOD BLOCKS?

Before getting to Zone Food Blocks, you need to learn a bit about nutrition first. For starters, just remember this little rhyme (which is a great oversimplification of nutrition) which says: Protein moves around, and carbohydrates grow in the ground.

Fish move around so they must be protein. Chickens move around, so they must be protein also. So far so good. Now here's the hard part: what's a carbohydrate? Most people will immediately say pasta and sweets. Pasta comes from wheat which grows in the ground, so it must be a carbohydrate. But then broccoli also grows in the ground and so do apple trees. The fact that vegetables and fruits are also carbohydrates is a startling revelation to most Americans. No wonder we are so confused as a nation as to what to eat, since we often don't know what we're eating.

And fat? We have been told that it is the evil incarnate. But actually, there are good fats and bad fats. Bad fats include saturated fat and artificial trans fatty acids. Everyone agrees these should be a minor part of your diet. On the other hand, good fats include monounsaturated fats (like olive oil) and Omega–3 fats (like fish oil). As I will explain later, adding the right type of fat to each meal and snack is critically important for the success of the Zone Diet.

Once you have a clearer conception of what protein, carbohydrate, and fats actually are (and there will always be some exceptions) then you have to deal with the facts that different food items contain at least one (if not more) of these macronutrients (i.e., protein, carbohydrate, and fat) in different densities even if the foods are related to one another. As an example, pasta and broccoli are both carbohydrates. But one cup of cooked pasta contains the same number of carbohydrates as 12 cups of steamed broccoli. Although there will be an obvious difference in the total volume of these items on your plate, they both contain the same amount of carbohydrates. Likewise, 4 ounces of chicken breast will contain the same amount of protein as 12 ounces of tofu. And that's why I developed Zone Food Blocks—so that you can compare the amount of a particular macronutrient in any food ingredient with the quantity of the same macronutrient in another food ingredient. Essentially, using the Zone Food Blocks, all the calculations are done for you. You no longer think about grams or calories but simply the amount of Zone Food Blocks contained in a typical food ingredient. Since most people are not likely to eat more than 20 food items in their entire lives, remembering the sizes of your favorite foods in terms of Zone Food Blocks becomes easier than remembering family birthdays. And because the Zone Food Block system normalizes nutrient density between many foods, you'll have an easy time making Zone meals.

Now let me show how each of these Zone Food Blocks is actually calculated and then why they let you make Zone meals with ease.

PROTEIN

One block of protein equals 7 grams of protein. Don't confuse this with the actual weight of the protein. Most animal protein is found in muscle tissue, and much of that muscle weight is water. As an example, 1 oz of chicken breast is approximately 28 g of total weight, but it contains only 7 grams of protein with the rest being primarily water and small amounts of fat. Using the Zone Food Block method, 1 oz of chicken breast would equal 1 protein block.

   1 oz of chicken breast = 7 g of protein
   7 g protein/7 g of protein per block = 1 protein block

Some sources of protein, however, contain lots of fat and very little protein. A good example is bacon. To get the same amount of protein as found in 1 oz of low-fat chicken breast, you would have to consume 3 oz of bacon. Unfortunately, that amount of bacon would also contain five times as much fat. Obviously, bacon is not a very good source of protein but a tremendous source of fat (and bad fat at that). How can you determine whether a protein is low-fat? In the following guide, all food blocks are rounded to the nearest whole number. Any protein with the number of fat blocks being zero is considered to be low-fat.

CARBOHYDRATES

Carbohydrate blocks are complicated by two factors. The first is the fiber content of the food, and the second is the food's water content. Carbohydrate Zone blocks are based upon the amount of carbohydrate that actually enters the bloodstream and thus stimulates the release of insulin.

Since fiber doesn't enter the bloodstream, you have to subtract out the fiber content of any food in order to determine the amount of insulin-stimulating carbohydrate actually in that food. This is why I define one carbohydrate block as 9 grams of insulin-stimulating carbohydrate. Now you can understand why 3 cups of steamed broccoli has the same amount of insulin-stimulating carbohydrate as ¼ cup of cooked pasta. Although each contains the same amount of insulin-stimulating carbohydrate, the broccoli has lots of water and lots of fiber, whereas the pasta doesn't. The water content also explains why it takes nearly two heads of lettuce to make one carbohydrate block. The lettuce is virtually all water with some fiber to hold it together. That's why it takes a lot of vegetables to make up one carbohydrate Zone Food Block. Fruits generally have less water and less fiber than vegetables, so they are intermediate in volume when calculated in terms of Zone Food Blocks. Finally, starches have very little fiber and virtually no water, so they are extremely carbohydrate-dense, and, as a result, it takes very small amounts of them to constitute one carbohydrate Zone Food Block.

While virtually no protein contains carbohydrates (except for some dairy products and tofu), some carbohydrates do contain small amounts of protein. Moreover, the amounts of protein are very low in comparison to the amount of carbohydrate also contained within the same carbohydrate. Another complicating factor is that the high-fiber content of vegetables prevents a good chunk of that protein from being absorbed. Therefore, you have to reduce the actual amount of protein contained in a carbohydrate source (like beans) to reflect the amount of protein that will be absorbed. On average only 70 to 75 percent of the vegetable protein will be absorbed. I have taken this correction factor into account when calculating the number of protein Zone blocks found in vegetable sources. Although I have incorporated these correction factors, it frankly is just easier to treat vegetables as a great carbohydrate source and plan to get your protein elsewhere. (Note for vegetarians: There are excellent sources of protein-rich vegetarian sources listed in the Protein Zone Food Block section.)

Being aware of the number of carbohydrate blocks in a meal is critical on the Zone Diet because carbohydrates are very potent stimulators of insulin. The Zone Diet is all about insulin control, so any excess consumption of carbohydrates in a meal is the real enemy of the Zone concept. Unfortunately, as if working with carbohydrates wasn't already tricky enough, you also have to take into account the concept known as the glycemic index.

The glycemic index of a carbohydrate measures the rate at which a carbohydrate enters the bloodstream. The faster the carbohydrate enters the bloodstream, the more insulin is secreted. Some simple carbohydrates, such as fructose, enter the bloodstream very slowly, while some complex carbohydrates, such as bread or potatoes, enter the bloodstream very quickly. The Zone Diet is based upon hormonal thinking which strives to keep insulin within a discrete zone throughout the day. Therefore, a Zone meal is not based on whether a carbohydrate is simple or complex but how that carbohydrate will affect insulin production. This is why I like to use the term glycemic load to describe Zone meals. The glycemic load is defined as the amount of total carbohydrate consumed at a meal times the overall composite glycemic index of each of the carbohydrate sources.

Glycemic Load = Total Insulin-Stimulating Carbohydrate
× Composite Glycemic Index

Understanding the concept of the glycemic load means that having small amounts of high-glycemic carbohydrates (like pasta or starches) at a meal is okay as long as most of the carbohydrates in that same meal are coming from low-density and low-glycemic carbohydrates, such as fruits and vegetables. This ensures that the overall composite glycemic load of a meal is not high enough to overstimulate insulin release. Let me give you an example. Black beans have a very low glycemic index, so that should be good for the Zone Diet. Unfortunately, they have a very high amount of total carbohydrates in a small volume. This means you can't eat massive amounts of black beans without causing a significant increase in the glycemic load of a meal. In other words, go easy on eating too many carbohydrates.

FAT

Ironically, although the role of fat has been scorned for the past 15 years, it is one of the most important components of the Zone Diet. Why? There are several hormonal reasons that no one ever appreciated as we began our national fat phobia in 1980s. First, fat supplies essential fatty acids to your diet. These fats are known as polyunsaturated fats and can be categorized in two distinct classes: Omega–6 and Omega–3 fats. Without these essential fatty acids, your body can't make another group of exceptionally powerful hormones called eicosanoids. These hormones exert a significant control on insulin production. Second, fat slows down the rate of entry of any carbohydrate into the bloodstream which further reduces insulin secretion. Third, fat causes the release of a hormonal signal from the gut to tell the brain to stop eating.

Finally, fat makes food taste better. Before you get too excited, let me tell you that like carbohydrates, not all fat is the same. In fact, there are some fats that you definitely want to minimize on the Zone Diet. The first of these is saturated fat. These are the fats that are solid at room temperature. Not surprisingly, excess consumption of saturated fat tends to make your cell membranes have a fluidity similar to molasses. As a result, the receptors for insulin don't work as well, and this forces your body to make even more insulin in order to drive nutrients into cells. And as you now know, the more insulin you make, the fatter you become. Another group of fats to be avoided are called trans fatty acids. These are artificial fats that have been developed by the food industry to improve the shelf life of processed foods. If you see the designation "partially hydrogenated vegetable oil" on a food label, you know it contains these trans fatty acids. The final group of fats you want to moderate are called Omega–6 essential fatty acids. Although these are critical for human health (because they are the building blocks for certain types of eicosanoids), an excess of Omega–6 essential fatty acids can increase insulin levels. By eating low-fat protein, you will consume more than adequate amounts of Omega–6 essential fats.

So when you add fat to your diet (and on the Zone Diet you will), you want it to come from either monounsaturated fats (like olive oil, slivered almonds, and avocados) or Omega–3 fatty acids such as those found in cold-water fish. It should be noted that fish is the only source of protein that is rich in Omega–3 fatty acids, while simultaneously low in Omega–6 fatty acids. This is one reason why a high percentage of fish in your diet is so protective against heart disease (4).

And before you start thinking that the Zone Diet is a high-fat diet, let me point out that a Zone Fat Food Block contains only 3 grams of fat, which isn't very much compared to the 7 grams for a protein block and 9 grams for a carbohydrate block. While fat is important to the Zone Diet, it is not a diet built upon fat gluttony.

So here is your summary of a Zone program: Carbohydrates rarely contain any significant amounts of fat, so consider them to be fat-free. They also contain very small amounts of protein relative to the amount of carbohydrate. So, just to make it simple, consider them also to be protein-free. On the other hand, protein almost always contains some fat. A good rule to follow is that every Zone block of low-fat protein will contain about one-half block of a "hidden" fat. As an example, take chicken breast in which 1 oz of meat will contain one block of protein (7 grams) less than one-half block of fat (1.4 grams). Because I have rounded all the Zone blocks to the nearest whole number, this would show in the following tables as containing zero fat blocks. This means that if you had four Zone Protein Blocks of low-fat protein, this portion would also contain about two Zone Fat Blocks of hidden fat. On the other hand, a high-fat source of protein, like bacon, will contain about 20 fat blocks for the same amount of protein. Not only is bacon a high-fat source of protein but also most of the fat is saturated. Two strikes against bacon. So you can see that bacon is obviously not a high priority item on the Zone Diet.

In my previous books, I took this hidden fat into account to try to make your calculations easier and set a fat block at 1½ grams of fat to counterbalance the same amount of hidden fat in low-fat protein. When the added fat and the hidden fat from the protein were combined, a total of one fat block of 3 grams in the meal would be achieved. With this book, I am being more rigorous and giving the actual amount of fat (at least rounded to the nearest whole number) contained within each protein block. Obviously, the higher the number of the fat blocks within a protein source, the less desirable it is on the Zone Diet.

CHOOSING THE BEST INGREDIENTS FOR ZONE MEALS

In each category of food ingredients I have marked off the preferred choices for Zone meals. This means using low-fat protein for the protein component, low–glycemic load carbohydrates for the carbohydrates, and fats rich in monounsaturated and Omega–3 fats for the fat component. This doesn't mean that other food ingredients can't be used, only that you will be the most successful by primarily using those with the check marks in the Zone-preferred category.

HOW TO MAKE ZONE MEALS

All you have to do is to keep the balance of protein, carbohydrate, and fat blocks in 1:1:1 balance at every meal and snack. You have an infinite number of choices, all based on the foods you like to eat and, therefore, will eat.

Using the Zone Food Block method makes constructing Zone meals easy. You simply keep the number of protein blocks equal to the number of carbohydrate blocks at every meal and snack. As I explained above, although fat has no effect on the hormone insulin, it does have the benefit of (1) making food taste better, (2) slowing down the rate of entry of any carbohydrate into the bloodstream and therefore lowering the insulin response, and (3) sending a hormonal off signal to the brain that says "stop eating." These are three good reasons why you add extra fat blocks to every meal, especially if they are good fats. Every Zone meal should consist of equal numbers of protein, carbohydrate, and fat blocks. It's that simple.

I have found that it may take about two weeks to get the hang of this program as you train your eyes to recognize what a Zone Food Block of your favorite food items actually looks like. I suggest that you go out and buy an inexpensive scale to weigh your protein and a set of inexpensive measuring cups to determine what volumes your carbohydrates actually take up. Once you learn to eyeball the volume of your favorite foods based on Zone Food Blocks, you'll find making Zone meals by sight alone becomes almost foolproof.

To make it even easier in the first couple of weeks, I recommend using the recipes in *Zone Perfect Meals in Minutes* to give you an idea what a four-block Zone meal looks like. One note of caution. The only problem with using low-density carbohydrates like vegetables as your primary source of carbohydrates is that you will have a hard time being able to eat the entire meal. As an example, here is the ingredient list for a four-block meal of Hungarian Chicken which is typical of a Zone meal.

> 4 ounces of chicken tenderloin
> 1¼ cups of chopped tomatoes
> 2¼ cups of green and red pepper strips
> 1 cup of chopped onions
> ¼ cup of chickpeas
> 1⅓ teaspoons of olive oil

Given that this is a serving for one, I'm sure it's not lost on you that given that quantity of vegetables to consume, this will not be an easy meal to finish. This is why your grandmother told you that you couldn't leave the table until you finished your vegetables.

Let's see how these ingredients for Hungarian Chicken can be divided into Zone Food Blocks.

> 4 ounces of chicken tenderloin = 4 Protein Blocks and 2 Fat Blocks
> 1¼ cups of chopped tomatoes = 1 Carbohydrate Block
> 2¼ cups of green and red pepper strips = 1 Carbohydrate Block
> 1 cup of chopped onions = 1 Carbohydrate Block
> ¼ cup of chickpeas = 1 Carbohydrate Block
> 1⅓ teaspoons of olive oil = 2 Fat Blocks

If you add up all of the Zone Food Blocks, here is what you get

Protein = 4 Blocks
Carbohydrate = 4 Blocks
Fat = 4 Blocks

In other words, it's a balanced Zone meal. More importantly, because Zone Food Blocks are interchangeable, you have the ability to make an infinite number of meals using the foods you like to eat. Just make the corresponding change of one Zone Food Block with another Zone Food Block from the same category, and you now have a new meal.

Using Zone Food Blocks you are finally in hormonal control of your diet. Each meal becomes a question of which drug you want to prepare to maintain insulin in the Zone for the next four to six hours. If you think that takes all of the enjoyment out of food, let me remind you that the one region of the world where Zone cooking is commonplace is called France. Gourmet French cooking is really very similar to the Zone in the balance of food blocks at each meal. And no one has ever accused the French of not eating well or not enjoying their food. Maybe that's why they have the lowest rate of heart disease in Europe and actually fit into French designer clothing.

EATING OUT IN THE ZONE

Once you have mastered the volume of various Zone Food Blocks, you can apply this knowledge when you eat out. From your own experience in your kitchen, you will know what the volume of a Zone Food Block looks like. Use that knowledge when you go to any restaurant and make slight adjustments to the meals you are served to transform them into Zone meals. In typical American restaurants, this might mean taking home much of the protein on your plate because there is simply too much of it. But this also means your next meal at home starts off with a great source of protein to which you can add the appropriate numbers of Zone carbohydrate and fat food blocks to make it a great Zone meal. Another good tip is to always ask to replace any starches on the menu with extra vegetables. A great Zone dessert is always fresh fruit. All of a sudden your mega-size American meal is looking more and more like a typical European meal.

FROZEN DINNERS AND FAST-FOOD MEALS

But there are times when you simply don't have time to make a meal at home or sit down at a restaurant. This is why frozen meals in supermarkets and fast-food restaurants are so popular. To make it easier for you, I have included separate sections in this book for frozen dinners and fast-food menus. Just remember that you have to try to maintain an equal number of protein and carbohydrate blocks at each meal. To do this well means learning how to read food labels on the back of any prepared meal.

Food labels are very useful once you convert frozen meals or fast-food meals into Zone Food Blocks. The conversion of a serving size of protein from the typical food label is pretty easy. First, just take the amount of protein and divide by 7 (remember a protein block is 7 grams), then round that number into the most appropriate whole number. As an example, if a serving size contains 7 grams of protein per serving, this means that each serving size contains one protein block. If it contained 10 grams of protein per serving, then divide 10 by 7 to get 1.4 protein blocks. Just round this down to 1 protein block. If the serving size contains 14 grams of protein, then it contains two protein blocks. You don't have to be obsessive about the calculations, just get a rough idea.

Next, divide the total fat content by 3 (3 grams of fat equals one Zone fat block) and then round to the nearest whole number. If you have less than one fat block for every protein block in prepared meals, then you will have to add some extra fat blocks. Just make sure that they are primarily monounsaturated fat because it is generally the easiest fat to add to a meal. Good sources are olive oil, slivered almonds, or guacamole.

Finally, you will have to calculate the carbohydrate blocks. Unfortunately, the food label will have the combination of both insulin-promoting carbohydrate and fiber contained on the total carbohydrate section of the label. Your first task is to subtract the amount of fiber from the total carbohydrate to get the amount of insulin-promoting carbohydrate in a typical serving size. Divide that number by 10 (for some reason dividing by 9 is a difficult process, so just use the number 10) to get the approximate number of carbohydrate blocks. As you did with the protein blocks, just round this number to the nearest whole number.

Now see if the approximate number of protein blocks is equal to the approximate number of carbohydrate blocks and fat blocks in that frozen meal. If so, you have a Zone meal (perhaps not a great tasting Zone meal, but at least a Zone meal). Unfortunately you will probably find that most frozen meals are primarily carbohydrates with small amounts of protein and not enough fat. So to make it a Zone meal you must make some additions, which I will demonstrate with a typical example.

Let's use the food label of the Weight Watchers Low-fat Ravioli to illustrate these points.

Figure 1 Nutritional Label for Low-fat Ravioli

<table>
<tr><td colspan="2">Nutrition Facts
Serving Size 1
Servings 1</td></tr>
<tr><td colspan="2">Amount Per Serving</td></tr>
<tr><td>Calories 220</td><td>Calories from Fat 15</td></tr>
<tr><td colspan="2" align="right">% Daily Value*</td></tr>
<tr><td colspan="2">Total Fat 2g</td></tr>
<tr><td colspan="2">   Saturated Fat 0g</td></tr>
<tr><td colspan="2">Cholesterol 5mg</td></tr>
<tr><td colspan="2">Sodium 450mg</td></tr>
<tr><td colspan="2">Potassium   mg</td></tr>
<tr><td colspan="2">Total Carbohydrate 43g</td></tr>
<tr><td colspan="2">   Dietary Fiber 4g</td></tr>
<tr><td colspan="2">   Sugars 10g</td></tr>
<tr><td colspan="2">Protein 9g</td></tr>
</table>

What a confusing mess. Now let's translate this food label into Zone blocks, starting with the protein first, since the protein content is the core around which every Zone meal is built.

If you divide the protein amount in the stated serving size (9 g) by the amount of protein in one block (7 g), you get approximately one protein block. Now divide the total fat content by 3 to get approximately one fat block. So at least the protein and fat blocks are in the correct ratio.

Finally let's calculate the number of carbohydrate blocks. Although the total carbohydrate content equals 43 grams, we have to subtract out the 4 grams of fiber to get the total amount of insulin-promoting carbohydrate in this serving size which will be 39 grams. Divide this by 10, and you get approximately four blocks of carbohydrate.

So let's look at our meal. This frozen dinner contains one block of protein, one block of fat, and four blocks of carbohydrate. Nowhere near a Zone meal. In fact, this low-fat, high-carbohydrate meal is a surefire way to increase insulin levels.

Now the challenge is to make this hormonal disaster of a meal into a Zone meal. First, you are going to add another three blocks of low-fat protein to it. That could be 3 oz of sliced chicken breast. These three added protein blocks to the one protein block already contained within the meal gives a total of four blocks of protein. So now you at least have an equal number of protein and carbohydrate blocks, even though all the carbohydrate blocks are high-glycemic carbohydrates and thus not the best choices.

Finally, we have to increase the fat content to make this a Zone meal. Since it originally contained only one fat block, you have to add another three fat blocks. Half of those needed extra fat blocks come from the extra 3 oz of chicken breast. So that means you have to add just a dash more of fat. You could add 1 teaspoon of olive oil or ¼ ounce of slivered almonds. This is not a great amount of extra fat, but enough to improve the taste of the meal and give a better hormonal response. Although this frozen dinner is improved hormonally, you probably realize by now that it is probably easier and cheaper to make a Zone meal yourself in your own kitchen.

In addition, there are some frozen dinners and fast-food meals that are pretty close to being in the Zone. These will have equal amounts of protein, carbohydrate, and fat blocks. Let's be frank—these won't be the best-tasting meals, but they can be used in a pinch.

And what about fast-food restaurants? Actually fast-food restaurants have been given a bad rap over the years. They do serve protein in defined sizes (although most of it contains a higher fat content). The only trouble is they also serve amazing amounts of carbohydrate at the same time. Knowing when to hold back the carbohydrates (and if necessary throw out some of them that come with the meal) is the key to eating fast food in the Zone. But there are many examples (especially grilled chicken sandwiches without the mayo) which are surprisingly good and very quick Zone meals. As for other menu items, you have to be a little creative. Let me give you two examples using McDonald's. One might buy two of the cheap hamburgers, then throw away one of the buns, put the two hamburger patties together, and surround them with the remaining bun. Voila. It's a little rich in the saturated fat, but at least it's quick. A better choice would be to purchase the McGrilled Chicken sandwich and a McDonald's salad. Throw away ¾ of the bun, put the grilled chicken breast on the salad, and use the remaining ¼ of the bun for your carbohydrate. Much less saturated fat, but still not the most appealing Zone meal.

Of course the best fast-food restaurant remains the supermarket salad bar where you can load up on precut fresh fruits and vegetables. Then walk over to the deli section to get some low-fat protein, and walk back to the salad bar to add a dash of oil and vinegar salad dressing for the necessary fat. It's quick, it's healthy, and it's in the Zone.

MAKING ADJUSTMENTS TO YOUR MEALS USING ZONE FOOD BLOCKS

Another powerful use of the Zone Food Blocks is to help you convert the meals you already like to eat into Zone meals compatible with your own unique biochemistry. In reality most people tend to eat only about 10 meals at home. How many meals do you really eat for breakfast? For most people, it's probably two. How many do you really eat for lunch? About three. And dinner? Maybe four. That's a total of nine meals. And when you go out to eat, it's probably the same. You eat at your favorite restaurants, eating only your favorite meals. It's just human nature. Using the Zone Food Blocks you can make human nature work in your favor.

First, don't be overly obsessive about how many Zone Food Blocks there are in a meal, but do be very observant about what that meal looked like and how you felt four hours after eating it. If after four hours you have good mental focus and have no hunger (both a consequence of maintaining adequate blood sugar levels), then you know that the meal you ate was a Zone meal. You can come back to that same meal in the same proportions in the future and experience the same druglike benefits of insulin control.

But what if you are hungry less than four hours after eating a meal? Obviously it wasn't a Zone meal. But with some simple adjustments using the Zone Food Blocks you can make it so. Before you make those adjustments you have to ask yourself one other question: Did you feel loopy after the meal or did you have good mental acuity? If you were unable to concentrate (i.e. loopy) or had a hard time staying awake after the meal, this means that the meal you ate four hours earlier had too many carbohydrate blocks for the number of protein blocks in the same meal. This imbalance of carbohydrate to protein blocks had increased insulin levels, and that resulted in reduced blood sugar levels and the corresponding mental fog. Here's the simple adjustment: make the same meal again keeping the same number of protein blocks but decrease the carbohydrate blocks by one. What you are doing is adjusting your hormonal carburetor, which is controlled by the ratio of protein to carbohydrate blocks in a meal.

On the other hand, if you were hungry four hours after a meal, but had good mental acuity, this means you pushed insulin too low with your previous meal. Your adjustment? Maintain the same amount of protein blocks but increase the carbohydrate blocks by one and have the same meal again in a few days. These simple rules are summarized in Figure 2.

By using Zone Food Blocks it becomes very easy to make every meal you eat, both inside and outside your home, hormonally correct.

ZONE COMMANDMENTS

Here are the basic ten Zone commandments. Not only are they easy to remember, but, more importantly, they are easy to follow.

Figure 2   Picture of Hormonal Adjustment Diagnostic

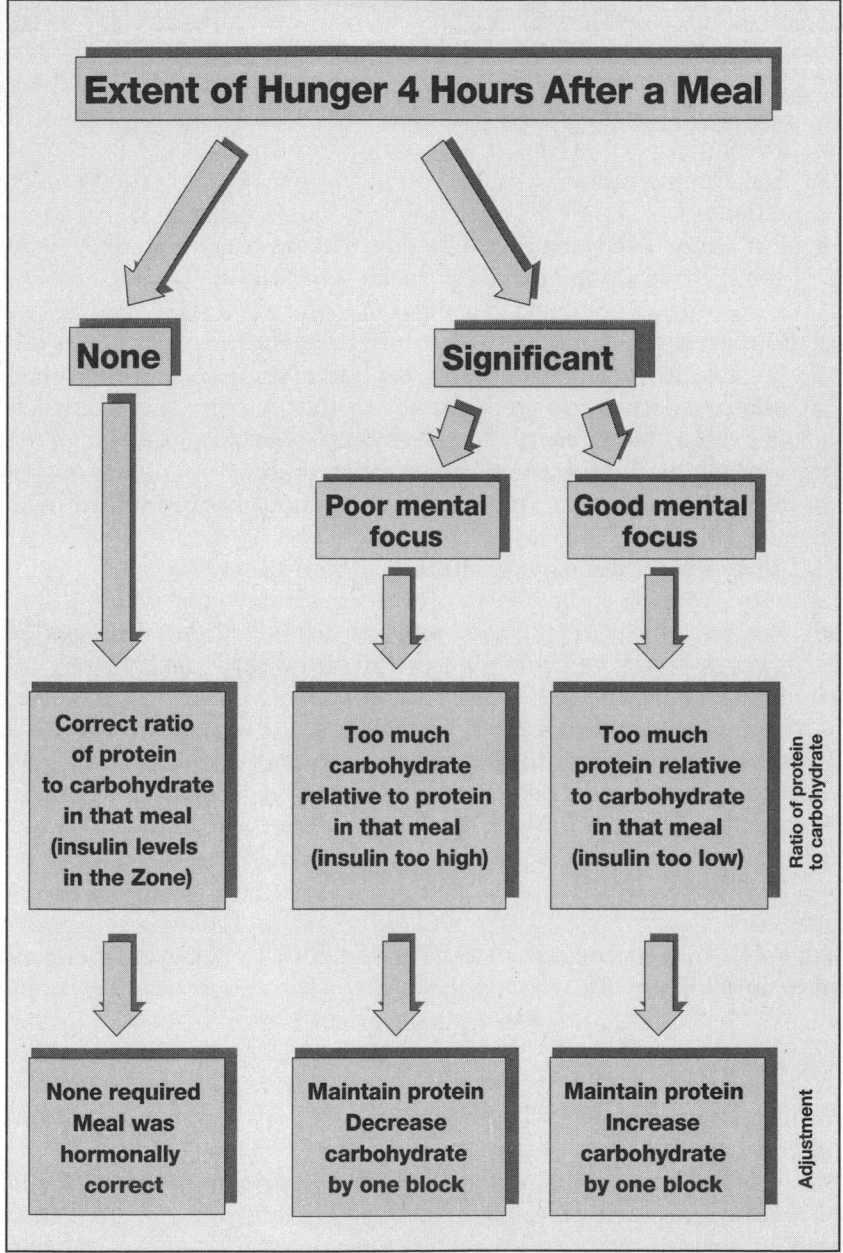

1. Try to make each meal with the same number of protein and carbohydrate Zone blocks. Add an equal number of Zone fat blocks remembering the low-fat protein you are using already contains one half hidden fat block for each block of protein.
2. Read food labels in terms of Zone Food Blocks and make the necessary adjustments with ingredients readily accessible in your kitchen.
3. Make adjustments in meals you like to eat by using the Zone Food Blocks.
4. Eat three Zone meals every day. The average female will need about three Zone blocks per meal, whereas the average male will need four Zone blocks per meal. A Zone meal will control insulin for about five hours.
5. Eat two Zone snacks (one in the late afternoon and the other 30 minutes before you go to bed) every day. A Zone snack consists of one Zone block each of protein, carbohydrate, and fat and will control insulin for approximately two hours.
6. Never let more than five hours pass without having a Zone meal or snack.
7. Always eat a Zone meal within one hour of waking.
8. Drink at least eight glasses of water each day.
9. Forget about guilt. If you make a mistake, then your next Zone meal or snack will get you right back into the Zone.
10. If all else fails, read *Zone Perfect Meals in Minutes*. Learn to use the eyeball method described in that book, and use the recipes like prescription drugs until you get the hang of the program. Then read *Mastering the Zone* that goes into even greater detail of how to use the Zone Food Block method. But continue to use this book as your reference guide for the Zone Food Blocks for virtually every food known.

Once you master the use of Zone Food Blocks, you can make every meal to be Zone appetit.

REFERENCES

1. Heini AF and Weinsier RL. "Divergent trends in obesity and fat intake patterns: the American paradox." *Am J Med* 102: 259–264 (1997).
2. Katan MB, Grundy SM, Willett WC. "Beyond low-fat diets." *N Engl J Med* 337: 563–566 (1997).

3. Jeppesen J, Schaaf P, Jones C, Zhou MY, and Reaven GM. "Effects of low-fat, high-carbohydrate diets on risk factors for ischemic heart disease in postmenopausal women." *Am J Clin Nutr* 65: 1027–1033 (1997).
4. Albert CM, Hennekens CH, O'Donnell CJ, Ajani UA, Carey VJ, Willett WC, Ruskin JN, and Manson JE. "Fish consumption and risk of sudden death." *JAMA* 279: 23–28 (1998).

PART II

Zone Food Blocks for Individual Food Ingredients

I have broken out individual food ingredients that might be a part of any Zone meal into their three respective classes: protein, carbohydrate, and fat. In each section, the size of the ingredient is normalized to provide one block of that particular macronutrient. Here are some helpful hints to make the use of this section easier.

First and foremost, don't be too obsessive about the volume or weight of a particular Zone Food Block. Primarily use them to increase your awareness of the relative amounts of different macronutrients within a food ingredient. In addition, use them to become comfortable with different densities of macronutrients in various food sources. Often you will be surprised at how little food (or in some cases how much as with vegetables) you will need to meet your block requirements for a particular Zone meal.

In the protein section I have included both dairy products and vegetarian sources that are rich in protein. Most proteins will be carbohydrate-free (except for dairy and vegetarian sources), but all protein will contain some fat. Since Zone Food Blocks are rounded to the nearest whole number, if you find a protein ingredient with zero associated fat blocks, then consider it to be a low-fat protein source. All of these low-fat proteins, however, will contain approximately one half block of hidden fat. Just take this into account when making a Zone meal. For vegetarians, any time you see a protein selection surrounded by quotation marks, this is your indication that it is the vegetarian equivalent of that form of animal protein.

For the carbohydrate section, I have taken into account the lowered absorption of vegetable protein compared to animal protein. Most carbohydrates can be considered to be both fat-free and protein-free. However, with the inclusion of the correction factor for decreased protein absorption, it is easier for vegetarians to ensure adequate intake of vegetable protein to meet their protein requirements. I have also included those sauces in this section which are primarily composed of carbohydrates.

Finally, in the fat section the majority of the listings are both protein-free and carbohydrate-free. Furthermore, as you can see, a Zone fat block is not very much in volume or weight. This is because of the high macronutrient density of most fat sources such as nuts and oils. Also included in this section are a number of traditional dips which tend to be very rich in fat.

As you will notice, some of the ingredients in every section can have vastly different volumes based on their nutrient density. Therefore, you may have to convert some of the listed measurements into easier to use amounts for day-to-day cooking. Here are the conversion factors for solid and liquid forms.

LIQUID

  1 cup = 8 fluid ounces
  1 cup = 16 tablespoons
  2 tablespoons = 1 fluid ounce
  1 tablespoon = 3 teaspoons

SOLID

  1 pound = 16 ounces

Please keep in mind there can be differences due to seasonal variations in natural ingredients. Even with the new food labeling laws, changes in packaging and recipes of items may change compared to the values in this book.

Protein Table

FOOD ITEM	SPECIFICATIONS	BRAND NAME	QUANTITY	SIZE	PROTEIN BLOCKS	CARBOHYDRATE BLOCKS	FAT BLOCKS
Abalone	meat only		1.4	oz.	1	0	0
Abruzzese sausage		Boar's Head Cinghiale	0.9	oz.	1	0	3
Anchovy, meat only	Fresh, European, raw		1.3	oz.	1	0	0
	canned, in olive oil drained		0.8	oz.	1	0	1
	canned, in olive oil		6.3	medium	1	0	1
Bacon, Canadian		Boar's Head	1.2	oz.	1	0	1
		Jones Dairy Farm Lean Choice	1.9	slices	1	0	1
Bacon, cooked		Agar Prestige	3.3	slices	1	0	3
		Black Label	2.9	slices	1	0	3
		Black Label Center Cut	5	slices	1	0	3
		Black Label low salt	2.9	slices	1	0	3
		Black Label thin/thin low salt	3.3	slices	1	0	3
		Boar's Head	3.3	slices	1	0	3
		Hormel Microwave	2.9	slices	1	0	3
		Hormel Layout Pack regular/low salt	2.9	slices	1	0	3
		John Morrell Hardwood Smoked	3.3	slices	1	0	5
		Jones Dairy Farm	3.3	slices	1	0	5
		Jones Dairy Farm Thick	2.5	slice	1	0	5
		Old Smokehouse	2.9	slices	1	0	3
		Oscar Mayer	3.3	slices	1	0	3
		Oscar Mayer Thick	1.7	slice	1	0	3
		Oscar Mayer Center Cut	3.3	slices	1	0	2
		Patrick Cudahy	3.3	slices	1	0	3
		Patrick Cudahy Rind	2.9	slices	1	0	4
		Red Label	2.9	slices	1	0	3
		Range Brand Thick	2	slices	1	0	3
		Rock River/Sinnissippi	5	slices	1	0	8
		Sweet Applewood Farms	3.3	slices	1	0	3
Bacon, Irish	precooked	Fast'N Easy	3.3	slices	1	0	3
	back		1.4	slices	1	0	2
"Bacon," vegetarian	frozen	Morningstar Farms Breakfast Strips	6.7	strips	1	0	7
	frozen	Worthington Stripples	6.7	strips	1	0	7

Food	Description	Brand	Amount	Unit			
Beef, round, tip	broiled, lean only		0.9	oz.	1	0	—
	roasted, lean w/fat		0.9	oz.	1	0	—
	roasted, lean only		0.9	oz.	1	0	—
Beef, round, top	broiled, lean w/fat		0.8	oz.	0	0	—
	broiled, lean only		0.8	oz.	1	0	—
	fried, lean w/fat		0.8	oz.	1	0	—
	fried, lean only		0.7	oz.	—	0	—
Beef, shank, crosscuts	braised, lean w/fat		0.8	oz.	0	0	—
	braised, lean only		0.7	oz.	5	0	—
Beef, shortribs	braised, lean w/fat		1.1	oz.	1	0	—
	braised, lean only		0.8	oz.	1	0	—
Beef, sirloin, top	broiled, lean w/fat		0.9	oz.	2	0	—
	broiled, lean only		0.8	oz.	1	0	—
	fried, lean w/fat		0.9	oz.	2	0	—
	fried, lean only		0.8	oz.	1	0	—
Beef, T-bone steak	broiled, lean w/fat		1	oz.	2	0	—
	broiled, lean only		0.9	oz.	1	0	—
Beef, tenderloin	broiled, lean w/fat		1	oz.	2	0	—
	broiled, lean only		0.9	oz.	1	0	—
Beef, top loin	broiled, lean w/fat		1	oz.	1	0	—
	broiled, lean only		0.9	oz.	1	0	—
Beef, canned	corned		1	oz.	1	0	—
	cubed	Goya	0.1	cup	0	0	—
	roast, w/gravy	Hormel	0.2	cup	0	0	—
	brisket, cooked	Libby's	1.3	oz.	1	0	—
	cured	Hormel	1.4	oz.	2	0	—
	sliced	Libby's	0.8	oz.	0	0	—
	rib eye, salted	Hormel	0.9	oz.	1	0	—
Beef, corned	canned	Hormel	1.7	oz.	5	0	—
Beef, dried	canned	Hebrew National	2.1	slices	2	0	—
Beef, refrigerated	canned	Worthington Savory Slices	0.8	pc.	2	0	—
		Worthington Prime Steaks	1	slices	0	0	—
		Worthington Vegetable Steaks			2	0	—
	frozen, corned	Worthington Roll	0.8	3/8" slice		0	—

FOOD ITEM	SPECIFICATIONS	BRAND NAME	QUANTITY	SIZE	PROTEIN BLOCKS	CARBOHYDRATE BLOCKS	FAT BLOCKS
Beef, lunch meat	frozen, corned	Worthington Slices	2.9	slices	1	0	2
	frozen, smoked	Worthington Roll	0.7	3/8" slice	1	0	1
	frozen, smoked	Worthington Sliced	3.8	slices	1	0	1
	corned, cooked	Hebrew National	1	oz.	1	0	0
	corned, cooked, brisket	Boar's Head	1.2	oz.	1	0	1
	corned, cooked, round	Healthy Deli	1.3	oz.	1	0	1
	corned, cooked, round	Hebrew National	1.3	oz.	1	0	1
	cut	Boar's Head Deluxe Low Sodium	1	oz.	1	0	1
	roast	Hormel	1.3	oz.	1	0	1
	roast	Hormel Chuck	1.3	oz.	1	0	2
	roast	Hormel Top Round	1.3	oz.	1	0	0
	roast	Hormel Light & Lean 97	1.4	oz.	1	0	1
	roast	Oscar Mayer Deli-Thin	2.5	slices	1	0	1
	Cajun	Boar's Head	1	oz.	1	0	1
	seasoned	Healthy Deli	1.2	oz.	1	0	1
	Italian	Healthy Deli	1.3	oz.	1	0	1
	top round	Boar's Head No Salt	1	2 oz.	1	0	1
	round	Boar's Head No Salt	1	2 oz.	1	0	1
	round, eye, pepper seasoned	Boar's Head	1	2 oz.	1	0	1
	round, top	Boar's Head Low Sodium	1	2 oz.	1	0	1
Beefalo	meat only, roasted		1.1	oz.	1	0	1
Blood sausage			2.5	oz.	1	0	8
Bluefish, meat only	raw		1.3	oz.	1	0	1
Boar, wild	baked, broiled, or microwaved		1		1	0	0
	meat only, roasted		0.9	oz.	1	0	0
Bologna		Boar's Head	2	oz.	1	0	4
		Boar's Head 28% lower sodium	1.8	oz.	1	0	4
		Healthy Deli Regular/German	1.8	oz.	1	0	1
		95% Fat Free John Morrell	2.2	oz.	1	0	6
		Oscar Mayer	2.5	1-oz. slice	1	0	8

Food	Description	Brand	Amount	Unit			
"Bologna," vegetarian, frozen	beef	Oscar Mayer Fat Free	2.2	slices	0	0	1
	beef	Oscar Mayer Light	2.5	1-oz. slice	3	8	1
	beef	Oscar Mayer Wisconsin Ring	2.2	oz.	6	0	1
	beef	Boar's Head	2	oz.	4	0	1
	beef	Hebrew National	2	oz.	5	0	1
	beef	Hebrew National Lean	1.8	oz.	2	0	1
	beef	Hebrew National Reduced Fat	2.2	oz.	4	0	1
	beef	Oscar Mayer	2.5	1-oz. slice	8	0	1
	beef	Oscar Mayer Light	2.5	1-oz. slice	3	0	1
	garlic	Boar's Head	2	1.5-oz. slice	4	0	1
	garlic	Oscar Mayer	1.4	1.5-oz. slice	6	0	1
	roll	Worthington Bolono	0.7	3/8" slice	1	0	1
	sliced	Worthington Bolono	2.1	slices	1	0	1
Bonito			1	oz.	0	0	1
Brains	meat only, raw		2	oz.	3	0	1
	beef, fried		1.9	oz.	3	0	1
	lamb, fried		3	oz.	2	0	1
	pork, braised		3	oz.	3	0	1
	veal, fried			oz.	3	0	1
Bratwurst	pork, cooked	Boar's Head	1.5	oz.	5	0	1
		Jones Dairy Farm Dinner	0.7	cooked link	3	0	1
Braunschweiger		Jones Dairy Farm Chub	1.5	oz.	3	0	1
		Jones Dairy Farm Chunck	1.8	oz.	5	0	1
	w/bacon	Oscar Mayer	1.7	1-oz. slice	5	0	1
	light	Jones Dairy Farm Chub	1.5	oz.	3	0	1
	light	Boar's Head	1.5	oz.	2	0	1
	light	Jones Dairy Farm Chub	1.4	oz.	1	1	1
	light	Jones Dairy Farm Chunck	1.4	oz.	1	1	1
		Jones Dairy Farm Chunck	1.4	oz.	3	0	1
	w/onion	Jones Dairy Farm Chub	1.5	oz.	4	0	1
	sliced	Jones Dairy Farm	1.7	1.2-oz. slice	5	0	1
	spread	Oscar Mayer	1.8	oz.			1
			1.4	oz.			
Butterfish, meat only	raw						
	baked, broiled, or microwaved		1.1	oz.	1	0	1

FOOD ITEM	SPECIFICATIONS	BRAND NAME	QUANTITY	SIZE	PROTEIN BLOCKS	CARBOHYDRATE BLOCKS	FAT BLOCKS
Carp, meat only	raw		1.4	oz.	1	0	1
	baked, broiled, or microwaved		1.1	oz.	1	0	1
Catfish, channel, meat only	farmed, raw		1.6	oz.	1	0	1
	farmed, baked, broiled, or microwaved		1.3	oz.	1	0	1
	wild, raw		1.5	oz.	1	0	0
	wild, baked, broiled, or microwaved		1.3	oz.	1	0	0
Catfish, frozen	fillets	Delta Pride	1.9	oz.	1	0	0
	nuggets	Delta Pride	1.7	oz.	1	0	2
	steaks	Delta Pride	1.7	oz.	1	0	2
	whole	Delta Pride	1.5	oz.	1	0	1
Caviar	black or red		1.7	Tbsp.	1	0	2
	carp roe	Krinos Tarama	2.5	1 Tbsp.	1	0	0
	lumpfish, black or red	Romanoff	10	2 Tbsp.	1	0	0
	salmon, red	Romanoff	2.5	3 Tbsp.	1	0	3
	whitefish, black	Romanoff	10	4 Tbsp.	1	0	10
Cheese	American processed	Boar's Head Loaf	1.1	oz.	1	0	3
	American processed	Borden	1.7	2/3-oz. slice	1	0	3
	American processed	Borden	1.7	3/4-oz. slice	1	0	3
	American processed	Borden Loaf	1.1	oz.	1	0	3
	American processed	Harvest Moon	1.7	2/3-oz. slice	1	0	3
	American processed	Kraft Deluxe Loaf	1.1	oz.	1	0	3
	American processed	Kraft Deluxe Slice	1.7	2/3-oz. slice	1	0	3
	American processed	Kraft Deluxe Slice	1.7	3/4-oz. slice	1	0	3
	American processed	Kraft Deluxe Slice	1.4	1-oz. slice	1	0	4
	American processed	Old English Loaf	1.1	oz.	1	0	3
	American processed	Old English Slice	1.1	1-oz. slice	1	0	3
	American processed, sharp	Borden	1.1	oz.	1	0	3
	Bel Paese	Medallions	1.9	oz.	1	0	5
	Bel Paese	flavored varieties	1.4	oz.	1	0	4

Food	Brand / Variety	Amount	Unit			PROTEIN
Bel Paese	w/basil, sun-dried tomatoes	1.1	oz.	3	0	1
blue	Kraft	1.1	oz.	3	0	1
blue, crumbled	Sargento	0.3	cup	3	0	1
brick	Kraft	1.1	oz.	3	0	1
Brie		1.3	oz.	4	0	1
butterkase, plain or smoked		1.1	oz.	3	0	1
Camembert		1.3	oz.	3	0	1
cheddar	Boar's Head	0.8	oz.	2	0	1
cheddar	Alpine Lace Reduced Fat	1	oz.	3	0	1
cheddar	Boar's Head Double Glouster	0.8	oz.	3	0	1
cheddar	Cracker Barrel 1/3 Less Fat	1	oz.	2	0	1
cheddar	Dorman	0.8	oz.	3	0	1
cheddar	Dorman Reduced Fat	1	oz.	2	0	1
cheddar	Heluva Good Low Sodium	1	oz.	3	0	1
cheddar	Kraft Cracker Barrel	0.8	oz.	3	0	1
cheddar, mild	Kraft 1/3 Less Fat	1	oz.	2	0	1
cheddar, mild	Heluva Good Reduced Fat	0.9	oz.	2	0	1
cheddar, mild	Weight Watchers Low Sodium	8	oz.	2	0	1
cheddar, mild, light, snack	MooTown Snackers	0.9	oz.	1	0	1
cheddar, mild or sharp	Weight Watchers	1.1	oz.	2	0	1
cheddar, mild or sharp	MooTown Snackers	1	oz.	4	0	1
cheddar, mild, sharp, or extra sharp	Heluva Good	1	oz.	3	0	1
cheddar, sharp	Boar's Head Slicing	1	oz.	3	0	1
cheddar, sharp	Kraft Less Fat	0.8	oz.	2	0	1
cheddar, sharp	Sargento Sliced	1.1	oz.	3	0	1
cheddar, nacho w/peppers	Kraft	1	oz.	3	0	1
cheddar, shredded	Kraft	0.3	cup	3	0	1
cheddar, shredded, fat free	Kraft Healthy Favorites	0.2	cup	0	0	1
cheddar, shredded, fine	Kraft	0.4	cup	4	0	1
cheddar, shredded, mild	Kraft 1/3 Less Fat	0.2	cup	1	0	1
cheddar, shredded, mild	Sargento Preferred Light	0.2	cup	2	0	1
cheddar, shredded, mild or sharp	Sargento	0.3	cup	3	0	1
cheddar, shredded, sharp	Cracker Barrel 1/3 Less Fat	0.2	cup	2	0	1
Cheshire		1.1	oz.	3	0	1
Colby	Alpine Lace Reduced Fat	0.8	oz.	2	0	1

FOOD ITEM	SPECIFICATIONS	BRAND NAME	QUANTITY	SIZE	PROTEIN BLOCKS	CARBOHYDRATE BLOCKS	FAT BLOCKS
Colby		Dorman Sandwich	1	oz.	1	0	3
		Kraft	1	oz.	1	0	3
		Kraft 1/3 Less Fat	0.8	oz.	1	0	2
		Sargento Sliced	1.1	oz.	1	0	3
	Colby, mild	Heluva Good Longhorn	1	oz.	1	0	3
	Colby Jack	Heluva Good	1.1	oz.	1	0	3
	Colby Jack, shredded	Sargento	0.3	cup	1	0	3
	Colby Jack, snack	MooTown Snackers	1.1	oz.	1	0	4
	Colby Monterey Jack	Kraft	1	oz.	1	0	3
	Colby Monterey Jack, shredded	Kraft	0.3	cup	1	0	3
	cottage, nonfat	Knudsen Free	0.2	cup	1	0	0
	cottage, nonfat	Light 'n Lively Free	0.3	cup	1	0	0
	cottage, 4%	Breakstone's	0.3	cup	1	0	1
	cottage, 4%	Sealtest	0.3	cup	1	0	1
	cottage, 4%, large curd	Knudsen	0.2	cup	1	0	1
	cottage, 4%, small curd	Knudsen	0.2	cup	1	0	1
	cottage, 4%, dry curd	Breakstone's	0.5	cup	1	0	0
	cottage, lowfat, 2%	Breakstone's	0.3	cup	1	0	1
	cottage, lowfat, 2%	Knudsen	0.2	cup	1	0	0
	cottage, lowfat, 2%	Sealtest	0.3	cup	1	0	1
	cottage, lowfat, 2%	Weight Watchers	0.3	cup	1	0	1
	cottage, lowfat, 1%	Light 'n Lively	0.3	cup	1	0	1
	cottage, lowfat, 1%	Weight Watchers	0.3	cup	1	0	0
	cottage, lowfat, garden salad 1 %	Light 'n Lively	0.3	cup	1	1	1
	cottage, lowfat, peach 1.5%	Knudsen	2.5	oz.	1	1	1
	cottage, lowfat, peach and pineapple, 1%	Light 'n Lively	0.6	oz.	1	1	0
	cottage, lowfat, pineapple 1.5%	Knudsen	2.5	oz.	1	1	1
	cottage, lowfat, strawberry 1.5%	Knudsen	2.5	oz.	1	1	1

Food	Brand	Amount	Unit			
cottage, lowfat, tropical fruit	Knudsen	2.5	oz.	1	1	1
Edam	Boar's Head	1	oz.	1	0	2
Edam	Dorman Sliced	1	oz.	1	0	2
farmer	Kraft	1.1	oz.	1	0	3
farmer	Western Creamy	2.6	oz.	1	0	3
farmer, dry	Western Creamy Fat Free	1.3	oz.	1	0	0
feta	Alpine Lace Reduced Fat	1.4	oz.	1	0	1
feta	Classika Portions	1.1	oz.	1	0	3
feta	Krinos Imported	1.4	oz.	1	0	4
fontina	Classica	1	oz.	1	0	3
goat, hard type		0.8	oz.	1	0	3
goat, semisoft type		1.1	oz.	1	0	3
goat, soft type		1.3	oz.	1	0	3
Gorgonzola	Galbani Dolcelatte	1.4	oz.	1	0	4
Gouda	Boar's Head	1.1	oz.	1	0	3
Gouda	Dorman Sliced	1	oz.	1	0	3
Gouda	Kraft	1	oz.	1	0	3
Gruyerre		0.8	oz.	1	0	3
Havarti	Boar's Head	1.1	oz.	1	0	3
Havarti	Dorman Sliced	1	oz.	1	0	4
Havarti	Kraft Casino	1.1	oz.	1	0	2
hot pepper	Alpine Lace	1.1	oz.	1	0	3
Italian	Classica Italian	1.1	oz.	1	0	0
Italian style, grated	Kraft 1/3 Less Fat	6.7	tsp.	1	0	2
Italian style, shredded	Sargento Recipe Blend	0.3	cup	1	0	2
Jarlsberg	Sargento	0.8	1.2-oz. slice	1	0	3
	Laughing Cow Babybel	7.8	oz.	1	0	3
	Laughing Cow Babybel Mini	1.4	oz.	1	0	3
	Laughing Cow Original Wedge	1.7	3/4-oz. pc.	1	0	3
limburger	Kraft Mohawk Valley	1.1	oz.	1	0	3
Mexican, 4, shredded	Sargento Recipe Blend	0.3	cup	1	0	3
Monterey Jack	Boar's Head	1.1	oz.	1	0	3
Monterey Jack	Dorman	1	oz.	1	0	3
Monterey Jack	Dorman	1.1	oz.	1	0	3
Monterey Jack	Dorman Reduced Fat	0.8	oz.	1	0	2
Monterey Jack	Dorman Reduced Fat	0.8	oz.	1	0	1

FOOD ITEM	SPECIFICATIONS	BRAND NAME	QUANTITY	SIZE	PROTEIN BLOCKS	CARBOHYDRATE BLOCKS	FAT BLOCKS
	Monterey Jack	Heluva Good	1.1	oz.	1	0	3
	Monterey Jack	Kraft	1.1	oz.	1	0	3
	Monterey Jack	Kraft 1/3 Less Fat	0.8	oz.	1	0	2
	Monterey Jack	Sargento Sliced	1.1	oz.	1	0	3
	Monterey Jack	Weight Watchers	0.9	cup	1	1	2
	Monterey Jack, shredded	Dorman	0.3	cup	1	0	2
	Monterey Jack, shredded	Kraft	0.3	cup	1	0	3
	Monterey Jack, shredded	Sargento	0.3	cup	1	0	3
	Monterey Jack, jalapeno	Boar's Head	1.1	oz.	1	0	3
	Monterey Jack, jalapeno	Heluva Good	1	oz.	1	0	3
	Monterey Jack, jalapeno	Kraft	1	oz.	1	0	3
	Monterey Jack, peppers	Kraft 1/3 Less Fat	0.9	oz.	1	0	2
	mozzarella	Boar's Head	1.1	oz.	1	0	2
	mozzarella	Polly-O Fat Free	1	oz.	1	0	2
	mozzarella	Polly-O Fior Di Latte	1.4	oz.	1	0	3
	mozzarella	Polly-O Lite	1	oz.	1	0	1
	mozzarella, whole milk	Heluva Good	1.1	oz.	1	0	2
	mozzarella, whole milk	Polly-O	1.1	oz.	1	0	2
	mozzarella, part skim	Alpine Lace Reduced Fat	1	oz.	1	0	2
	mozzarella, part skim	Dorman	0.9	oz.	1	0	2
	mozzarella, part skim	Heluva Good	1.1	oz.	1	0	2
	mozzarella, part skim	Kraft	0.9	oz.	1	0	2
	mozzarella, part skim	Polly-O	0.2	cup	1	0	2
	mozzarella, sliced	Sargento	1	oz.	1	0	2
	mozzarella, sliced	Sargento Preferred Light	1	oz.	1	0	1
	mozzarella, shredded	Sargento	0.3	cup	1	0	2
	mozzarella, shredded	Sargento Preferred Light	0.2	cup	1	0	1
	mozzarella, shredded, whole milk	Kraft	0.3	cup	1	0	2
	mozzarella, shredded, whole milk	Polly-O	0.3	cup	1	0	2
	mozzarella, shredded, part skim	Kraft	0.2	cup	1	0	2

	Brand	Amount	Unit			
mozzarella, shredded, part skim	Kraft 1/3 Less Fat	0.2	cup	1	0	2
mozzarella, shredded, part skim	Polly-O	0.2	cup	1	0	2
mozzarella, shredded, part skim, fine	Kraft	0.3	cup	1	0	2
mozzarella, shredded, fat free	Kraft Healthy Favorites	0.2	cup	1	0	0
mozzarella, shredded, fat free	Polly-O	0.2	cup	1	0	0
mozzarella, shredded, light	Polly-O Lite	0.2	cup	1	0	1
Muenster	Alpine Lace Reduced Sodium	1	oz.	1	0	3
Muenster	Boar's Head	1.1	oz.	1	0	3
Muenster	Boar's Head Low Sodium	1.1	oz.	1	0	3
Muenster	Dorman	1.1	oz.	1	0	3
Muenster	Dorman	1.1	oz.	1	0	3
Muenster	Dorman Reduced Fat	0.9	oz.	1	0	2
Muenster	Dorman Reduced Sodium	1.1	oz.	1	0	3
Muenster	Heluva Good	1.1	oz.	1	0	3
Muenster	Kraft	1.1	oz.	1	0	3
Muenster	Sargento Sliced	1.1	oz.	1	0	3
Neufchatel	Philadelphia Brand	2.5	oz.	1	0	5
Parmesan, grated	Classica	3.3	Tbsp.	1	0	3
Parmesan, grated	Kraft	3.3	Tbsp.	1	0	0
Parmesan, grated	Kraft Italian Blend	6.7	tsp.	1	0	3
Parmesan, grated	Polly-O	5	tsp.	1	0	3
Parmesan, grated	Sargento	6.7	tsp.	1	0	3
Parmesan, shredded	Classica	0.8	cup	1	0	3
Parmesan, shredded	Kraft	3.3	Tbsp.	1	0	3
Parmesan, shredded	Sargento	6.7	tsp.	1	0	0
Parmesan-Romano, grated	Sargento	0.2	cup	1	0	3
Parmesan-Romano, shredded	Sargento	3.3	Tbsp.	1	0	2
pimiento, processed	Kraft Deluxe	0.2	oz.	1	0	3
pizza, shredded	Sargento	1.1	cup	1	0	2
pizza, shredded	Sargento Pizza Double Cheese	0.3	cup	1	0	2

PROTEIN

FOOD ITEM	SPECIFICATIONS	BRAND NAME	QUANTITY	SIZE	PROTEIN BLOCKS	CARBOHYDRATE BLOCKS	FAT BLOCKS
	pizza, shredded, cheddar, mild, and mozzarella	Kraft	0.3	cup	1	0	2
	pizza, shredded, four cheese	Kraft	0.3	cup	1	0	2
	pizza, shredded, mozzarella and cheddar	Kraft	0.3	cup	1	0	3
	pizza, shredded, mozzarella and smoke provolone	Kraft	0.3	cup	1	0	2
	Port du Salut		1	oz.	1	0	3
	provolone	Alpine Lace Reduced Fat	0.8	oz.	1	0	2
	provolone	Boar's Head	1	oz.	1	0	3
	provolone	Dorman	1	oz.	1	0	3
	provolone	Dorman Reduced Fat	0.8	oz.	1	0	1
	provolone	Sargento Sliced	1	oz.	1	0	3
	provolone, smoke flavor	Kraft	1	oz.	1	0	2
	ricotta	Breakstone's	0.3	cup	1	0	3
	ricotta	Polly-O Light	0.2	cup	1	0	1
	ricotta	Sargento Light	0.4	cup	1	0	1
	ricotta	Sargento Old Fashioned	0.3	cup	1	0	2
	ricotta, whole milk		0.3	cup	1	0	3
	ricotta, whole milk	Polly-O	0.3	cup	1	0	3
	ricotta, part skim	Polly-O	0.2	cup	1	0	2
	ricotta, part skim	Sargento	0.3	cup	1	0	2
	ricotta, fat free	Polly-O	0.2	cup	1	0	0
	Romano, grated	Kraft	6.7	tsp.	1	0	3
	Romano, grated, dry	Classica Pecorino	10	Tbsp.	1	0	10
	Romano, grated, fresh	Classica Pecorino	10	Tbsp.	1	0	10
	Romano, shredded	Classica Pecorino	10	Tbsp.	1	0	10
	Romano-Parmesan, grated	Polly-O	6.7	tsp.	1	0	3
	Roquefort		1.1	oz.	1	0	3
	string	Polly-O	1	oz.	1	0	2
	string	Polly-O Light Mozzarella	1	oz.	1	0	1
	string, snack	Polly-O	0.8	oz.	1	0	1
	string, snack	Handi-Snacks/Kraft	1	pc.	1	0	2

		Amount	Unit			PROTEIN
string, snack	MooTown Snackers	0.9	oz.	1	0	2
string, snack, light	MooTown Snackers	0.8	oz.	1	0	1
Swiss	Alpine Lace Reduced Fat	0.9	oz.	1	0	2
Swiss	Boar's Head Domestic	0.9	oz.	1	0	3
Swiss	Boar's Head Gold Label Imported	0.9	oz.	1	0	3
Swiss	Boar's Head No Salt	0.9	oz.	1	0	3
Swiss	Borden	1	oz.	1	0	3
Swiss	Dorman	0.9	oz.	1	0	2
Swiss	Dorman Low Sodium	0.9	oz.	1	0	2
Swiss	Dorman Reduced Fat	0.8	oz.	1	0	1
Swiss	Dorman Sandwich	0.9	oz.	1	0	3
Swiss	Dorman Very Low Sodium	0.9	oz.	1	0	3
Swiss	Kraft	0.9	oz.	1	0	3
Swiss	Sargento Sliced	0.8	oz.	1	0	2
Swiss	Sargento Preferred Light Sliced	0.8	oz.	1	0	1
Swiss	Sargento Wafer Thin Sliced	1.8	slices	1	0	3
Swiss, baby	Boar's Head	1	oz.	1	0	3
Swiss, baby	Kraft Cracker Barrel	1	oz.	1	0	3
Swiss, processed	Kraft Deluxe	1.4	3/4-oz. slice	1	0	2
Swiss, processed	Kraft Deluxe	1	oz.	1	0	3
Swiss, shredded	Kraft	0.2	cup	1	0	3
Swiss, shredded	Sargento	0.2	cup	1	0	3
taco, shredded	Sargento	0.3	cup	1	0	2
taco, shredded	Sargento Preferred Light	0.2	cup	1	0	3
taco, shredded, cheddar and Monterey Jack	Kraft	0.2	cup	1	0	3
taco, shredded, nacho and taco	Sargento	0.3	cup	1	0	3
"Cheese," nondairy substitute						
all varieties	Tal-Fino Taleggio	0.4	cup	1	0	4
all varieties	Sandwich Mate	2.5	.7 oz. slice	1	0	5
all varieties	Smart Beat	1.1	oz.	1	0	0
all varieties	AlmondRella	1.4	oz.	1	0	1
all varieties	TofuRella	1.4	oz.	1	0	3
all varieties	Zero-FatRella	1	oz.	1	0	0
American flavor	Borden	2.5	slice	1	0	5

FOOD ITEM	SPECIFICATIONS	BRAND NAME	QUANTITY	SIZE	PROTEIN BLOCKS	CARBOHYDRATE BLOCKS	FAT BLOCKS
	American flavor	Cheeztwo/Sandwich-Mate	2.5	slice	1	0	5
	American flavor	Golden Image	1.1	oz.	1	0	3
	American flavor	Lunchwagon	1.7	oz.	1	0	5
	American flavor	Lunchwagon	1.3	oz.	1	0	3
	American flavor	Smart Beat Fat Free	1.1	oz.	1	0	0
	American flavor, shredded	Harvest Moon	0.3	cup	1	0	3
	cheddar flavor, mellow	Smart Beat	1.1	oz.	1	0	0
	cheddar flavor, sharp	Smart Beat	1.1	oz.	1	0	0
	cheddar flavor, shredded	Harvest Moon	0.3	cup	1	0	3
	cheddar flavor, shredded	Sargento	0.4	cup	1	0	3
	Jamaican Jack style	HempRella	1	oz.	1	0	1
	Monterey Jack	Borden	1.1	oz.	1	0	2
	mozzarella, shredded	Borden	1.1	oz.	1	0	2
	mozzarella, shredded	Harvest Moon	0.2	cup	1	0	3
	mozzarella, shredded	Sargento	0.3	cup	1	0	2
	mozzarella, shredded, imitation	Borden	1.7	oz.	1	0	5
	Swiss	Borden	2.5	slice	1	0	5
	American	Heluva Good	1.7	oz.	1	0	3
	American	Kraft Singles	1.7	2/3-oz. slice	1	0	3
	American	Kraft Singles	1.7	3/4-oz. slice	1	0	3
	American	Kraft Singles	1.1	1.2-oz. slice	1	0	3
	American, grated	Kraft	10	Tbsp.	1	0	10
	American, sharp	Borden	1.4	oz.	1	0	4
	cheddar, sharp	Cracker Barrel	2.9	Tbsp.	1	0	4
	cheddar, sharp	Kaukauna Premium Blend	1.4	oz.	1	0	3
	cheddar, sharp	Kaukauna Lite 50	1.4	oz.	1	1	1
	cheddar, sharp or extra sharp	Kaukauna	1.4	oz.	1	0	3
	cheddar, extra sharp	Cracker Barrel	2.9	Tbsp.	1	0	4
	w/garlic	Kraft	1.4	oz.	1	0	3
	w/jalapenos	Kraft	1.4	oz.	1	0	3
	w/jalapenos	Kraft Mexican Singles	1.7	3/4-oz. slice	1	0	3

Category	Description	Item			Protein		
	w/jalapenos, shredded, hot	Velveeta Mexican	0.2	cup	1	0	3
	w/jalapenos, shredded, mild	Velveeta Mexican	0.2	cup	1	0	3
	Monterey	Kraft Singles	1.7	3/4-oz. slice	1	0	3
	w/pimento	Kraft Singles	1.7	2/3-oz. slice	1	0	3
	w/pimento	Kraft Singles	1.7	3/4-oz. slice	1	0	3
	port wine	Kaukauna	1.4	oz.	1	0	3
	port wine	Kaukauna Premium Blend	1.4	oz.	1	0	3
	port wine	Kaukauna Lite	1.4	oz.	1	1	1
	port wine	Wispride Cup	3.3	Tbsp.	1	0	3
	port wine	Wispride Light Cup	2.9	Tbsp.	1	1	1
	sharp	Kraft Singles	1.7	3/4-oz. slice	1	0	3
	shredded	Velveeta	0.2	cup	1	0	3
	smoke flavor	Kaukauna Smokey	1.4	oz.	1	0	3
	smoke flavor	Kaukauna Lite 50 Smokey	1.4	oz.	1	1	1
	Swiss	Borden	1.7	slice	1	0	3
	Swiss	Kraft Singles	1.7	3/4-oz. slice	1	0	3
	Swiss, almond	Kaukauna	1.4	oz.	1	0	3
	Swiss, almond	Kaukauna Lite 50	1.4	oz.	1	1	1
	sharp	Wispride	3.3	Tbsp.	1	0	5
Cheese nut log	all varieties	Borden Fat Free	1.1	slice	1	1	0
Cheese products		Cheez Whiz Light	3.3	Tbsp.	1	0	0
		Kraft Free Singles	1.4	2/3-oz. slice	1	0	0
		Kraft Free Singles	1.4	3/4-oz. slice	1	0	1
		Velveeta Light	1.1	oz.	1	1	0
	all varieties	Lite-Line	1.7	7-oz. slice	1	0	2
	American flavor	Alpine Lace	1.1	oz.	1	0	0
	American flavor	Alpine Lace Nonfat	0.9	oz.	1	2	0
	American flavor	Alpine Lace Nonfat	1.4	3/4-oz. slice	1	0	0
	American flavor	Borden Fat Free	1.4	3/4-oz. slice	1	1	1
	American flavor	Borden Light	1.4	3/4-oz. slice	1	0	0
	American flavor	Borden Lowfat	1.7	slice	1	1	2
	American flavor	Harvest Moon	1.1	oz.	1	0	3
	American flavor	Kraft Deluxe 25% Less Fat	1.7	3/4-oz. slice	1	0	1
	American flavor	Kraft Singles Less Fat	1.4	3/4-oz. slice	1	0	1
	American flavor	Light n' Lively 50% Less Fat	1.4	3/4-oz. slice	1	0	1
	American flavor	Light n' Lively White 50% Less Fat	1.4	3/4-oz. slice	1	0	1

PROTEIN

FOOD ITEM	SPECIFICATIONS	BRAND NAME	QUANTITY	SIZE	PROTEIN BLOCKS	CARBOHYDRATE BLOCKS	FAT BLOCKS
	cheddar flavor	Alpine Lace Nonfat	0.9	oz.	1	0	0
	cheddar flavor, all varieties	Spreadery	2.9	Tbsp.	1	0	3
	cheddar flavor, sharp	Kraft Singles 1/3 Less Fat	1.4	3/4-oz. slice	1	0	1
	cheddar flavor, sharp	Kraft Free Singles	1.4	3/4-oz. slice	1	0	0
	mozzarella	Alpine Lace Nonfat	0.9	oz.	1	0	0
	Neufchatel, garlic herb	Spreadery	5	Tbsp.	1	0	5
	Neufchatel, ranch	Spreadery	5	Tbsp.	1	0	5
	Neufchatel, vegetable	Spreadery	5	Tbsp.	1	0	5
	pimiento	Spreadery	3.3	Tbsp.	1	0	5
	Swiss flavor	Kraft Singles Less Fat	1.4	3/4-oz. slice	1	0	1
	Swiss flavor	Kraft Free Singles	1.4	3/4-oz. slice	1	0	0
	zesty	Manischewitz Gold/Brine	1.4	ball	1	0	1
Chicken, fresh	broiler-fryer, roasted, w/skin		0.9	oz.	1	0	1
	broiler-fryer, roasted, w/skin		1	oz.	1	0	1
	broiler-fryer, roasted, meat only		0.8	oz.	1	0	1
	broiler-fryer, roasted, meat only, chopped or diced		0.2	cup	1	0	1
	broiler-fryer, roasted, skin only		1	oz.	1	0	4
	broiler-fryer, roasted, dark meat only		0.3	oz.	1	0	1
	broiler-fryer, roasted, light meat only		0.2	oz.	1	0	0
	broiler-fryer, roasted, breast, w/skin		0.9	oz.	1	0	1
	broiler-fryer, roasted, drumstick, w/skin		0.9	oz.	1	0	1
	broiler-fryer, roasted, leg w/skin		1	oz.	1	0	1
	broiler-fryer, roasted, thigh w/skin		1.1	oz.	1	0	2
	broiler-fryer, roasted, wing, w/skin		1.2	oz.	1	0	2

Category	Description	Brand	Amount	Unit			
	capon roasted w/skin		0.1	lbs.	1	0	1
	capon roasted w/skin		0.8	oz.	1	0	1
	roaster, roasted, w/skin		0.1	lb.	1	0	1
	roaster, roasted, meat w/skin		1	oz.	1	0	2
	stewing, stewed, w/skin		0.9	oz.	1	0	2
	stewing, stewed, meat w/skin		1	oz.	1	0	1
	stewing, stewed, meat only		0.8	oz.	1	0	1
	stewing, stewed, meat only, chopped or diced		0.2	cup	1	0	1
Chicken, canned, chunk	breast	Hormel	1	oz.	1	0	1
	breast	Swanson	2	oz.	1	0	1
	broth	Hormel	1	oz.	1	0	1
	broth	Hormel No Salt	1	oz.	1	0	1
	water	Swanson Mixin'	2	oz.	1	0	1
	white	Swanson Premium	5	oz.	1	0	1
	white	Swanson	5	oz.	1	0	2
	white, in water	Swanson Premium	2	oz.	1	0	2
Chicken, ground	raw	Perdue	1.3	oz.	1	0	1
	raw	Perdue Burger	2	oz.	1	0	2
	cooked	Perdue	2	oz.	1	0	2
	cooked	Perdue Burger	1.5	oz.	1	0	3
Chicken, refrigerated or frozen	whole, cooked, dark meat	Perdue Oven Stuffer	1	oz.	1	0	2
	whole, cooked, white meat	Perdue	1	oz.	1	0	1
	whole, cooked, white meat	Perdue Oven Stuffer	1.3	oz.	1	0	1
	barbecued	Empire Kosher	1.3	oz.	1	0	2
	breast raw, halves	Tyson	1	oz.	1	0	1
	breast raw, halves, skinless	Tyson	1.3	oz.	1	0	0
	breast raw, quarters	Tyson	1	oz.	1	0	2
	breast, raw, boneless	Perdue	1	oz.	1	0	0
	breast, raw, boneless	Perdue Family Pack	1	oz.	1	0	0
	breast, raw, boneless	Perdue Oven Stuffer	1	oz.	1	0	0
	breast, raw, boneless, tenderloins	Perdue	1	oz.	1	0	0
	breast, raw, boneless, tenderloins	Tyson	1	oz.	1	0	0

FOOD ITEM	SPECIFICATIONS	BRAND NAME	QUANTITY	SIZE	PROTEIN BLOCKS	CARBOHYDRATE BLOCKS	FAT BLOCKS
	breast, raw, boneless, thin sliced	Perdue	1	oz.	1	0	0
	breast, raw, seasoned, boneless, barbeque	Perdue	1.3	oz.	1	0	0
	breast, raw, seasoned, boneless, lemon pepper	Perdue	1.3	oz.	1	0	0
	breast, raw, seasoned, boneless, Italian	Perdue	1.3	oz.	1	0	0
	breast, raw, seasoned, boneless, Italian, Oriental	Perdue	1.3	oz.	1	0	0
	breast, cooked, whole	Perdue	1	oz.	1	0	1
	breast, cooked, whole	Perdue Oven Stuffer	1	oz.	1	0	1
	breast, cooked, boneless	Perdue	0.8	oz.	1	0	0
	breast, cooked, boneless	Perdue Oven Stuffer	1	oz.	1	0	0
	breast, cooked, quartered	Perdue	1	oz.	1	0	1
	breast, cooked, roundelet	Tyson	2.6	oz.	1	1	3
	breast, cooked, tenderloins	Perdue	1	oz.	1	0	0
	breast, cooked, thin sliced	Perdue	1	oz.	1	0	0
	breast, cooked, seasoned, boneless, barbeque	Perdue	1	oz.	1	0	0
	breast, cooked, seasoned, boneless, lemon pepper	Perdue	1	oz.	1	0	0
	breast, cooked, seasoned, boneless, Italian	Perdue	1	oz.	1	0	0
	breast, cooked, seasoned, boneless, Oriental	Empire Kosher	1	oz.	1	0	0
	breast, fried, battered and breaded		1	oz.	1	0	1
	breast, roasted	Perdue	1	oz.	1	0	1
	breast, roasted	Tyson	0.1	breast	1	0	1
	breast, roasted, boneless	Perdue	0.9	oz.	1	0	0
	breast, roasted, boneless	Perdue Fit 'n Easy	0.9	oz.	1	0	0
	breast, roasted, skinless	Perdue	0.8	oz.	1	0	0

breast, seasoned, Cajun	Chicken By George	1.3	oz.	1	0	0
breast, seasoned, Caribbean grill	Chicken By George	1.3	oz.	1	0	0
breast, seasoned, garlic and herb	Chicken By George	1.3	oz.	1	0	0
breast, seasoned, Italian bleu cheese	Chicken By George	1.3	oz.	1	0	1
breast, seasoned, lemon herb	Chicken By George	1.3	oz.	1	0	0
breast, seasoned, lemon oregano	Chicken By George	1.3	oz.	1	0	0
breast, seasoned, mesquite barbeque	Chicken By George	1.3	oz.	1	0	0
breast, seasoned, mustard dill	Chicken By George	1.3	oz.	1	0	1
breast, seasoned, roasted	Chicken By George	1.3	oz.	1	0	0
breast, seasoned, teriyaki	Chicken By George	1.3	oz.	1	0	0
breast, seasoned, tomato herb w/basil	Chicken By George	1.3	oz.	1	0	1
cutlet, battered or breaded	Empire Kosher	1.1	oz.	1	0	1
diced	Tyson	2.3	oz.	1	0	0
drumstick and thigh, fried	Empire Kosher	1.5	oz.	1	1	3
drumstick, roasted	Perdue	1.1	oz.	1	0	1
drumstick, roasted	Perdue Oven Stuffer	0.9	oz.	1	0	1
drumstick, roasted	Tyson	0.8	pcs.	1	0	1
drumstick, roasted, skinless	Perdue Pick	0.5	pcs.	1	0	1
leg, whole, roasted	Perdue	1.1	oz.	1	0	2
leg, quarters, raw	Perdue Jumbo Family/Value	1.1	oz.	1	0	2
leg, quarters, raw	Tyson	1.3	oz.	1	0	2
leg, quarters, cooked	Perdue	1	oz.	1	0	2
nuggets	Empire Kosher	2.5	pcs.	1	0	2
sticks	Empire Kosher Stix	1.3	pcs.	1	1	2
thigh, raw	Tyson	2	oz.	1	0	4
thigh, raw, boneless, skinless	Tyson	1.3	oz.	1	0	1
thigh, roasted	Perdue	1.1	pc.	1	0	2
thigh, roasted, boneless	Perdue	0.9	oz.	1	0	1
thigh, roasted, boneless	Perdue Fit 'n Easy	0.5	pcs.	1	0	1

FOOD ITEM	SPECIFICATIONS	BRAND NAME	QUANTITY	SIZE	PROTEIN BLOCKS	CARBOHYDRATE BLOCKS	FAT BLOCKS
	thigh, roasted, boneless	Perdue Oven Stuffer	0.8	oz.	1	0	1
	thigh, roasted, skinless	Perdue	0.9	oz.	1	0	1
	thigh, roasted, skinless	Tyson	1	oz.	1	0	2
	wing, raw, whole	Tyson	1.3	oz.	1	0	2
	wing, roasted	Perdue	0.7	pcs.	1	0	2
	wing, roasted	Perdue Wingettes	1	pcs.	1	0	2
	wing, roasted	Perdue Oven Stuffer Drummettes	1	pcs.	1	0	2
	wing, roasted	Perdue Oven Stuffer Wingettes	1	pcs.	1	0	2
"Chicken," vegetarian	canned, diced	Worthington Chik	0.3	cup	1	0	1
	canned, fried	Loma Linda Chik'n	0.7	pcs.	1	0	3
	canned, fried	Worthington FriChik	2	pcs.	1	0	3
	canned, sliced	Worthington Chik	3	slices	1	0	2
	frozen	Worthington ChikStiks	1	pc.	1	0	2
	frozen, diced	Worthington Meatless	0.3	cup	1	0	2
	frozen, fried	Loma Linda Chik'n	0.5	pc.	1	0	3
	frozen, nuggets	Worthington Chik-Nuggets	2.5	pcs.	1	0	3
	frozen, patties	Morningstar Farms Chik	1	patty	1	1	3
	frozen, patties	Worthington Crispy Chik	1	patty	1	1	3
	frozen, roll	Worthington	1	3/9" slice	1	0	2
	frozen, roll	Worthington Chic-Ketts 1 lb.	1	slices	1	0	1
	frozen, roll	Worthington Chic-Ketts 56 oz.	0.5	1/2" slice	1	1	1
	frozen, sliced	Worthington	2	slices	1	0	2
	mix	Loma Linda Supreme	0.2	cup	1	0	0
Chicken frankfurter	simmered	Empire Kosher	1	2-oz. link	1	0	2
Chicken giblets	simmered, chopped		0.2	cup	1	0	1
Chicken lunch meat	breast, baked, grilled, or honey glazed	Louis Rich Carving Board	2	slices	1	0	0
	breast, honey glazed	Oscar Mayer Deli-Thin	4	slices	1	0	0
	breast, oven roasted	Boar's Head Golden	1	oz.	1	0	0
	breast, oven roasted	Hebrew National	2	oz.	1	0	0
	breast, oven roasted	Hebrew National	5	slices	1	0	0
	breast, oven roasted	Louis Rich Deluxe	1	1-oz. slice	1	0	0

Food	Description	Brand	Amount	Unit			
	breast, oven roasted	Louis Rich Deli-Thin	4	slices	1	0	1
	breast, oven roasted	Oscar Mayer Fat Free	4	slices	0	0	1
	breast, oven roasted, peppered	Tyson	1.5	slices	0	0	1
	breast, smoked	Boar's Head Hickory	1	oz.	0	0	1
	breast, smoked	Tyson Hickory	3	slices	0	0	1
	roll, light meat		1	oz.	1	0	1
	white, sliced	Tyson	3	slices	2	1	1
	white, sliced, oven roasted	Louis Rich	1	1-oz. slice	1	0	1
Chicken sausage	and apricot	Bilinski	2.2	link	1	0	1
	and broccoli	Bilinski	2.2	link	1	0	1
	Italian, w/pepper and onion	Bilinski	1.7	link	1	0	1
	and jalapeno	Bilinski	1.6	link	1	0	1
	and pesto	Bilinski	1.9	link	1	0	1
	and spinach	Bilinski	2.2	link	1	0	1
	and sun-dried tomato w/basil	Bilinski	1.9	link	1	0	1
Chicken spread	chunky	Underwood	0.3	cup	3	0	1
Chorizo		Goya	0.9	1.6-oz. stick	4	0	1
Cisco			1.3	oz.	0	0	1
Clam, meat only	meat only, raw		2.7	oz.	0	0	1
	raw		3.9	large	0	0	1
Clam, canned	boiled, poached, or steamed		1.4	oz.	0	0	1
	baby, whole	S&W	0.3	cup	0	0	1
	chopped	S&W	0.6	cup	1	1	1
	chopped or minced	Doxsee	0.6	cup	0	1	1
	chopped or minced	Progresso	0.6	cup	0	0	1
	minced	S&W	0.3	cup	0	0	1
	smoked	S&W	0.3	cup	0	0	1
Clam, fried	frozen	Gorton's Crunchy	3.3	oz.	4	2	1
		Mrs. Paul's	1.3	oz.	6	1	1
Cod, meat only	Atlantic, raw		1	oz.	0	0	1
	Atlantic, baked, broiled, or microwaved		1.3	oz.	0	0	1
	Pacific, raw		1.3	oz.	0	0	1
	Pacific, baked, broiled, or microwaved		1	oz.	0	0	1

FOOD ITEM	SPECIFICATIONS	BRAND NAME	QUANTITY	SIZE	PROTEIN BLOCKS	CARBOHYDRATE BLOCKS	FAT BLOCKS
Cod, canned	Atlantic, w/liquid		1	oz.	1	0	0
Cod, dried	Atlantic salted		0.3	oz.	1	0	0
Cod, frozen	Pacific, loins	Peter Pan	1.3	oz.	1	0	0
Cod, entree	frozen, breaded	Mrs. Paul's Premium	0.5	fillet	1	1	2
	frozen, breaded	Van de Kamp's Light	0.5	fillet	1	1	2
Cornish hen	cooked, dark meat	Perdue	1.8	oz.	1	0	3
	cooked, white meat	Perdue	1.4	oz.	1	0	1
	roasted, half, dark meat	Perdue	3.6	oz.	1	0	3
	roasted, half, white meat	Perdue	2.7	oz.	1	0	2
Crab, meat only	Alaska King, raw		1.3	oz.	1	0	0
	Alaska King, boiled, poached or steamed		1.3	oz.	1	0	0
	blue, raw		1.3	oz.	1	0	0
	blue, boiled, poached, or steamed		1.3	oz.	1	0	0
	dungeness, raw		1.3	oz.	1	0	0
	dungeness, boiled, poached, steamed		1	oz.	1	0	0
	queen, raw		1.3	oz.	1	0	0
	queen, boiled, poached, or steamed		1	oz.	1	0	0
Crab, canned	blue		1.3	oz.	1	0	0
	dungeness	S&W	1	oz.	1	0	0
		Peter Pan	3	oz.	1	1	0
"Crab," imitation	from surimi		2	oz.	1	1	0
	flaked	Captain Jac Crab Tasties	3	oz.	1	2	1
	flaked	Louis Kemp Crab Delights	3	oz.	1	1	0
	flaked	Pacific Mate	3	oz.	1	2	0
	flaked	Pacific Mate Fat Free	3	oz.	1	2	0
	flaked	Seafest	3	oz.	1	1	0
	flaked, or chunk	Louis Kemp Crab Delights	3	oz.	1	1	1
	leg style	Louis Kemp Crab Delights	3	oz.	1	1	0
	leg style	Captain Jac Crab Tasties	3	oz.	1	2	1
	leg style w/crab	Captain Jac Easy Shreds	3	oz.	1	1	0

Food	Description	Brand	Amount	Unit	Protein	Carb.	Fat
Crab cake	deviled, frozen	Mrs. Paul's	0.5	pc.	1	1	1
Crayfish, meat only	deviled, frozen, miniature	Mrs. Paul's	3	pcs.	1	2	2
	wild, raw		1.3	oz.	1	0	0
	wild, raw		8	medium	1	0	0
	wild, boiled or steamed		1.3	oz.	1	0	0
	farmed, boiled or steamed		1.3	oz.	1	0	0
Croaker, meat only	raw, Atlantic		1.3	oz.	1	0	0
Cusk, meat only	raw		1.8	oz.	1	0	0
	baked, broiled or microwaved		1.4	oz.	1	0	0
Cuttlefish, meat only	raw		2.2	oz.	1	0	0
	boiled or steamed		1.1	oz.	1	0	0
Cuttlefish, canned	in ink	Goya	0.3	cup	1	0	4
Dolphinfish, meat only	raw		1.9	oz.	1	0	0
	baked, broiled, or microwaved		1.1	oz.	1	0	0
Duck, domesticated, roasted	meat w/skin		1.8	oz.	1	0	5
	meat only		1.5	oz.	1	0	2
Duck, wild, raw	meat w/skin		2	oz.	1	0	3
	breast meat		1.7	oz.	1	0	1
Eel, meat only	raw		1.9	4 oz.	1	0	2
	baked, broiled, or microwaved		1.5	4 oz.	1	0	2
Egg, chicken	raw, whole		1	large egg	1	0	2
	raw, white only		1	large egg	1	0	0
	raw, yolk only (includes a small portion of white)		2.5	large egg	1	0	4
	cooked, hard boiled, chopped		0.5	cup	1	0	3
	cooked, poached		1	large egg	1	0	2
	dried, whole		0.5	oz.	1	0	2
	dried, whole, stabilized		0.5	oz.	1	0	2
	dried, whole, stabilized, flakes		0.3	oz.	1	0	0
	dried, yolk		1	oz.	1	0	6

FOOD ITEM	SPECIFICATIONS	BRAND NAME	QUANTITY	SIZE	PROTEIN BLOCKS	CARBOHYDRATE BLOCKS	FAT BLOCKS
Egg, duck			1	egg	1	0	3
Egg, goose			0.3	egg	1	0	2
Egg, quail			5	egg	1	0	2
Egg, turkey			0.5	egg	1	0	0
Egg, substitute or imitation		Egg Beaters	0.3	cup	1	0	0
		Egg Watchers	0.3	cup	1	0	0
		Morningstar Farms Better'n Eggs	0.3	cup	1	0	0
		Morningstar Farms Scramblers	0.3	cup	1	0	0
		Second Nature	0.3	cup	1	0	0
"Fish" vegetarian	frozen	Worthington	1	fillets	1	0	2
	mix	Loma Linda Ocean Platter	0.2	cup	1	0	0
Flatfish, meat only	raw		1.3	oz.	1	0	0
	baked, broiled, or microwaved		1	oz.	1	0	0
Frankfurter	frozen	Van de Kamp's	1.3	oz.	1	0	0
		Boar's Head	1	link	1	0	5
		Hormel 10	1.6	oz.	1	0	4
		Hormel 8	2	oz.	1	0	6
		Hormel Big 8	2	oz.	1	0	6
		Hormel Light & Lean 97	1.6	oz.	1	0	0
		Hormel Light & Lean 97 Jumbo	2	oz.	1	1	1
		John Morrell Fat Free	1.4	oz.	1	1	0
		John Morrell Lite	1	link	1	1	2
		Oscar Mayer Weiners	1	link	1	0	4
		Oscar Mayer Weiners Light	1	link	1	0	3
		Oscar Mayer Weiners Littles	6	links	1	0	6
		Oscar Mayer Big Juicy Wieners	1	link	1	0	7
		Oscar Mayer Bun Length Wieners	1	link	1	0	6
	beef	Boar's Head Lite	1	link	1	0	2
	beef	Boar's Head Giant	1	link	1	0	5
	beef	Boar's Head Skinless	1	link	1	0	4
	beef	Hebrew National	1.7	oz.	1	0	5

Modifier	Brand/Name	Amount	Unit	Protein	Carbohydrate	Fat
beef	Hebrew National	8	oz.	1	0	4
beef	Hebrew National Bulk	2.7	oz.	1	0	7
beef	Hebrew National Family Pack	2	oz.	1	0	5
beef	Hebrew National Picnic Pack	1.6	oz.	1	0	4
beef	Hebrew National Reduced Fat	1.7	oz.	1	0	3
beef	Hebrew National Reduced Fat 3 lb.	1.4	oz.	1	0	3
beef	Hebrew National Quarter Pound/Jumbo	0.5	link	1	0	6
beef	Hormel 8	1	link	1	0	5
beef	Hormel Light & Lean 97	1	link	1	0	0
beef	Oscar Mayer	1	link	1	0	4
beef	Oscar Mayer Light	1	link	1	0	3
beef	Oscar Mayer Big & Juicy	2.7	oz.	1	0	7
beef	Oscar Mayer Big & Juicy 1/4 lb.	0.5	link	1	0	6
beef	Oscar Mayer Big & Juicy Deli	2.7	oz.	1	0	7
beef	Oscar Mayer Bun Length	1	link	1	0	6
beef	Wranglers	1	link	1	0	5
cocktail	Hormel	5	links	1	0	5
cocktail, beef	Boar's Head	5	links	1	0	5
cocktail, beef	Hebrew National	4	links	1	0	5
cocktail, beef	Hebrew National 32 oz.	6	links	1	0	5
cocktail, smoked	Hormel Smokies	5	links	1	0	5
cheese	Oscar Mayer	1	link	1	0	4
cheese	Wranglers	1	link	1	0	5
hot and spicy	Oscar Mayer Big & Juicy	1	link	1	0	7
smoked	Oscar Mayer Big & Juicy Smokie	1	link	1	0	6
smoked	Wranglers	1	link	1	0	5
"Frankfurter," vegetarian	New Menu VegiDog	1	link	1	0	0
canned	Loma Linda Big	1	link	1	0	2
canned	Loma Linda Linketts	1	link	1	0	2
canned	Worhington VegaLinks	1	link	1	0	1
canned	Worthington SuperLinks	1	link	1	0	3
frozen	Morningstar Farms Deli Franks	1	link	1	0	2
frozen	Natural Touch Vege	1	link	1	0	2
frozen	Worthington Leanies	1	link	1	0	3
frozen, corn battered	Loma Linda Corn Dog	1	link	1	2	3

PROTEIN

FOOD ITEM	SPECIFICATIONS	BRAND NAME	QUANTITY	SIZE	PROTEIN BLOCKS	CARBOHYDRATE BLOCKS	FAT BLOCKS
	refrigerated, chili	Yves Veggie Cuisine Dogs	0.5	link	1	0	0
	refrigerated, tofu	Yves Veggie Cuisine Wieners	1	link	1	0	0
Frog's legs	meat only, raw		1.3	oz.	1	0	2
Gefilte fish, drained		Manischewitz Gold/Jelled Broth	1	ball w/jell	1	1	1
		Manischewitz Gold/Vegetable Medley	1	ball, 1/6 carrot	1	0	1
		Manischewitz Gold w/Olives/Carrots	1	ball, 1/4 carrot	1	0	1
	zesty	Manischewitz Gold/Brine	1	ball	1	0	1
Gelatin	unflavored	Knox	1	pkt.	1	0	0
Gelatin drink mix	orange	Knox	1	pkt.	1	0	0
Goat	meat only, roasted		0.9	oz.	1	0	3
Goose, roasted	meat w/skin		1.4	oz.	1	0	1
	meat only		1.2	oz.	1	0	0
Grouper, meat only	raw		1.3	oz.	1	0	0
	baked, broiled, or microwaved		1	oz.	1	0	0
Guinea hen, raw	meat w/skin		1.1	oz.	1	0	1
	meat only		1.2	oz.	1	0	0
Haddock, meat only	raw		1.3	oz.	1	0	0
	baked, broiled, or microwaved		1	oz.	1	0	0
	smoked		1	oz.	1	0	0
Halibut, meat only	Atlantic and Pacific, raw		1.2	oz.	1	0	0
	Atlantic and Pacific, baked, broiled, or microwaved		0.9	oz.	1	0	0
	Greenland, raw		1.7	oz.	1	0	2
	Greenland, baked, broiled, or microwaved		1.3	oz.	1	0	2
Halibut, frozen	fillet or steaks	Peter Pan	1.4	oz.	1	0	0
Ham, fresh, meat only	whole leg, roasted, lean w/fat		1	oz.	1	0	2
	whole leg, roasted, lean w/fat, chopped or diced		0.2	cup	1	0	2
	whole leg, roasted, lean only		0.9	oz.	1	0	1

	Amount	Unit	P	C	F
whole leg, roasted, lean only, chopped, or diced	0.2	cup	1	0	1
rump half, roasted, lean w/fat	0.9	oz.	1	0	2
rump half, roasted, lean only	0.9	oz.	1	0	1
shank half, roasted, lean w/fat	1	oz.	1	0	2
shank half, roasted, lean only	0.9	oz.	1	0	1
Ham cured					
whole leg, lean w/fat, unheated	1.3	oz.	1	0	2
whole leg, lean w/fat, roasted	1.1	oz.	1	0	2
whole leg, lean w/fat, roasted, chopped or diced	0.2	cup	1	0	2
whole leg, lean only, unheated	1.1	oz.	1	0	1
whole leg, lean only, roasted	1	oz.	1	0	0
whole leg, lean only, roasted, chopped or diced	0.2	cup	1	0	1
boneless (11% fat), unheated	1.4	oz.	1	0	1
boneless (11% fat), roasted	1.1	oz.	1	0	1
boneless (11% fat), roasted, chopped or diced	0.2	cup	1	0	1
boneless, extra lean (5% fat), unheated	1.3	oz.	1	0	1
boneless, extra lean (5% fat), roasted	1.2	oz.	1	0	1
boneless, extra lean (5% fat), roasted, chopped or diced	0.2	cup	1	0	1
Ham, canned or refrigerated					
Black Label Refrigerated	1.5	oz.	1	0	1
Black Label Shelf	1.5	oz.	1	0	1
Curemaster Half	1.5	oz.	1	0	1
Hormel Light & Lean	1.5	oz.	1	0	1
John Morrell Boneless	1.6	oz.	1	0	2

FOOD ITEM	SPECIFICATIONS	BRAND NAME	QUANTITY	SIZE	PROTEIN BLOCKS	CARBOHYDRATE BLOCKS	FAT BLOCKS
		Jones Dairy Farm Country Carved Family/Dainty	1.3	oz.	1	0	0
	baked	Jones Dairy Farm Country Club	1.3	oz.	1	0	0
	Black Forest	Jones Dairy Farm Family/Dainty	1.3	oz.	1	0	0
	chunk	Jones Dairy Farm Homestead	1.3	oz.	1	0	1
	fully cooked	Jones Dairy Farm Old Fashioned	1.4	oz.	1	0	3
	honey	Louis Rich Dinner	1.4	oz.	1	0	0
		Boar's Head Baby	1.3	oz.	1	0	0
		Hormel	1.5	oz.	1	0	2
		Jones Dairy Farm	1.6	oz.	1	0	4
		Jones Dairy Farm Country Carved Family	1.3	oz.	1	0	0
	honey	Patrick Cudahy Real Lean	1.9	oz.	1	1	1
	maple	Boar's Head Baby Honey Coat	1.3	oz.	1	0	0
	maple	Jones Dairy Farm Country Carved Family	1.4	oz.	1	0	0
	semi-boneless	Jones Dairy Farm	1.3	oz.	1	0	2
	skinless, shankless	Jones Dairy Farm	1.3	oz.	1	0	2
	slice	Oscar Mayer	1.5	oz.	1	0	1
	slice, smoke flavor	Patrick Cudahy Real Lean	1.9	oz.	1	0	1
	slice, smoked or maple glaze	Boar's Head Sweet Slice	1.4	oz.	1	0	1
	slice, smoked, semi-boneless	Boar's Head	1.4	oz.	1	0	1
	spiral sliced	Jones Dairy Farm	1.3	oz.	1	0	2
	spiral sliced	Spiral Cure 81 Half	1.4	oz.	1	0	1
	steak	Jones Dairy Farm Lean Choice/ Rock River	1.3	oz.	1	0	0
	steak	Oscar Mayer	1.4	oz.	1	0	1
	steak, honey	Patrick Cudahy	1.5	oz.	1	0	1
	steak, smoke flavor	Patrick Cudahy	1.5	oz.	1	0	1
	Virginia	Boar's Head Ready-to-Eat	1.5	oz.	1	0	1
	Virginia, smoked	Boar's Head Baby Gourmet	1.3	oz.	1	0	0

Food	Preparation	Brand	Amount	Unit			
"Ham" vegetarian, frozen	roll	Worthingham Wham	0.8	3/8" slice	1	0	2
Ham bologna	sliced	Worthingham Wham	2	slices	1	0	2
Ham lunch meat	baked	Boar's Head	1.5	oz.	1	0	1
	baked	Boar's Head Deluxe	1.5	oz.	1	0	0
	baked	Boar's Head Lower Sodium Extra Lean	1.4	oz.	1	0	0
	baked, Virginia	Healthy Deli Cinnamon Apple Grove	1.5	oz.	1	0	1
	baked, Virginia	Healthy Deli Deluxe	1.5	oz.	1	0	1
	Black Forest	Healthy Deli Less Sodium	1.5	oz.	1	0	1
	Black Forest	Healthy Deli Old Tyme Tavern	1.4	oz.	1	0	1
	boiled	Hormel Light & Lean 97	1.7	oz.	1	0	1
	boiled	Hormel Light & Lean 97 Deli	1.5	oz.	1	0	0
	boiled	Jones Dairy Farm Lean Choice	1.5	slices	1	0	1
	cappacola	Menumaster	1.7	oz.	1	0	0
	cappacola	Old Tyme	1.4	oz.	1	0	1
	chopped	Oscar Mayer Lower Sodium	2.1	slices	1	0	0
	chopped	Louis Rich Carving Board	1.8	slices	1	0	1
	cooked	Oscar Mayer	1.9	slices	1	0	1
	cooked	Oscar Mayer Healthy Favorites	3.1	slices	1	0	0
	cooked	Healthy Deli	1.5	oz.	1	0	1
	cooked	Healthy Deli Less Sodium	1.5	oz.	1	0	1
	honey	Boar's Head	1.4	oz.	1	0	0
	honey	Healthy Deli	1.4	oz.	1	0	1
		Oscar Mayer	2.1	slices	1	0	1
		Oscar Mayer Deli-Thin	3.1	slices	1	0	0
		Patrick Cudahy	1.4	oz.	1	0	1
		Boar's Head Cappy	1.4	oz.	1	0	1
		Healthy Deli Cappi	1.5	oz.	1	0	0
		Black Label	2	oz.	1	0	1
		Oscar Mayer	1.7	oz.	1	0	1
		Alpine Lace	1.5	oz.	1	0	4
		Hormel Deli	1.8	oz.	1	0	2
		Hormel Low Salt	1.8	oz.	1	0	1
		Patrick Cudahy Less Sodium	1.4	oz.	1	0	1
		Healthy Deli Honey Valley Farms	1.5	oz.	1	0	1
		Louis Rich Carving Board Thin	3.8	slices	1	0	0

FOOD ITEM	SPECIFICATIONS	BRAND NAME	QUANTITY	SIZE	PROTEIN BLOCKS	CARBOHYDRATE BLOCKS	FAT BLOCKS
	honey	Louis Rich Carving Board Traditional	1.8	oz.	1	0	1
	honey	Oscar Mayer	2.1	slices	1	0	1
	honey	Oscar Mayer Deli-Thin	3.1	slices	1	0	1
	honey	Oscar Mayer Healthy Favorites	3.1	slices	1	0	1
	honey	Patrick Cudahy	1.4	oz.	1	0	0
	hot	Healthy Deli Rodeo	1.5	oz.	1	0	1
	jalapeno	Healthy Deli	1.8	oz.	1	0	0
	maple	Boar's Head Honey Coat	1.4	oz.	1	0	0
	maple	Healthy Deli Vermont	1.5	oz.	1	0	0
	maple	Patrick Cudahy	1.4	oz.	1	0	0
	minced		1.4	oz.	1	0	3
	pepper	Boar's Head	1.5	oz.	1	0	1
	pepper	Healthy Deli	1.5	oz.	1	0	1
	smoked	Boar's Head Gourmet	1.4	oz.	1	0	0
	smoked	Hormel Light & Lean 97 Deli	1.8	oz.	1	0	1
	smoked	Louis Rich Carving Board	1.8	oz.	1	0	1
	smoked	Oscar Mayer	2.1	slices	1	0	1
	smoked	Oscar Mayer Deli-Thin	3.1	slices	1	0	1
	smoked	Oscar Mayer Healthy Favorites	3.1	slices	1	0	1
	smoked, double	Healthy Deli	1.4	oz.	1	0	1
	spiced	Boar's Head	2	oz.	1	0	3
	Virginia	Boar's Head	1.5	oz.	1	0	0
	Virginia	Healthy Deli	1.5	oz.	1	0	1
Ham patty		Hormel	2	oz.	1	0	6
Ham and cheese loaf		Oscar Mayer	1.7	oz.	1	0	3
Ham and cheese patty		Hormel	1	2-oz. patty	1	0	6
"Hamburger" vegetarian		New Menu Vegiburger	1.6	oz.	1	0	0
	canned	LaLoma RediBurger	0.4	5/8" slice	1	1	1
	canned	Loma Linda VegeBurger	0.2	cup	1	0	1
	canned	Worthington	0.2	cup	1	0	1
	frozen	Amy's California	1.7	patty	1	3	2
	frozen	Amy's Chicago	0.8	patty	1	2	2

	Product	Amount	Unit			
frozen	Green Giant Harvest Burgers Original	0.4	patty	1	0	0
frozen	Ken & Robert's Veggie Burger	1.4	patty	1	4	0
frozen	Morningstar Farms Better'n Burgers	0.6	patty	1	0	0
frozen	Morningstar Farms Grillers	0.5	patty	1	0	1
frozen	Natural Touch Vegan Burger	0.6	patty	1	0	0
frozen	Natural Touch Vege Burger	0.5	patty	1	0	1
frozen, black bean, spicy	Morningstar Farms	0.9	patty	1	1	0
frozen, garden grain	Morningstar Farms	1.1	patty	1	2	1
frozen, garden vegetable	Morningstar Farms	0.7	patty	1	1	1
frozen, garden vegetable	Natural Touch	0.7	patty	1	0	1
frozen, Italian	Green Giant Harvest Burgers	0.4	patty	1	0	0
frozen, Southwestern	Green Giant Harvest Burgers	0.4	patty	1	0	1
frozen, tofu	Natural Touch Okra	0.6	patty	1	1	1
frozen, ground	Worthington	0.3	cup	1	1	0
refrigerated	Hempeh Burger	0.7	patty	1	0	0
refrigerated	Yves Veggie Cuisine	0.6	patty	1	0	0
mix, dry	Worthington Granburger	2.1	Tbsp.	1	0	0
mix, dry, chunks	Loma Linda Vita-Burger	0.2	cup	1	1	1
mix, dry, granules	LaLoma Vita-Burger	2.1	Tbsp.	1	0	0
mix	Fantastic Nature's Burger Original	0.9	patty, prepared	1	0	1
mix	Fantastic Nature's Burger BBQ	1	patty, prepared	1	3	1
Hash, canned	Mary Kitchen Fiesta	0.3	cup	1	3	3
Head cheese	Oscar Mayer	1.4	1-oz. slice	1	1	1
Heart, braised or simmered — beef		0.9	oz.	1	0	0
chicken, broiler-fryer		0.9	oz.	1	0	1
lamb		1	oz.	1	0	0
pork		1.1	oz.	1	0	1
turkey		0.9	oz.	1	0	0
veal		0.9	oz.	1	0	0
Herring, fresh — Atlantic, meat only, raw		1.4	oz.	1	0	1
Atlantic, meat only, baked, broiled, or microwaved		1.1	oz.	1	0	1
Atlantic, meat only, kippered		1	oz.	1	0	1
Atlantic, meat only, pickled		1.7	oz.	1	0	3

FOOD ITEM	SPECIFICATIONS	BRAND NAME	QUANTITY	SIZE	PROTEIN BLOCKS	CARBOHYDRATE BLOCKS	FAT BLOCKS
Herring, in jars, drained	Pacific, meat only, raw		1.5	oz.	1	0	2
	Pacific, meat only, baked, broiled, or microwaved		1.2	oz.	1	0	2
	lunch, sliced	Vita Homestyle	1.5	oz.	1	1	2
	in sour cream	Vita Party Snacks	1.5	oz.	1	1	2
	roll mops	Vita	1.5	oz.	1	1	2
		Vita	0.3	cup	1	1	2
		Vita	1.6	oz.	1	1	1
Ice cream	almond praline	Edys Grand	1.7	cup	1	7	9
	amaretto	Haagen Dazs DiSaronno	1.3	cup	1	7	13
	banana split	Edys Grand	1.7	cup	1	7	11
		Ben & Jerry's Chubby Hubby	0.6	cup	1	4	10
		Ben & Jerry's Chunky Monkey	1.3	cup	1	8	15
		Ben & Jerry's Rainforest Crunch	1	cup	1	5	15
		Ben & Jerry's Wavy Gravy	0.8	cup	1	5	13
	brownie, batter	Edys Grand	1.7	cup	1	7	9
	brownie, fudge	Healthy Choice	1.7	cup	1	8	2
	brownie, fudge, double	Edys Grand	2.5	cup	1	11	15
	brownie 'n fudge	Edys Grand Light	1.7	cup	1	7	4
	Brownie's a la Mode	Haagen-Dazs Extraas	1	cup	1	6	12
	butter pecan	Ben & Jerry's	1	cup	1	4	17
	butter pecan	Edy's Grand	1.7	cup	1	6	10
	butter pecan	Edy's Grand Light	1.7	cup	1	6	6
	butter pecan	Haagen-Dazs	1	cup	1	4	16
	butter pecan crunch	Healthy Choice	1.7	cup	1	8	2
	cappuccino chocolate chunk	Healthy Choice	1.7	cup	1	22	2
	Cappuccino Commotion	Haagen-Dazs Extraas	1	cup	1	5	14
	Caramel Cone Explosion	Haagen-Dazs Extraas	1	cup	1	6	13
	caramel cream, dreamy	Edy's Grand Light	1.7	cup	1	6	4
	caramel praline crunch	Edy's Fat Free	1.7	cup	1	9	0
	cheesecake chunk	Edy's Grand Light	1.7	cup	1	6	6
	cherry chocolate chip	Ben & Jerry's Cherry Garcia	1.7	cup	1	9	18
	cherry chocolate chip	Edy's Grand	1.7	cup	1	7	9

Food	Brand	Amount	Unit			
cherry vanilla, black	Edy's Grand No Sugar	1.7	cup	1	5	4
cherry vanilla, black, swirl	Edy's Fat Free	1.3	cup	1	6	0
chocolate	Edy's Grand	1.7	cup	1	6	10
chocolate	Edy's Grand No Sugar	1.7	cup	1	5	4
chocolate	Haagen Dazs	1	cup	1	5	12
chocolate, triple	Edy's Grand No Sugar	1.7	cup	1	6	6
chocolate, triple	Weight Watchers Tornado	1.3	cup	1	7	3
chocolate, almond	Edy's Grand Light	1.3	cup	1	4	4
chocolate chip	Edy's Grand Chips!	1.7	cup	1	6	9
chocolate chip	Edy's Grand No Sugar	1.7	cup	1	5	6
chocolate chip, cookie dough	Ben & Jerry's	1.7	cup	1	11	17
chocolate chip, chocolate	Edy's Grand	2.5	cup	1	10	17
chocolate chip, chocolate	Haagen Dazs	1	cup	1	5	13
chocolate chip, chunk	Healthy Choice	1.7	cup	1	7	2
chocolate chip, mint	Healthy Choice	1.7	cup	1	8	2
chocolate chip, mint	Edy's Grand Chips!	1.7	cup	1	6	10
chocolate cookie, mint	Ben & Jerry's	1.3	cup	1	7	14
chocolate fudge	Edy's Fat Free	1.3	cup	1	7	0
chocolate fudge	Edy's No Sugar	1.3	cup	1	6	0
chocolate fudge, chunk	Edy's Low Fat	1.7	cup	1	8	2
chocolate fudge, mousse	Edy's Grand Light	1.7	cup	1	6	4
chocolate fudge, mousse	Healthy Choice	1.7	cup	1	7	2
chocolate fudge, sundae	Edy's Grand	1.7	cup	1	7	11
coffee	Ben & Jerry's Café Ole	1.3	cup	1	6	13
coffee	Edy's Grand	1.7	cup	1	6	9
coffee	Haagen-Dazs	1	cup	1	5	12
coffee fudge	Edy's Fat Free	1.7	cup	1	9	0
coffee fudge	Edy's No Fat/Sugar	1.7	cup	1	7	0
coffee fudge, almond	Ben & Jerry's	0.8	cup	1	4	11
coffee toffee crunch	Ben & Jerry's	1.3	cup	1	8	16
cookie chink	Edy's Fat Free	1.3	cup	1	7	0
cookies and cream	Edy's Grand	1.7	cup	1	8	9
cookies and cream	Edy's Low Fat	1.7	cup	1	7	9
cookies and cream	Haagen Dazs	1	cup	1	8	2
cookies and cream	Healthy Choice	1.7	cup	1	5	12
cookies and cream, mint	Edy's Grand Light	1.7	cup	1	6	4

FOOD ITEM	SPECIFICATIONS	BRAND NAME	QUANTITY	SIZE	PROTEIN BLOCKS	CARBOHYDRATE BLOCKS	FAT BLOCKS
	cookie dough	Edy's Grand	1.7	cup	1	7	10
	cookie dough	Edy's Grand Light	1.7	cup	1	7	6
	cookie dough	Weight Watchers Craze	1.7	cup	1	9	4
	Cookie Dough Dynamo	Haagen Dazs Extraas	1.3	cup	1	8	16
	espresso chip	Edy's Grand	1.7	cup	1	6	9
	espresso chip	Edy's Low Fat	1.7	cup	1	7	2
	espresso chip, fudge	Edy's Grand Light	1.7	cup	1	7	4
	French silk	Edy's Grand Light	1.7	cup	1	7	6
	fudge chunk	Ben & Jerry's New York	1.3	cup	1	7	17
	ice cream sandwich	Edy's Grand	1.7	cup	1	5	9
	Irish cream	Haagen Dazs Baileys	1.3	cup	1	7	15
	macadamia brittle	Haagen Dazs	1.3	cup	1	7	17
	marble fudge	Edy's Fat Free	1.7	cup	1	9	0
	marble fudge	Edy's Grand No Sugar	1.7	cup	1	6	4
	mint fudge	Edy's Fat Free	1.7	cup	1	9	0
	mint fudge	Edy's Grand No Sugar	1.7	cup	1	6	4
	mocha fudge	Ben & Jerry's	1	cup	1	6	12
	mocha fudge	Edy's Grand No Sugar	1.7	cup	1	6	4
	mocha fudge	Edy's Grand Light	1.7	cup	1	6	4
	mocha fudge almond	Haagen Dazs Extraas	0.8	cup	1	5	12
	Peanut Butter Burst	Ben & Jerry's	0.6	cup	1	4	11
	peanut butter cup	Edy's Grand Light	1.7	cup	1	6	6
	peanut butter cup	Weight Watchers Positively Crunch	1.7	cup	1	6	6
	praline	Edy's Grand Light	1.7	cup	1	9	3
	praline caramel	Healthy Choice	1.7	cup	1	7	4
	praline caramel	Edy's No Fat/Sugar	1.3	cup	1	9	2
	raspberry vanilla swirl	Edy's Grand	1.7	cup	1	5	0
	rocky road	Edy's Grand	1.7	cup	1	6	11
	rocky road	Edy's Grand Light	1.7	cup	1	6	4
	rocky road	Edy's Low Fat	1.7	cup	1	8	2
	rocky road	Healthy Choice	1.7	cup	1	10	2
	rocky road	Weight Watchers Reckless	1.3	cup	1	6	3
	rum raisin	Haagen Dazs	1.3	cup	1	6	14
	strawberry	Edy's Grand	2.5	cup	1	10	10

strawberry	Edy's Grand No Sugar	1.7	cup	1	5	4
strawberry	Haagen Dazs	1.3	cup	1	7	13
strawberry cheesecake chunk	Edy's Grand	1.7	cup	1	7	9
Strawberry Cheesecake Craze	Haagen Dazs Extraas	1.3	cup	1	8	15
strawberry shortcake	Edy's Fat Free	1.7	cup	1	8	0
toffee n' caramel	Edy's Heath Low Fat	2.5	cup	1	13	4
toffee crunch, English	Ben & Jerry's	1.7	cup	1	10	21
Triple Brownie Overload	Haagen-Dazs Extraas	1	cup	1	6	13
vanilla	Ben & Jerry's	1.3	cup	1	6	14
vanilla	Edy's Fat Free	1.3	cup	1	6	0
vanilla	Edy's No Fat/Sugar	1.3	cup	1	5	0
vanilla	Edy's Grand	2.5	cup	1	8	17
vanilla	Edy's Grand Light	1.7	cup	1	5	4
vanilla	Edy's Grand No Sugar	1.7	cup	1	5	4
vanilla	Edy's Low Fat	1.7	cup	1	6	2
vanilla	Haagen-Dazs	1	cup	1	5	12
vanilla	Healthy Choice	1.7	cup	1	6	2
vanilla	Weight Watchers Oh So Very	1.3	cup	1	5	2
vanilla, French	Edy's Grand	2.5	cup	1	9	17
vanilla bean	Edy's Grand	2.5	cup	1	9	15
vanilla caramel	Edy's No Fat/Sugar	1.7	cup	1	7	0
vanilla caramel	Edy's Grand No Sugar	1.7	cup	1	6	4
vanilla caramel, fudge swirl	Ben & Jerry's	1.3	cup	1	9	14
vanilla chocolate strawberry	Edy's Grand	1.7	cup	1	6	8
vanilla chocolate swirl	Edy's No Fat/Sugar	1.3	cup	1	5	0
vanilla fudge	Haagen Dazs	1	cup	1	6	12
vanilla Swiss almond	Haagen Dazs	0.8	cup	1	4	12
"Ice cream," imitation						
bar, chocolate	Rice Dream	5	bar	1	17	25
bar, nutty, chocolate or vanilla	Rice Dream	2.5	bar	1	6	15
bar, strawberry	Rice Dream	10	bar	1	33	43
cappuccino	Rice Dream	5	cup	1	20	17
carob	Rice Dream	5	cup	1	21	17
carob almond	Rice Dream	5	cup	1	20	20
carob chip	Rice Dream	5	cup	1	21	20

FOOD ITEM	SPECIFICATIONS	BRAND NAME	QUANTITY	SIZE	PROTEIN BLOCKS	CARBOHYDRATE BLOCKS	FAT BLOCKS
	cocoa marble fudge	Rice Dream	5	cup	1	22	20
	cookies 'n dream	Rice Dream	5	cup	1	22	20
	lemon	Rice Dream	5	cup	1	20	17
	mint carob ship	Rice Dream	5	cup	1	21	20
	Neapolitan	Rice Dream	5	cup	1	20	17
	peanut butter fudge	Rice Dream	2.5	cup	1	11	10
	pie, cookie, chocolate or mint	Rice Dream	3.3	pie	1	14	20
	pie, cookie, mocha	Rice Dream	3.3	pie	1	14	19
	pie, cookie, vanilla	Rice Dream	3.3	pie	1	13	1
	strawberry	Rice Dream	5	cup	1	19	17
	vanilla or vanilla fudge	Rice Dream	5	cup	1	20	17
	vanilla Swiss almond	Rice Dream	5	cup	1	21	20
"Ice cream," tofu	all fruit flavors	Tofutti Fruitti	2.5	cup	1	11	0
	butter pecan	Tofutti	5	cup	1	24	43
	chocolate	Tofutti	1.7	cup	1	7	12
	chocolate cake	Tofutti	1.7	cup	1	9	12
	chocolate fudge	Tofutti Low Fat	2.5	cup	1	14	4
	coffee marshmallow	Tofutti Low Fat	5	cup	1	27	3
	passion island fruit	Tofutti Low Fat	5	cup	1	23	3
	peach mango	Tofutti Low Fat	5	cup	1	26	3
	sandwich, chocolate	Tofutti Cuties	5	pc.	1	9	9
	sandwich, vanilla or wildberry	Tofutti Cuties	5	pc.	1	10	9
	soft serve, all flavors	Tofutti	2.5	cup	1	11	7
	soft serve, all flavors	Tofutti Light	2.5	cup	1	11	2
	sticks, chocolate	Tofutti Fruitti	10	bar	1	17	17
	sticks, fudge	Tofutti Teddy	10	bar	1	21	3
	sticks, fudge	Tofutti Treats	10	bar	1	7	0
	strawberry banana	Tofutti Low Fat	5	cup	1	26	3
	vanilla	Tofutti	2.5	cup	1	11	19
	vanilla	Tofutti Cutie Slice	10	slice	1	17	27
	vanilla, almond bark	Tofutti	1.7	cup	1	8	14
	vanilla, chocolate covered	Tofutti Cutie	10	pie	1	20	63
	vanilla, fudge	Tofutti	2.5	cup	1	14	15

Ice cream bar	vanilla, fudge	Tofutti Low Fat	2.5	cup	1	14	4
	wildberry	Tofutti	2.5	cup	1	14	15
	wildberry	Tofutti Slice	10	slice	1	20	7
	wildberry, chocolate covered	Tofutti Slice	10	slice	1	20	33
	almond	DoveBar	2	bar	1	5	13
	almond	DoveBar Single	1.7	bar	1	5	13
	almond praline	Edy's Grand	2.5	bar	1	8	14
		Butterfinger	5	bar	1	9	22
		Knondike Original	3.3	bar	1	9	22
	Caramel Cone Explosion	Haagen-Dazs Extraas	2.5	bar	1	8	18
	Caramel Cone Explosion	Haagen-Dazs Extraas Singles	2.5	bar	1	9	19
	caramel creme w/toffee chips	Dovebar	3.3	bar	1	11	18
	caramel nut	Weight Watchers	5	bar	1	8	14
	chocolate	Nestle Crunch	5	bar	1	10	24
	chocolate	3 Musketeers	5	bar	1	9	14
	chocolate	3 Musketeers Single	5	bar	1	12	19
	chocolate	Weight Watchers Treat	3.3	bar	1	7	1
	chocolate, dark	Haagen-Dazs	2.5	bar	1	7	18
	chocolate, dark	Haagen-Dazs Single	2	bar	1	6	18
	chocolate, double	Dove Bite Size	12.5	bar	1	10	19
	chocolate cookie dough	Ben & Jerry's	2	bar	1	10	17
	chocolate dip	Weight Watchers	5	bar	1	6	10
	cookies 'n cream	Edy's Grand	2.5	bar	1	8	14
	Cookie Dough Dynamo	Haagen-Dazs Extraas	2.5	bar	1	9	21
	coffee w/almond crunch	Haagen Dazs	2.5	bar	1	6	18
	coffee w/almond crunch	Haagen Dazs Single	2	bar	1	6	17
	eggnog, dark chocolate	Dove Bite Size	16.7	bar	1	13	24
	fudge chunk	Ben & Jerry's New York	1.7	bar	1	4	17
	Iced Cappuccino	Haagen-Dazs Extraas	2.5	bar	1	6	18
	Iced Cappuccino		2	bar	1	5	16
		Milky Way	5	bar	1	11	12
	mocha cashew crunch	DoveBar	3.3	bar	1	9	19
		Nestle Crunch Crunch King	3.3	bar	1	8	21
		Nestle Crunch Reduced Fat	3.3	bar	1	5	8
	rocky road	Edy's Grand	2.5	bar	1	7	16

FOOD ITEM	SPECIFICATIONS	BRAND NAME	SIZE	QUANTITY	PROTEIN BLOCKS	CARBOHYDRATE BLOCKS	FAT BLOCKS
	toffe crunch, English	Ben & Jerry's	bar	2.5	1	9	18
	mousse, chocolate	Weight Watchers	bar	5	1	4	1
	mousse, berries 'n cream	Weight Watchers	bar	6.7	1	6	2
	orange vanilla	Weight Watchers Treat	bar	5	1	4	1
	peppermint w/dark chocolate	DoveBar	bar	3.3	1	11	19
	peppermint w/dark chocolate	Dove Bite Size	bar	16.7	1	14	24
	pralines 'n cream crispy	Weight Watchers	bar	5	1	9	12
		Snickers	bar	3.3	1	7	13
		Snickers Snack	bar	5.7	1	5	12
	toffee crunch	Weight Watchers	bar	5	1	7	12
	Triple Brownie Overload	Haagen-Dazs Extraas	bar	2.5	1	6	19
	Triple Brownie Overload	Haagen-Dazs Extraas	bar	2	1	6	18
	vanilla	Ben & Jerry's	bar	2.5	1	8	19
	vanilla	Dove Bite Size	bar	12.5	1	10	20
	vanilla	Nestle Crunch	bar	5	1	9	24
	vanilla	3 Musketeers	bar	5	1	12	17
	vanilla, brownie	Ben & Jerry's	bar	2.5	1	12	14
	vanilla, French	Dove Bite Size	bar	2.5	1	10	19
	vanilla, white coated	DoveBar	bar	3.3	1	10	19
	vanilla, w/almonds	Edy's Grand	bar	2	1	5	13
	vanilla, w/almonds	Haagen-Dazs	bar	2	1	4	15
	vanilla, w/almonds	Haagen-Dazs Single	bar	1.7	1	5	15
	vanilla, dark chocolate	Dove Bar	bar	3.3	1	10	19
	vanilla, dark chocolate	Dove Bar Single	bar	2.5	1	9	18
	vanilla, dark chocolate	Haagen-Dazs	bar	2.5	1	7	18
	vanilla, dark chocolate	Haagen-Dazs Single	bar	2	1	6	18
	vanilla, milk chocolate	Dove Bar	bar	3.3	1	9	19
	vanilla, milk chocolate	Dove Bar Single	bar	2.5	1	9	18
	vanilla, milk chocolate	Haagen-Dazs	bar	2.5	1	6	17
	vanilla, milk chocolate	Haagen-Dazs Single	bar	2	1	5	16
		Weight Watchers Arctic D'Lites	bar	3.3	1	5	8
Ice cream cone, filled	caramel almond crunch	Edy's Grand	cone	1.7	1	7	11
	chocolate	Drumstick	cone	1.7	1	6	10

	Food	Brand	Amount	Unit			
	chocolate dipped	Drumstick	2	cone	1	9	11
	chocolate fudge	Edy's Grand	1.4	cone	1	5	13
	cookies 'n cream	Drumstick	2	cone	1	6	13
	vanilla	Drumstick	1.7	cone	1	6	11
	vanilla, caramel	Drumstick	1.7	cone	1	7	11
	vanilla, fudge	Drumstick	2	cone	1	8	13
	vanilla, fudge sundae	Edy's Grand	2	cone	1	9	13
Ice cream cup, filled	chocolate	Carnation	15	fl. oz.	1	9	14
	chocolate malt	Carnation	17.1	fl. oz.	1	7	3
	chocolate sundae	Carnation	25	fl. oz.	1	16	15
	vanilla	Carnation	30	fl. oz.	1	12	20
	vanilla	Carnation	25	fl. oz.	1	11	17
	strawberry	Carnation	15	fl. oz.	1	16	14
	strawberry sundae	Carnation	25	fl. oz.	1	16	14
Ice cream frozen desserts	bananas Foster	Healthy Choice	1.7	cup	1	7	2
	Black Forest	Healthy Choice	1.7	cup	1	8	2
	brownie, a la mode	Weight Watchers	2	pc.	1	7	3
	brownie, chocolate frosted	Weight Watchers	5	pc.	1	11	4
	brownie, double fudge parfait	Weight Watchers	1.7	pc.	1	7	1
	brownie fudge, a la mode	Healthy Choice	3.3	pc.	1	8	2
	peanut butter fudge	Weight Watchers	5	pc.	1	10	4
	cappuccino mocha fudge	Healthy Choice	3.3	pc.	1	8	2
	caramel fudge a la mode	Weight Watchers	7.4	oz.	1	8	3
	cheesecake, brownie	Weight Watchers	1.1	pc.	1	4	2
	cheesecake, chocolate, triple	Weight Watchers	1.4	pc.	1	5	2
	cheesecake, French	Weight Watchers	1.4	pc.	1	4	2
	cheesecake, New York	Weight Watchers	1.7	pc.	1	4	3
	cherry chocolate	Healthy Choice	3.3	pc.	1	7	2
	chocolate, caramel mousse	Weight Watchers	2	pc.	1	7	3
	chocolate chip cookie dough sundae	Weight Watchers	3.3	pc.	1	11	4
	chocolate eclair	Weight Watchers	5	pc.	1	13	7
	chocolate eclair, triple	Weight Watchers	3.3	pc.	1	9	6
	chocolate malt	Milky Way	1.4	cup	1	7	1

FOOD ITEM	SPECIFICATIONS	BRAND NAME	QUANTITY	SIZE	PROTEIN BLOCKS	CARBOHYDRATE BLOCKS	FAT BLOCKS
	chocolate mocha pie	Weight Watchers	1.7	pc.	1	5	2
	chocolate mousse	Weight Watchers	1.7	pc.	1	5	3
	chocolate raspberry royale	Weight Watchers	2	pc.	1	8	2
	fudge cake, double	Weight Watchers	2.5	pc.	1	10	4
	loaf, cappuccino	Vienetta	0.7	of 12 oz. pkg.	1	7	13
	loaf, chocolate, mint, or vanilla	Vienetta	0.7	of 12 oz. pkg.	1	7	13
	mud pie, Mississippi	Weight Watchers	2.5	pc.	1	7	4
	nuggets, w/chocolate	Bon-Bons	20	pcs.	1	7	18
	nuggets, w/chocolate dark	Bon-Bons	25	pcs.	1	9	22
	nuggets, w/chocolate dark	Bon-Bons	26.7	pcs.	1	10	23
	nuggets, w/chocolate milk	Bon-Bons	25	pcs.	1	10	24
	nuggets, w/chocolate milk	Bon-Bons	26.7	pcs.	1	10	26
	praline, caramel cluster	Healthy Choice	3.3	pc.	1	9	2
	praline, pecan mousse	Weight Watchers	6.8	oz.	1	9	3
	praline, toffee crunch parfait	Weight Watchers	10.2	fl. oz.	1	8	2
	strawberry parfait royale	Weight Watchers	10.5	fl. oz.	1	8	1
	turtle fudge cake	Healthy Choice	3.3	pc.	1	9	2
Ice cream sandwich	chocolate chip cookie	Chipwich Jr.	3.3	pc.	1	13	11
	cookies and cream	Cool Creations	5	pc.	1	19	19
		Klondike Big Bear	3.3	pc.	1	11	8
		Klondike Krispy	3.3	pc.	1	10	22
		Cool Creations	10	pc.	1	18	17
Kidney's	mini		1.4	oz.	1	0	0
	beef		1.5	oz.	1	0	1
	lamb		1.4	oz.	1	0	1
	pork		0.3	cup	1	0	1
	pork, chopped		1.3	oz.	1	0	1
	veal		2.2	oz.	1	0	4
Kielbasa		Boar's Head	2.7	oz.	1	0	6
Knockwurst, beef		Boar's Head	1	3-oz. link	1	0	8
		Hebrew National	0.7	oz.	1	0	1
Lamb, choice grade, meat only	cubed, leg/shoulder, braised or stewed		0.9	oz.	1	0	1
	cubed, leg/shoulder, broiled						

	Amount	Unit	Protein	Carbohydrate	Fat
foreshank, braised, lean w/fat	0.9	oz.	1	0	1
foreshank, braised, lean only	0.8	oz.	1	0	0
ground, raw	1.5	oz.	1	0	3
ground, broiled	1	oz.	1	0	2
ground, broiled	0.2	cup	1	0	2
leg, whole, roasted, lean	1	oz.	1	0	1
leg, whole, roasted, lean w/fat	1	slice, 3" diam.x1/4	1	0	2
leg, whole, roasted, lean only	0.9	oz.	1	0	1
leg, whole, roasted, lean only	0.9	3" slice	1	0	1
leg, shank, roasted, lean	0.9	oz.	1	0	1
leg, shank, roasted, lean w/fat	0.9	slice, 3" diam.x1/4	1	0	1
leg, shank, roasted, lean only	0.9	oz.	1	0	1
leg, shank, roasted, lean only	0.9	3" slice	1	0	2
leg, sirloin, roasted, lean	1	oz.	1	0	2
leg, sirloin, roasted, lean w/fat	1	slice, 3" diam.x1/4	1	0	2
leg, sirloin, roasted, lean only	0.9	oz.	1	0	1
leg, sirloin, roasted, lean only	0.9	slice	1	0	2
loin chop, broiled, lean w/fat	1	oz.	1	0	2
loin chop, broiled, lean w/fat	0.8	oz.	1	0	1
loin chop, broiled, lean only	0.8	oz.	1	0	1
loin chop, broiled, lean only	1.1	oz.	1	0	2
loin, roasted, lean w/fat	0.9	oz.	1	0	1
loin, roasted, lean only	1.1	oz.	1	0	3
rib, broiled, lean w/fat	1.1	oz.	1	0	1
rib, broiled, lean only	0.9	oz.	1	0	3
rib, roasted, lean w/fat	1.2	oz.	1	0	1
rib, roasted, lean only	1	oz.	1	0	3
shoulder, whole, braised, lean w/fat	0.9	oz.	1	0	2
shoulder, whole, braised, lean only	0.8	oz.	1	0	1

PROTEIN

FOOD ITEM	SPECIFICATIONS	BRAND NAME	QUANTITY	SIZE	PROTEIN BLOCKS	CARBOHYDRATE BLOCKS	FAT BLOCKS
	shoulder, whole, roasted, lean w/fat		1.1	oz.	1	0	2
	shoulder, whole, roasted, lean only		1	oz.	1	0	1
Lamb, New Zealand, frozen, meat only	foreshank, braised, lean w/fat		0.9	oz.	1	0	1
	foreshank, braised, lean only		0.8	oz.	1	0	0
	leg, whole, roasted, lean w/fat		1	oz.	1	0	2
	leg, whole, roasted, lean only		0.9	oz.	1	0	1
	loin chop, broiled, lean w/fat		1.1	oz.	1	0	2
	loin chop, broiled, lean only		0.9	oz.	1	0	1
	rib, roasted, lean w/fat		1.3	oz.	1	0	4
	rib, roasted, lean only		1	oz.	1	0	1
	shoulder, braised, lean w/fat		0.9	oz.	1	0	2
	shoulder, braised, lean only		0.7	oz.	1	0	1
Ling, meat only	raw		1.3	oz.	1	0	0
	baked, broiled or microwaved		1	oz.	1	0	0
Ling cod	raw		1.4	oz.	1	0	0
	baked, broiled or microwaved		1.1	oz.	1	0	0
Liver	beef, pan-fried		0.9	oz.	1	0	1
	chicken, raw	Tyson	1.5	oz.	1	0	1
	chicken, simmered		1	oz.	1	0	1
	chicken, simmered, chopped		0.2	cup	1	0	1
	duck, raw		1.3	oz.	1	0	1
	goose, raw		1.4	oz.	1	0	0
	lamb, pan-fried		1	oz.	1	0	0
	pork, braised		1	oz.	1	0	1
	turkey, simmered		1	oz.	1	0	0
	turkey, simmered, chopped		0.2	cup	1	0	1
	veal (calves), braised		1.1	oz.	1	0	1

Food	Brand	Description	Amount	Unit	Protein	Carbohydrate	Fat
Liver cheese	Oscar Mayer		1.1	oz. slice	1	0	3
Liverwurst	Boar's Head Strassburger/Smoked		1.8	oz.	1	0	5
	Underwood	pate	2	oz.	1	0	5
	Boar's Head	spread	1.5	oz.	1	0	3
	Hormel	raw	1.8	oz.	1	0	3
Lobster, northern, meat only		boiled or steamed	1.3	oz.	1	0	0
		boiled or steamed	1.2	cup	1	0	0
"Lobster," imitation		chunks	0.2	cup	1	1	0
		chunks	0.4	cup	1	1	0
		salad style	0.5	cup	1	1	0
		tail style	0.5	4-oz. tail	1	1	0
Lunch meat	Oscar Mayer	spiced loaf	0.9	oz.	1	0	3
Lunch meat, canned	Spam		1.7	oz.	1	0	3
	Spam Less Salt		2	oz.	1	0	5
	Spam Light		2	oz.	1	0	5
	Spam		1.5	oz.	1	0	2
Lunch "meat," vegetarian		spread	1.8	oz.	1	0	4
	Loma Linda Nuteena	canned	1.1	3/8" slice	1	0	4
Lupin		boiled	0.3	cup	1	1	1
Mackerel, meat only		Atlantic, raw	1.3	oz.	1	0	2
		Atlantic, baked, broiled, or microwaved	1	oz.	1	0	2
		king, raw	1.2	oz.	1	0	0
		king, baked, broiled, or microwaved	1	oz.	1	0	0
		Pacific and jack, raw	1.2	oz.	1	0	1
		Pacific and jack, baked, broiled, or microwaved	1	oz.	1	0	1
		Spanish, raw	1.3	oz.	1	0	1
		Spanish, baked, broiled, or microwaved	1.1	oz.	1	0	1
	Spence & Co.	smoked	1.1	oz.	1	0	3
Mackerel, canned		jack	1.1	oz.	1	0	1
	Reese	skinless	0.3	4.375 oz. can	1	0	2
	Peter Pan	frozen, fillet	1.2	oz.	1	0	0

FOOD ITEM	SPECIFICATIONS	BRAND NAME	QUANTITY	SIZE	PROTEIN BLOCKS	CARBOHYDRATE BLOCKS	FAT BLOCKS
"Meat" vegetarian, ground	frozen	Morningstar Farms Ground Meatless	0.4	cup	1	0	0
"Meat" loaf, vegetarian mix	vegetarian	Natural Touch	0.1	cup	1	0	0
"Meatball" vegetarian	w/gravy, canned	Loma Linda Tender Rounds	3	pcs.	1	0	1
Milk	buttermilk, cultured		6.7	fl. oz.	1	1	1
	whole, 3.3% fat		7.3	fl. oz.	1	1	3
	lowfat, 2% fat		6.7	fl. oz.	1	1	2
	lowfat, 2%, protein fortified		5.7	fl. oz.	1	1	1
	lowfat, 1% fat		7.3	fl. oz.	1	1	1
	lowfat, 1%, protein fortified		5.7	fl. oz.	1	1	1
	skim		6.7	fl. oz.	1	1	0
Milk, canned	condensed, sweetened	Borden	5	Tbsp.	1	8	3
	condensed, sweetened	Carnation	5	Tbsp.	1	5	3
	condensed, sweetened	Eagle/Magnolia Brand/Meadow Gold/Star	5	Tbsp.	1	8	3
	condensed, sweetened	Goya	5	Tbsp.	1	5	3
	condensed, sweetened, lowfat	Borden	5	Tbsp.	1	8	3
	condensed, sweetened, lowfat	Eagle	5	Tbsp.	1	8	3
	condensed, sweetened, skim	Borden Fat Free	20	fl. oz.	1	8	0
	condensed, sweetened, skim	Eagle Fat Free	20	fl. oz.	1	8	0
	evaporated	Carnation	26.7	fl. oz.	1	0	3
	evaporated	Pet	26.7	fl. oz.	1	0	3
	evaporated, lowfat	Carnation	26.7	fl. oz.	1	0	0
	evaporated, skim	Carnation	26.7	fl. oz.	1	0	0
	evaporated, skim	Pet	26.7	fl. oz.	1	0	0
Milk, dry	buttermilk, sweet cream		0.2	cup	1	1	0
	buttermilk, sweet cream		3.3	Tbsp.	1	0	0
	whole		0.9	oz.	1	1	3
	whole		0.2	cup	1	1	2
	nonfat, regular		0.2	cup	1	1	0

Food	Description	Brand	Amount	Unit			PROTEIN
Milk, goat's	nonfat, instant	Carnation	0.9	pkg.	1	1	0
Milk, sheep's			0.3	cup	1	1	0
"Milk," nondairy			0.8	cup	1	1	3
			0.7	cup	1	3	4
		EdenBlend	11.4	fl. oz.	1	23	1
		EdenRice	8.0	fl. oz.	1	28	10
		Rice Dream Original	8.0	fl. oz.	1	39	7
	chocolate	Rice Dream	8.0	fl. oz.	1	31	8
	vanilla	Rice Dream	8.0	fl. oz.	1	5	7
Milk beverage, flavored	shake, root beer	Nestle Killer	10.8	oz.	1	4	4
	Butterfinger	Nestle Quick	10	fl. oz.	1	0	2
Milkfish, meat only	raw		1.2	oz.	1	0	1
	baked, broiled, or microwaved		0.9	oz.	1	2	1
Miso, soy		Eden Hacho	3.3	oz.	1	2	2
	w/barley	Eden Organic Mugi	0.3	cup	1	0	2
	w/rice	Eden Kome	3.3	Tbsp.	1	1	2
	w/rice, brown	Eden Genmani	5	Tbsp.	1	2	2
	w/rice, white	Eden Shiro	5	Tbsp.	1	2	2
Monkfish, meat only	raw		1.7	oz.	1	0	0
	baked, broiled, or microwaved		1.3	oz.	1	0	0
Mortadella		Boar's Head Cinghiale	1.5	oz.	1	0	4
	w/pistachios	Boar's Head Cinghiale	1.5	oz.	1	0	4
Mullet, striped, meat only	raw		1.3	oz.	1	0	0
	baked, broiled, or microwaved		1	oz.	1	0	0
Mussel, blue, meat only	raw		2.1	oz.	1	0	1
	boiled or steamed		0.4	cup	1	0	0
Ocean perch, Atlantic, meat only	raw		1	oz.	1	0	1
	baked, broiled, or microwaved		1.3	oz.	1	0	0

FOOD ITEM	SPECIFICATIONS	BRAND NAME	QUANTITY	SIZE	PROTEIN BLOCKS	CARBOHYDRATE BLOCKS	FAT BLOCKS
Octopus, meat only	raw		1.7	oz.	1	0	0
	boiled, or steamed		0.8	oz.	1	0	0
Octopus, canned	in garlic sauce	Goya	0.2	cup	1	0	2
	a la marinara	Goya	0.1	cup	1	0	2
	in olive oil	Goya	0.2	cup	1	0	4
	spiced, in red sauce	Goya	0.2	cup	1	0	2
Opossum	meat only, roasted	Reese	2	oz.	1	0	3
Oyster, meat only	Eastern, wild, raw		1.2	oz.	1	0	1
	Eastern, wild, raw		0.2	lb. fruit	1	0	1
	Eastern, wild, baked, broiled, or microwaved		7.5	medium	1	1	1
	Eastern, wild, steamed or poached		3.1	oz.	1	0	1
			1.7	oz.	1	0	1
Oyster	Eastern, farmed, raw		5	oz.	1	1	1
	Eastern, farmed, baked, broiled, or microwaved		3.6	oz.	1	1	1
	Pacific, raw		2.7	oz.	1	1	0
	Pacific, boiled or steamed		1.4	medium	1	0	1
	Pacific, boiled or steamed		1.3	oz.	1	0	1
Oyster, canned	Eastern, wild, w/liquid		3.6	oz.	1	0	1
	Eastern, wild, w/liquid		0.4	cup	1	1	1
	whole	S&W	1.8	oz.	1	0	1
	smoked	Reese Petite	1.8	oz.	1	0	2
	smoked	S&W	1.4	oz.	1	1	1
Quail, raw	meat w/skin		0.5	quail, 3.8 oz.	1	0	2
	meat w/skin		1.7	oz.	1	0	2
	meat only		0.5	quail, 3.2 oz.	1	0	1
	meat only		1.7	oz.	1	0	1
	breast meat only		0.8	breast, 2 oz.	1	0	0
	breast meat only		1.7	oz.	1	0	0
Pancreas, braised	beef		0.9	oz.	1	0	2
	lamb		1.1	oz.	1	0	2

Food	Description	Brand	Amount	Unit			
Pastrami	pork		0.9	oz.	1	0	1
	veal (calf)		0.9	oz.	1	0	1
	brisket or Romanian	Healthy Deli	1.3	oz.	1	0	1
	round	Hebrew National	1.2	oz.	1	0	1
	round	Boar's Head	1.2	oz.	1	0	1
Pepperoni		Boar's Head	1.4	oz.	1	0	4
		Hormel/Leoni/Rosa Grande	1.1	oz.	1	0	6
		Oscar Mayer	16.7	slices	1	0	4
		Patrick Cudahy 3 oz.	17.8	slices	1	0	6
		Patrick Cudahy 6 oz.	16.7	pcs.	1	0	6
		Patrick Cudahy Stick	1.1	oz.	1	0	4
"Pepperoni" vegetarian		Yves Veggie Cuisine	1.8	slices	1	0	0
Perch, meat only	raw		1.3	oz.	1	0	0
	baked, broiled, or microwaved		1	oz.	1	0	0
Pheasant, raw	meat w/skin		1.1	oz.	1	0	1
	meat only		1.1	oz.	1	0	0
	meat only, breast		1	oz.	1	0	0
	meat only, leg		1.1	oz.	1	0	1
Pickle and pepper loaf		Boar's Head	3.3	oz.	1	0	7
Pickle and pimiento loaf		Oscar Mayer	3.3	oz. slice	1	0	7
Pike	northern, meat only, raw		1.8	oz.	1	0	0
	northern, meat only, baked, broiled or microwaved		1.4	oz.	1	0	0
	walleye, meat only, raw		1.8	oz.	1	0	0
	walleye, meat only, baked, broiled or microwaved		1.4	oz.	1	0	0
Pig's feet	simmered		1.3	oz.	1	0	2
	pickled, cured		2	oz.	1	0	4
Polish sausage	pickled	Hormel	2	oz.	1	0	2
	beef	Hebrew National	1.8	oz.	1	0	4
	beef	Hebrew National	1.7	oz.	1	0	4
	skinless	John Morrell	2	oz.	1	0	5

FOOD ITEM	SPECIFICATIONS	BRAND NAME	QUANTITY	SIZE	PROTEIN BLOCKS	CARBOHYDRATE BLOCKS	FAT BLOCKS
Pollack, meat only	Atlantic, raw		1.3	oz.	1	0	0
	Atlantic, baked, broiled, or microwaved		1	oz.	1	0	0
	walleye, raw		1.4	oz.	1	0	0
	walleye, baked, broiled, or microwaved		1.1	oz.	1	0	0
Pompano, Florida, meat only	raw		1.3	oz.	1	0	1
Pork, cured	arm (picnic), roasted, lean w/fat		1.2	oz.	1	0	2
	arm (picnic), roasted, lean only		1	oz.	1	0	1
	blade roll, lean w/fat, roasted		1.4	oz.	1	0	3
	loin, whole, braised, lean only		0.8	oz.	1	0	1
	loin, whole, broiled, lean only		1.1	oz.	1	0	3
	loin, whole, broiled, lean w/fat		0.9	oz.	1	0	1
	loin, whole, roasted, lean only		1.1	oz.	1	0	2
	loin, whole, roasted, lean w/fat		0.9	oz.	1	0	1
	loin, blade, braised, lean only		1	oz.	1	0	3
	loin, blade, braised, lean w/fat		0.8	oz.	1	0	2
	loin, blade, broiled, lean only		1.2	oz.	1	0	4
	loin, blade, broiled, lean w/fat		1	oz.	1	0	2
	loin, blade, roasted, lean w/fat		1.2	oz.	1	0	4

Item	Amount	Unit			
loin, blade, roasted, lean only	1	oz.	1	0	2
loin, center, braised, lean w/fat	0.8	oz.	1	0	2
loin, center, braised, lean only	0.7	oz.	1	0	1
loin, center, broiled, lean w/fat	0.9	oz.	1	0	2
loin, center, broiled, lean only	0.8	oz.	1	0	1
loin, center, roasted, lean w/fat	1	oz.	1	0	2
loin, center, roasted, lean only	0.9	oz.	1	0	1
loin, center rib, braised, lean w/fat	0.9	oz.	1	0	2
loin, center rib, braised, lean only	0.7	oz.	1	0	1
loin, center rib, broiled, lean w/fat	1	oz.	1	0	3
loin, center rib, broiled, lean only	0.9	oz.	1	0	1
loin, center rib, roasted, lean w/fat	1	oz.	1	0	2
loin, center rib, roasted, lean only	0.9	oz.	1	0	1
loin, top, braised, lean w/fat	0.9	oz.	1	0	2
loin, top, braised, lean only	0.7	oz.	1	0	1
loin, top, broiled, lean w/fat	1.1	oz.	1	0	3
loin, top, broiled, lean only	0.9	oz.	1	0	1
loin, top, roasted, lean only	0.9	oz.	1	0	1
shoulder, whole, roasted, lean w/fat	1.1	oz.	1	0	3
shoulder, whole, roasted, lean only	1	oz.	1	0	1
shoulder, arm (picnic), roasted, lean w/fat	1.1	oz.	1	0	3

PROTEIN

FOOD ITEM	SPECIFICATIONS	BRAND NAME	QUANTITY	SIZE	PROTEIN BLOCKS	CARBOHYDRATE BLOCKS	FAT BLOCKS
	shoulder, arm (picnic), roasted, lean w/fat, diced		0.2	cup	1	0	3
	shoulder, arm (picnic), roasted, lean only		0.9	oz.	1	0	1
	shoulder, arm (picnic), roasted, lean only, diced		0.2	cup	1	0	1
	shoulder, Boston, blade, braised, lean w/fat		0.9	oz.	1	0	3
	shoulder, Boston, blade, braised, lean only		0.8	oz.	1	0	1
	shoulder, Boston, blade, broiled, lean w/fat		1.1	oz.	1	0	3
	shoulder, Boston, blade, broiled, lean only		1	oz.	1	0	2
	shoulder, Boston, blade, roasted, lean only		1	oz.	1	0	2
	sirloin, braised, lean w/fat		0.9	oz.	1	0	2
	sirloin, braised, lean only		0.7	oz.	1	0	1
	sirloin, broiled, lean w/fat		1	oz.	1	0	3
	sirloin, broiled, lean only		0.9	oz.	1	0	1
	sirloin, roasted, lean w/fat		1	oz.	1	0	2
	sirloin, roasted, lean only		0.9	oz.	1	0	1
	spareribs, lean w/fat, braised		0.5	oz.	1	0	2
	tenderloin, lean only, roasted		0.9	oz.	1	0	0
Pork, pickled	hocks	Hormel	1.5	oz.	1	0	2
	tidbits	Hormel	1.8	oz.	1	0	3
Pork, refrigerated	loin, center	John Morrell Table Trim	1.5	oz.	1	0	1
	smoked shoulder butt	Oscar Mayer Sweet Morsel	1.9	oz.	1	0	3
	tenderloin	John Morrell Table Trim	1.4	oz.	1	0	1
Pork batter	frying	House of Tsang	10	Tbsp.	1	0	0
Pork belly	raw		2.5	oz.	1	0	13
Pork lunch meat		Hormel Deli Pork Roast	1.2	oz.	1	0	1
	seasoned	Boar's Head	1	oz.	1	0	1

Food	Description	Brand	Amount	Unit			
Pork rind snack		Old Dutch Bac'n Puffs	0.5	oz.	1	0	2
		Baken-ets	0.5	oz.	1	0	2
		Baken-ets Cracklins	0.5	oz.	1	0	2
	hot and spicy	Baken-ets	0.5	oz.	1	0	2
	hot and spicy	Baken-ets Cracklins	0.5	oz.	1	0	2
Pout, ocean, meat only	raw		1.5	oz.	1	0	0
	baked, broiled, or microwaved		1.1	oz.	1	0	0
Proscuitto		Primissimo	1.8	oz.	1	0	5
Rabbit, meat only	domesticated, roasted		0.9	oz.	1	0	1
	domesticated, stewed		0.8	oz.	1	0	1
	domesticated, stewed, diced		0.2	cup	1	0	1
	wild, stewed		0.8	oz.	1	0	0
	wild, stewed, diced		0.2	cup	1	0	0
Rockfish	raw		1.3	oz.	1	0	0
	baked, broiled, or microwaved		1	oz.	1	0	0
Roe, see also "Caviar"			1.1	oz.	1	0	1
			2	Tbsp.	1	0	0
Roughy, orange, meat only	raw		0.9	oz.	1	0	1
			1.7	oz.	1	0	1
			1.3	oz.	1	0	0
Sablefish, meat only	raw		1.8	oz.	1	0	3
	baked, broiled, or microwaved		1.4	oz.	1	0	3
Salami	smoked		1.4	oz.	1	0	3
	beef	Boar's Head Chub	1.4	oz.	1	0	2
	beef	Hebrew National	1.8	oz.	1	0	5
	beef	Hebrew National Lean	1.5	oz.	1	0	2
	beef	Hebrew National Reduced Fat	1.8	oz.	1	0	3
	beef	Oscar Mayer Machiach	2.2	slices	1	0	3
	beer	Oscar Mayer	2.2	slices	1	0	3
	cooked	Boar's Head	1.8	oz.	1	0	4
	cotto	Oscar Mayer	2.2	slices	1	0	3

FOOD ITEM	SPECIFICATIONS	BRAND NAME	QUANTITY	SIZE	PROTEIN BLOCKS	CARBOHYDRATE BLOCKS	FAT BLOCKS
	beef	Oscar Mayer	2.2	oz.	1	0	2
	beef, dry or hard	Boar's Head	1.1	oz.	1	0	3
	beef, dry or hard	Hormel Homeland/Sandwich Maker	1.4	oz.	1	0	4
	beef, dry or hard	Oscar Mayer	3.3	oz.	1	0	3
	Genoa	Boar's Head	1.2	oz.	1	0	3
	Genoa	Di Lusso	1.1	oz.	1	0	3
	Genoa	Hormel Pillow Pack	1.4	oz.	1	0	4
	Genoa	Hormel Sandwich Maker	1.4	oz.	1	0	6
	Genoa	Oscar Mayer	1.4	oz.	1	0	4
	Genoa	San Remo Brand	1.1	oz.	1	0	3
"Salami," vegetarian, frozen	roll	Worthington	1.8	slices	1	0	2
	sliced	Worthington	0.6	3/8" slice	1	1	2
Salmon, fresh, meat only	Atlantic, farmed, raw		1.3	oz.	1	0	1
	Atlantic, farmed, baked, broiled, or microwaved		1.1	oz.	1	0	1
	Atlantic, wild, raw		1.3	oz.	1	0	1
	Atlantic, wild, baked, broiled, or microwaved		1	oz.	1	0	1
	Chinook, raw		1.2	oz.	1	0	1
	Chinook, baked, broiled, or microwaved		1	oz.	1	0	1
	chum, raw		1.2	oz.	1	0	0
	chum, baked, broiled, or microwaved		1	oz.	1	0	0
	coho, farmed, raw		1.2	oz.	1	0	1
	coho, farmed, baked, broiled, or microwaved		1	oz.	1	0	1
	coho, wild, raw		1.1	oz.	1	0	1
	coho, wild, baked, broiled, or microwaved		1.1	oz.	1	0	1
	coho, wild, boiled, poached, or steamed		0.9	oz.	1	0	1

Sausage, cooked

Item	Brand	Amount	Unit			
beef	Hormel Special Recipe	2.5	link	1	0	10
beef, roll	Hormel Special Recipe	1.4	patty	1	0	9
beef, smoked	Jones Dairy Farm Golden Brown	2	links	1	0	5
	Jones Dairy Farm All Natural	1.2	oz.	1	0	2
brown and serve	Oscar Mayer Smokies	1.4	link	1	0	0
brown and serve	Little Sizzlers	2.7	links	1	0	6
brown and serve, beef, smoked	Little Sizzlers	2	patties	1	0	6
	Jones Dairy Farm	2.2	links	1	0	7
brown and serve, light	Jones Dairy Farm	2	links	1	0	3
brown and serve, pork	Jones Dairy Farm	2.9	links	1	0	9
brown and serve, pork and smoked / pork and bacon	Jones Dairy Farm	2.2	links	1	0	7
cheese, smoked	Oscar Mayer Smokies	1.1	link	1	0	4
cheese, smoked	Oscar Mayer Smokies	6	links	1	0	5
dinner	Jones Dairy Farm	0.8	link or patty	1	0	5
dinner	Jones Dairy Farm All Natural	1.1	link or patty	1	0	6
dinner, Italian	Jones Dairy Farm	0.7	link or patty	1	0	4
dinner, sandwich patty	Jones Dairy Farm	1.4	link or patty	1	0	7
Italian, pork		1.3	oz.	1	0	3
pickled, smoked or hot	Hormel	5.5	links	1	0	4
pork, fresh		1.3	oz.	1	0	3
pork	Jones Dairy Farm All Natural Light	1.8	links	1	0	4
pork	Jones Dairy Farm All Natural Little Links	2.7	links	1	0	5
pork	Little Sizzlers	2.7	links	1	0	6
pork	Oscar Mayer	1.5	links	1	0	4
pork, hot and spicy	Little Sizzlers	2.7	links	1	0	6
pork, light	Jones Dairy Farm Golden Brown	2	links	1	0	3
pork, maple	Jones Dairy Farm Golden Brown	2.9	links	1	0	9
pork, mild or milk	Jones Dairy Farm Golden Brown	2.2	links	1	0	7
pork, spicy	Jones Dairy Farm Golden Brown	2.2	links	1	0	7
pork, patty	Jones Dairy Farm All Natural	1.4	patty	1	0	7
pork, patty	Jones Dairy Farm Golden Brown	1.4	patty	1	0	6
pork, patty	Little Sizzlers	1.4	patties	1	0	7
pork roll, regular or hot	Jones Dairy Farm All Natural	1.5	oz.	1	0	5

FOOD ITEM	SPECIFICATIONS	BRAND NAME	QUANTITY	SIZE	PROTEIN BLOCKS	CARBOHYDRATE BLOCKS	FAT BLOCKS
	smoked	Boar's Head	1.9	oz.	1	0	5
	smoked	John Morrell Bun Size	0.7	link	1	0	6
	smoked	John Morrell Bun Size Less Fat	0.7	link	1	1	3
	smoked	Light & Lean 97 Dinner Link	0.9	link	1	0	1
	smoked	Oscar Mayer Little Smokies	6	links	1	0	5
	smoked	Oscar Mayer Smokie Links	1.4	link	1	0	6
	smoked, hot	Boar's Head	1.9	oz.	1	0	5
Sausage, canned		Diana Salchichas	4.3	links	1	0	6
Sausage hash	canned	Mary Kitchen	0.5	cup	1	1	4
"Sausage" vegetarian			1.4	.9-oz. link	1	0	3
			1	1.3-oz. patty	1	0	2
	canned	Loma Linda	1.8	links	1	0	2
		Worthington Saucettes	1.1	link	1	0	2
	frozen	Green Giant Breakfast	1.8	links	1	0	1
	frozen	Green Giant Breakfast	1.4	patties	1	0	1
	frozen	Morningstar Farms Breakfast	1.8	links	1	0	1
	frozen	Morningstar Farms Breakfast	0.9	patty	1	0	1
	frozen	Worthington Prosage Links	1.8	links	1	0	1
	frozen	Worthington Prosage Patties	0.8	patty	1	0	1
	frozen, ground	Worthington Vegetarian	0.3	cup	1	0	1
	frozen, roll	Worthington Prosage	0.7	5/8" slice	1	0	2
	mix, prepared	Fantasic Nature's Sausage	1.1	patty	1	1	1
Sausage stick		Tombstone Snappy Sticks	1.7	pc.	1	0	5
	beef	Boar's Head	1.5	oz.	1	0	8
		Old Dutch	1.1	oz.	1	0	3
		Rustlers Roundup Jerky	3.3	pc.	1	0	3
		Tombstone Jerky	1.1	pc.	1	0	0
		Tombstone Stick	2.5	pc.	1	0	8
	hot	Rustlers Roundup	3.3	pc.	1	0	3
	smoked, mild or spicy	Slim Jim	0.8	1.4-oz. box	1	0	5
	smoked	Rustlers Roundup Steak Stick	0.9	pc.	1	0	1
	spicy	Rustlers Roundup	3.3	pc.	1	0	3
	summer sausage	Old Dutch	1	oz.	1	0	3

Food	Preparation	Brand	Amount	Unit			
Scallop, meat only	raw		1.5	oz.	1	0	0
Scallop, fried, frozen	raw		1.6	oz.	1	0	0
"Scallop," vegetarian		Mrs. Paul's	7.1	pcs.	1	1	2
	canned	Loma Linda Tender Bits	1.9	oz.	1	0	0
	canned	Worthington Vegetable Scallops	3.8	pcs.	1	0	1
Scup, meat only	raw		0.2	cup	1	0	0
	baked, broiled, or microwaved		1.3	oz.	1	0	0
Sea bass, meat only	raw		1.3	oz.	1	0	0
	baked, broiled, or microwaved		1.1	oz.	1	0	0
Sea trout, meat only	raw		1.5	oz.	1	0	0
	baked, broiled, or microwaved		1.1	oz.	1	0	1
Shad, meat only	raw		1.5	oz.	1	0	2
	baked, broiled, or microwaved		1.1	oz.	1	0	2
Shark	meat only, raw		1.2	oz.	1	0	1
Sheepshead, meat only	raw		1.2	oz.	1	0	0
	baked, broiled, or microwaved		1	oz.	1	0	0
Shrimp, meat only	raw		1.2	oz.	1	0	0
Shrimp, canned	raw		1.3	oz.	1	0	0
	drained	S&W	0.2	cup	1	0	0
	deveined, small/medium	Goya	0.2	cup	1	0	0
	all sizes	Sau-Sea	1.4	oz.	1	0	0
		Sau-Sea	5	oz.	1	2	0
		Vita	5.5	oz.	1	2	0
Shrimp cocktail			5	oz.	1	2	0
"Shrimp," imitation	from surimi		2	oz.	1	1	1
	frozen, jumbo	Captain Jac Shrimp Tasties	3.3	oz.	1	0	0
Smelt, rainbow, meat only	raw		1.4	oz.	1	0	0
	baked, broiled, or microwaved		1.1	oz.	1	0	0
	frozen	Van de Kamp's Natural	1.2	oz.	1	0	0

FOOD ITEM	SPECIFICATIONS	BRAND NAME	QUANTITY	SIZE	PROTEIN BLOCKS	CARBOHYDRATE BLOCKS	FAT BLOCKS
Snapper, meat only	raw		1.7	oz.	1	0	0
	baked, broiled, or microwaved		1.7	oz.	1	0	0
Sole entree	frozen, breaded	Mrs. Paul's Premium	0.3	fillet	1	1	1
	frozen, breaded	Van de Kamp's Light	0.5	fillet	1	1	2
Sopressata		Boar's Head Cinghiale Mini	0.9	oz.	1	0	3
Soy beverage	milk		8.9	fl. oz.	1	0	2
		EdenSoy	8	fl. oz.	1	1	1
		EdenSoy Extra	8.9	fl. oz.	1	1	2
		Soy Moo Fat Free	13.3	fl. oz.	1	4	0
	carob	EdenSoy	13.3	fl. oz.	1	4	2
	vanilla	EdenSoy	13.3	fl. oz.	1	4	2
	vanilla	EdenSoy Extra	13.3	fl. oz.	1	4	2
Soy beverage mix, dry	all purpose	Loma Linda Soyagen No Sucrose	0.4	cup	1	2	3
	carob	Loma Linda Soyagen	0.4	cup	1	2	3
		Loma Linda Soyagen	0.4	cup	1	2	3
Soy meal	defatted, raw		0.1	cup	1	1	0
Soy protein	concentrate, w/alcohol		0.4	oz.	1	0	0
	concentrate, acid/water wash		0.4	oz.	1	0	0
Soybean	green, raw, shelled		0.2	cup	1	0	1
	green, boiled, drained		0.3	cup	1	0	1
	dried, raw		0.1	cup	1	0	1
	dried, boiled		0.3	cup	1	0	2
	dried, dry-roasted		0.1	cup	1	0	1
	dried, roasted		0.1	cup	1	0	2
Soybean kernels	roasted, toasted		0.7	oz.	1	1	1
	roasted, toasted, whole		0.2	cup	1	1	2
	roasted, toasted, salted, whole		0.2	cup	1	1	2
Soybean sprouts		Jonathan's	0.6	cup	1	1	1
			1.9	oz.	1	1	1

Food	Brand	Preparation	Amount	Unit	Protein	Carbohydrate	Fat
Spiny lobster, meat only		raw	1.2	oz.	1	0	0
		boiled or steamed	0.2	2 lb. lobster w/shell	1	0	0
Spot, meat only		boiled or steamed	0.9	oz.	1	0	0
		raw	1.3	oz.	1	0	1
		baked, broiled, or microwaved	1.1	oz.	1	0	1
Squab		fresh, raw, meat w/skin	1.3	oz.	1	0	3
		fresh, raw, breast meat only	1.4	oz.	1	0	1
Squid		meat only, raw	1.6	oz.	1	0	0
	Goya	canned	0.1	can	1	0	0
	Goya	canned, in juice	0.2	cup	1	0	3
Stomach		pork, raw	1.4	oz.	1	0	1
Sturgeon, meat only		raw	1.5	oz.	1	0	1
		baked, broiled, or microwaved	1.2	oz.	1	0	1
		smoked	0.8	oz.	1	0	0
Sucker, white, meat only		raw	1.5	oz.	1	0	0
		baked, broiled, or microwaved	1.1	oz.	1	0	0
Summer sausage	Old Smokehouse		1.7	oz.	1	0	5
	Oscar Mayer	beef	2	slices, 1.6 oz.	1	0	4
	Oscar Mayer		2	slices, 1.6 oz.	1	0	4
Sunfish, pumpkinseed, meat only		baked, broiled, or microwaved	1.3	oz.	1	0	0
		raw	1	oz.	1	0	0
Surimi		pollock	1.6	oz.	1	0	0
Swordfish, fresh, meat only		raw	1.3	oz.	1	0	1
		baked, broiled, or microwaved	1	oz.	1	0	0
Swordfish, frozen	Peter Pan	steaks	1	oz.	1	0	0
Thymus		beef, braised	1.1	oz.	1	0	3
		veal, braised	0.8	oz.	1	0	0
Tilefish, meat only		raw	1.4	oz.	1	0	0

FOOD ITEM	SPECIFICATIONS	BRAND NAME	QUANTITY	SIZE	PROTEIN BLOCKS	CARBOHYDRATE BLOCKS	FAT BLOCKS
Tofu	baked, broiled, or microwaved		1	oz.	1	0	1
	fresh		3.3	oz.	1	0	0
	fresh		0.4	cup	1	0	1
	fresh, extra firm	Nasoya	0.1	of 1-lb. block	1	0	1
	fresh, firm		1.7	oz.	1	0	2
	fresh, firm		0.2	cup	1	0	1
	fresh, firm	Nasoya	0.2	of 1-lb. block	1	0	1
	fresh, silken	Nasoya	0.3	of 1-lb. block	1	0	1
	fresh, soft	Nasoya	0.2	of 1-lb. block	1	0	1
	flavored, 5-spice	Nasoya	0.2	block	1	0	1
	flavored, French	Nasoya	0.2	block	1	0	1
	salted and fermented	Fuyu	3.3	oz.	1	0	3
Tofu dishes, mix, dry	burger	Fantastic	0.3	cup	1	3	3
	chow mein, mandarin	Fantastic	0.7	cup	1	3	1
	shells 'n curry	Fantastic	0.5	cup	1	4	1
	Stroganoff, creamy	Fantastic	0.4	cup	1	3	1
Tongue, braised	beef		1.1	oz.	1	0	2
	lamb		1.1	oz.	1	0	2
	pork		1	oz.	1	0	2
	veal (calf)		1	oz.	1	0	1
Tongue lunch meat	beef, corned	Hebrew National	1.4	oz.	1	0	2
Trout, meat only	mixed species, raw		1.2	oz.	1	0	1
	mixed species, baked, broiled, or microwaved		0.9	oz.	1	0	1
	rainbow, farmed, raw		1.2	oz.	1	0	1
	rainbow, farmed, baked, broiled, or microwaved		1	oz.	1	0	1
	rainbow, wild, raw		1.2	oz.	1	0	0
	rainbow, wild, baked, broiled, or microwaved		1.1	oz.	1	0	1
	smoked, peppered, rainbow	Spence & Co.	1	oz.	1	0	1

Food	Description	Brand	Amount	Unit			
Tuna, meat only	bluefin, raw		1.1	oz.	1	0	1
	bluefin, baked, broiled, or microwaved		0.8	oz.	0	0	1
	skipjack, raw		1.1	oz.	0	0	1
	skipjack, baked, broiled, or microwaved		0.9	oz.	0	0	1
	yellowfin, raw		1.1	oz.	0	0	1
	yellowfin, baked, broiled, or microwaved		0.8	oz.	0	0	1
Tuna, canned, drained	chunk light, oil	Bumble Bee	1.1	oz.	1	0	1
	chunk light, oil	Chicken of the Sea	1.1	oz.	1	0	1
	chunk light, oil	S&W	1	oz.	1	0	1
	chunk light, oil	Star-Kist	1.1	oz.	1	0	1
	chunk light, water	Bumble Bee	1.1	oz.	0	0	1
	chunk light, water	S&W	1	oz.	0	0	1
	solid, olive oil	Progresso	1.1	oz.	2	0	1
	solid light, water	Star-Kist/Star-Kist Prime Catch	1.1	oz.	0	0	1
	solid white, oil	Bumble Bee	1	oz.	1	0	1
	solid white, oil	Chicken of the Sea	1	oz.	0	0	1
	solid white, oil	S&W	0.8	oz.	0	0	1
	solid white, oil	Star-Kist	1	oz.	0	0	1
	solid white, water	Bumble Bee	1	oz.	0	0	1
	yellowtail	Peter Pan	1.1	oz.	0	0	1
Tuna, frozen	frozen, drained		0.6	cup	2	0	1
"Tuna," vegetarian		Worthington Tuno	0.3	cup	3	0	1
Tuna salad spread		Libby's Spreadables	1.5	oz.	0	0	1
Turbot, European, meat only	raw					0	
	baked, broiled, or microwaved		1.2	oz.	0	0	1
Turkey, fresh, roasted	meat w/skin		0.9	oz.	1	0	1
	meat only		8	oz.	4	0	1
	meat only, diced		0.2	cup	0	0	1
	skin only		1.3	oz.	5	0	1
	dark meat, w/skin		0.9	oz.	1	0	1
	dark meat, meat only		0.9	oz.	1	0	1
	dark meat, meat only, diced		0.2	cup	1	0	1

FOOD ITEM	SPECIFICATIONS	BRAND NAME	QUANTITY	SIZE	PROTEIN BLOCKS	CARBOHYDRATE BLOCKS	FAT BLOCKS
	light meat, w/skin		0.9	oz.	1	0	1
	light meat, meat only		0.8	oz.	1	0	0
	light meat, meat only, diced		0.2	cup	1	0	0
	breast, meat w/skin		0.1	lb., 1/2 breast, .42 lbs raw w/bone	1	0	1
	breast, meat w/skin		0.9	oz.	1	0	1
	leg, meat w/skin		0.1	lb., .5 lbs. raw w/bone	1	0	1
	leg, meat w/skin		0.9	oz.	1	0	1
	wing, meat w/skin		0.9	oz., 9.9 oz. raw w/bone	1	0	1
	wing, meat w/skin		0.9	oz.	1	0	1
Turkey, canned, chunk	white	Hormel	1.3	oz.	1	0	1
	white	Swanson Premium	2.2	oz.	1	0	0
		Hormel	1.1	oz.	1	0	3
		Swanson Premium	5	oz.	1	0	1
Turkey, frozen or refrigerated	whole, raw, young	Norbest Family Tradition, 8-16 lbs.	1.2	oz.	1	0	1
	whole, raw, young	Norbest Family Tradition, 16-24 lbs.	1.2	oz.	1	0	1
	whole, raw, young, basted	Norbest, 8-16 lbs.	1.3	oz.	1	0	1
	whole, raw, young, basted	Norbest, 16-24 lbs.	1.3	oz.	1	0	2
	whole, cooked, dark meat	Perdue	1.1	oz.	1	0	1
	whole, cooked, white meat	Perdue	1	oz.	1	0	1
	whole, cooked, barbecued	Empire Kosher	1	oz.	1	0	1
	breast, raw, basted	Norbest	1.3	oz.	1	0	0
	breast, raw, boneless	Perdue	1	oz.	1	0	0
	breast, raw, cutlets, thin sliced	Perdue	1.1	oz.	1	0	0
	breast, raw, fillets	Perdue	1	oz.	1	0	1
	breast, raw, roast, boneless	Norbest	1.4	oz.	1	0	0
	breast, raw, tenderloins	Perdue	1	oz.	1	0	0
	breast, cooked	Perdue Whole	0.9	oz.	1	0	0

Item		Brand	Amount	Unit			
	breast, cooked	Perdue Half	0.9	oz.	1	0	0
	breast, cooked, boneless or tenderloins	Perdue	0.8	oz.	1	0	1
	breast, cooked, cutlets, thin sliced	Perdue	0.8	oz.	1	0	0
	breast, cooked, fillets	Perdue	0.8	oz.	1	0	0
	breast, cooked, honey roasted	Louis Rich	1.2	oz.	1	0	0
	breast, oven roasted	Louis Rich	1.2	oz.	1	0	0
	breast, oven roasted	Hebrew National	1.1	oz.	1	0	0
	breast, oven roasted, skinless	Hebrew National	1.3	oz.	1	0	0
	breast, smoked	Hebrew National	1.2	oz.	1	0	0
	breast, smoked	Hormel Light & Lean 97	1.3	oz.	1	0	0
	breast, smoked	Louis Rich Hickory	1.2	oz.	1	0	0
	breast, smoked	Perdue	1	oz.	1	0	0
	maple glaze	Boar's Head Honey Coat	1	oz.	1	0	0
	roast, boneless	Norbest	1.5	oz.	1	0	1
	smoked, hickory	Norbest Young	1.3	oz.	1	0	0
	steak, cubed, raw	Perdue	1.2	oz.	1	0	1
	thigh, cooked	Perdue			1	0	0
	wing, cooked	Perdue Tom	0.9	oz.	1	0	1
	wing, cooked, portion	Perdue	1	oz. wing	1	0	0
	wing, cooked, roasted	Perdue	1	oz. pc.	1	0	1
	wing, cooked, roasted	Perdue Drummettes	1		1	0	1
Turkey, ground	raw	Louis Rich	1.4	oz.	1	0	1
	raw	Norbest	1.7	oz.	1	0	1
	raw	Perdue	1.3	oz.	1	0	1
	raw	Shady Brook Farms	1.3	oz.	1	0	1
	raw, breast	Perdue	1	oz.	1	0	1
	raw, breast	Shady Brook Farms			1	0	1
	cooked, breast	Perdue	0.9	oz.	1	0	0
	cooked, regular or burger	Perdue	1	oz.	1	0	0
"Turkey," vegetarian	canned	Worthington Turkee	1.6	slices	1	0	3
	frozen, smoked, roll	Worthington	0.7	3/8" slice	1	0	2
	frozen, smoked, sliced	Worthington	2.1	slices	1	0	2

FOOD ITEM	SPECIFICATIONS	BRAND NAME	QUANTITY	SIZE	PROTEIN BLOCKS	CARBOHYDRATE BLOCKS	FAT BLOCKS
Turkey bacon		Louis Rich	1.7	oz. slice	1	0	3
Turkey bologna		Empire	2.7	slices	1	0	2
		Louis Rich	2.5	oz. slice	1	0	3
Turkey frankfurter		Norbest	2	oz.	1	0	4
	and beef	Empire Kosher	0.8	link	1	0	2
	and chicken	Oscar Mayer Hot Dogs	1	link	1	0	0
	and chicken	Louis Rich 8/12 oz.	1.1	1.5 oz. link	1	0	2
		Louis Rich 10/16 oz.	1.4	1.6 oz. link	1	0	3
		Louis Rich Bun-Length	1	link	1	0	3
	cheese	Louis Rich	1.4	link	1	0	3
Turkey giblets	simmered		0.9	oz.	1	0	0
	simmered, diced		0.2	cup	1	0	0
Turkey ham		Healthy Deli	1.4	oz.	1	0	1
		Louis Rich	1.3	oz.	1	0	1
		Louis Rich Round	1.4	oz. slice	1	0	0
		Louis Rich Square	1.9	slices 2.2 oz.	1	0	1
		Louis Rich Deli-Thin	2.9	slices 2 oz.	1	0	1
		Norbest Tavern Ham	1.5	oz.	1	0	1
	canned	Hormel	1.5	oz.	1	0	1
	chopped	Louis Rich	1.4	oz. slice	1	0	1
	honey cured	Louis Rich	1.9	slices	1	0	1
Turkey hash		Mary Kitchen	0.3	cup	1	1	0
	roast	Boar's Head Premium Lower Sodium	1.3	oz.	1	0	1
Turkey lunch meat, breast		Boar's Head Premium Lower Sodium Skinless	1.2	oz.	1	0	0
		Boar's Head Ovengold	1.2	oz.	1	0	1
		Boar's Head Ovengold Skinless	1.1	oz.	1	0	0
		Boar's Head Salsalito	1.1	oz.	1	0	0
		Hormel Deli No Salt	1	oz.	1	0	0
		Hormel Deli Premium	1.3	oz.	1	0	0
		Hormel Light & Lean 97	1.4	oz.	1	0	0
		Hormel Light & Lean 97	1.4	oz. slice	1	0	0

	Brand	Amount	Unit			
barbecued	Hormel Sandwich Maker	1.8	oz.	1	○	0
Black Forest	Norbest Bronze Label	2	oz.	1	○	1
cured	Norbest Gold Label	1.4	oz.	1	○	1
honey roasted	Norbest Gold Label Golden Browned	1.4	oz.	1	○	1
honey roasted	Norbest Silver Label	2	oz.	1	○	1
honey roasted	Louis Rich	6.7	oz.	1	○	0
honey roasted	Healthy Deli	1.3	oz.	1	○	0
lemon garlic	Norbest Gourmet	2	oz.	1	○	2
maple honey	Healthy Deli	1.4	oz.	1	○	0
oven roasted	Hormel Light & Lean 97	1.3	oz.	1	○	0
oven roasted	Louis Rich	1.3	oz.	1	○	0
oven roasted	Hebrew National	3.1	slices, thin	1	○	0
oven roasted	Boar's Head	1	oz.	1	○	0
oven roasted	Alpine Lace	1.2	oz.	1	○	0
oven roasted	Boar's Head Golden	1.3	oz.	1	○	1
oven roasted	Boar's Head Golden Skinless	1.1	oz.	1	○	0
oven roasted	Empire	2.1	slices	1	○	0
oven roasted	Healthy Deli Gourmet	1.3	oz.	1	○	0
oven roasted	Healthy Deli Gourmet Brick Oven	1.3	oz.	1	○	0
oven roasted	Healthy Deli Less Sodium	1.4	oz.	1	○	0
oven roasted	Healthy Deli Natural Shape	1.3	oz.	1	○	0
oven roasted	Hebrew National	3.1	slices, thin	1	○	0
oven roasted	Louis Rich	1.3	oz.	1	○	0
oven roasted	Louis Rich Fat Free	1.7	oz. slice	1	○	0
oven roasted	Louis Rich Carving Board Thin	3.5	slices	1	○	0
oven roasted	Louis Rich Carving Board Traditional	1.5	slices	1	○	0
oven roasted	Louis Rich Deli-Thin Fat Free	3.6	slices	1	○	0
oven roasted	Oscar Mayer	1.4	oz. slice	1	○	0
oven roasted	Oscar Mayer Fat Free	3.6	slices	1	○	0
oven roasted, glazed	Healthy Deli Gourmet	1.3	oz.	1	○	0
oven roasted, Italian	Healthy Deli	1.4	oz.	1	○	0
oven roasted, white	Oscar Mayer	1.7	oz. slice	1	○	0
oven roasted, and white	Louis Rich	1.5	oz.	1	○	0
oven roasted, and white	Louis Rich	1.4	oz. slice	1	○	0
oven roasted, and white	Oscar Mayer Deli-Thin	3.1	slices	1	○	0
roast	Oscar Mayer Deli-Thin	3.1	slices	1	○	0

FOOD ITEM	SPECIFICATIONS	BRAND NAME	QUANTITY	SIZE	PROTEIN BLOCKS	CARBOHYDRATE BLOCKS	FAT BLOCKS
	skinless	Hormel	1.4	oz.	1	0	0
	skinless	Hormel Deli	1.3	oz.	1	0	0
	smoked	Boar's Head Hickory	1.2	oz.	1	0	1
	smoked	Boar's Head Cracked Pepper Mill	1.1	oz.	1	0	0
	smoked	Empire	2.7	slices	1	0	0
	smoked	Healthy Deli Mesquite	1.3	oz.	1	0	0
	smoked	Hebrew National	3.1	slices, thin	1	0	0
	smoked	Hebrew National Hickory	1.3	oz.	1	0	0
	smoked	Hormel Mesquite	1.3	oz.	1	0	0
	smoked	Hormel Light & Lean 97 Mesquite	1.4	oz.	1	0	0
	smoked	Louis Rich Hickory	1.3	oz.	1	0	0
	smoked	Louis Rich Hickory	1.4	oz. slice	1	0	0
	smoked	Louis Rich Fat Free Hickory	1.7	oz. slice	1	0	0
	smoked	Louis Rich Carving Board	1.5	slices	1	0	0
	smoked	Louis Rich Deli-Thin Hickory	3.1	slices	1	0	0
	smoked	Norbest Gold Label	1.4	oz.	1	0	1
	smoked	Oscar Mayer Fat Free	3.6	slices 1.8 oz.	1	0	0
	smoked, honey roasted	Oscar Mayer Deli-Thin	2.9	slices 1.8 oz.	1	0	0
	smoked, white	Louis Rich	1.4	oz. slice	1	0	0
Turkey nuggets	breaded	Louis Rich	2.1	pcs. 3.25 oz.	1	1	3
Turkey pastrami		Boar's Head	1	oz.	1	0	0
		Empire	2.3	slices	1	0	1
		Louis Rich	1.3	oz.	1	0	1
		Louis Rich Square	1.8	slices	1	0	1
		Healthy Deli	1.4	oz.	1	0	1
		Hebrew National	1.4	oz.	1	0	1
		Norbest	1.4	oz.	1	0	1
Turkey patty	breaded	Empire Kosher	0.5	pc.	1	1	2
	breaded	Louis Rich	0.6	pc.	1	1	2
Turkey salad spread		Libby's Spreadables	0.3	cup	1	0	3
Turkey salami		Empire	2.3	slices	1	0	1
		Louis Rich	1.8	oz.	1	0	3
		Louis Rich	1.4	oz. slice	1	0	1

Item	Brand	Amount	Unit	Protein	Carbohydrate	Fat
cooked	Norbest	1.5	oz.	1	0	2
cotto		1.4	oz.	1	0	1
raw		1.4	oz. slice	1	0	1
Turkey sausage raw	Louis Rich	1.3	links, 2 oz.	1	0	1
breakfast, raw	Louis Rich Links	1.4	oz.	1	0	1
breakfast, raw	Shady Brook Farms Old World	1.5	links	1	0	2
breakfast, cooked	Perdue	1.4	oz.	1	0	1
Italian, hot, raw	Shady Brook Farms	1.5	links	1	0	2
Italian, hot or sweet, raw	Perdue	1.4	oz.	1	0	1
Italian, hot or sweet, raw or cooked	Shady Brook Farms	1.5	links	1	0	2
Italian, sweet, raw	Shady Brook Farms	0.5	link	1	0	1
smoked, raw	Louis Rich	1.4	oz.	1	0	1
smoked, raw	Louis Rich Polska	1.5	oz.	1	0	2
smoked, w/cheese, raw	Louis Rich	1.5	oz.	1	0	2
Turkey sticks breaded	Louis Rich	1.5	oz.	1	1	2
Veal, meat only cubed, lean only, braised or stewed		1.8	pcs.	1	0	3
ground, broiled		0.7	oz.	1	0	0
leg, braised, lean w/fat		1	oz.	1	0	1
leg, braised, lean only		0.7	oz.	1	0	0
leg, roasted, lean w/fat		0.7	oz.	1	0	0
leg, roasted, lean only		0.9	oz.	1	0	0
loin, braised, lean w/fat		0.9	oz.	1	0	0
loin, braised, lean only		0.8	oz.	1	0	0
loin, roasted, lean w/fat		0.7	oz.	1	0	1
loin, roasted, lean only		1	oz.	1	0	1
rib, braised, lean w/fat		0.9	oz.	1	0	1
rib, braised, lean only		0.8	oz.	1	0	1
rib, roasted, lean w/fat		0.7	oz.	1	0	1
rib, roasted, lean only		1	oz.	1	0	1
shoulder, whole, braised, lean w/fat		0.8	oz.	1	0	1
shoulder, whole, braised, lean only		0.7	oz.	1	0	0

FOOD ITEM	SPECIFICATIONS	BRAND NAME	QUANTITY	SIZE	PROTEIN BLOCKS	CARBOHYDRATE BLOCKS	FAT BLOCKS
	shoulder, whole, roasted, lean w/fat		1	oz.	1	0	1
	shoulder, whole, roasted, lean only		1	oz.	1	0	1
	shoulder, arm, braised, lean w/fat		0.7	oz.	1	0	1
	shoulder, arm, braised, lean only		0.7	oz.	1	0	0
	shoulder, arm, roasted, lean w/fat		1	oz.	1	0	1
	shoulder, arm, roasted, lean only		1	oz.	1	0	0
	shoulder, blade, braised, lean w/fat		0.8	oz.	1	0	1
	shoulder, blade, braised, lean only		0.8	oz.	1	0	0
	shoulder, blade, roasted, lean w/fat		1	oz.	1	0	1
	shoulder, blade, roasted, lean only		1	oz.	1	0	1
	sirloin, braised, lean w/fat		0.8	oz.	1	0	1
	sirloin, braised, lean only		0.7	oz.	1	0	0
	sirloin, roasted, lean w/fat		1	oz.	1	0	1
	sirloin, roasted, lean only		0.9	oz.	1	0	0
"Veal," vegetarian	frozen	Worthington Veelets	0.5	patty	1	1	2
Venison, meat only	roasted		0.8	oz.	1	0	0
Vienna sausage, canned		Goya	4	links	1	0	5
		Hormel	2.2	oz.	1	0	4
		Libby's	4.3	links	1	0	6
	w/barbecue sauce	Libby's BBQ	4.3	links	1	0	6
	w/hot sauce	Goya	4.3	links	1	0	6
	chicken	Hormel	2.2	oz.	1	0	3
	chicken	Libby's	3.3	links	1	0	3

Food	Description	Brand	Amount	Unit			
Welsh rarebit	frozen	Stouffer's	4.4	oz.	1	1	6
Whelk	meat only, raw		1	oz.	1	0	0
Whitefish, meat only	raw		1.3	oz.	1	0	1
	baked, broiled, or microwaved		1	oz.	1	0	1
	smoked		1.1	oz.	1	0	0
Whiting, meat only	raw		1.3	oz.	1	0	0
	baked, broiled, or microwaved		1.1	oz.	1	0	0
Wolf fish, Atlantic, meat only	raw		1.4	oz.	1	0	0
Yellowtail, meat only	raw		1.1	oz.	1	0	1
	baked, broiled, or microwaved		0.8	oz.	1	0	1
Yogurt	plain	Breyers	0.6	cup	1	1	1
	plain	Colombo Lowfat	0.9	cup	1	1	1
	plain	Colombo Nonfat	0.6	cup	1	1	0
	plain	Dannon Lowfat	4.7	oz.	1	1	1
	plain	Dannon Lowfat	0.5	cup	1	1	1
	plain	Dannon Nonfat	4.7	oz.	1	1	0
	plain	Dannon Nonfat	0.5	cup	1	1	0
	plain	Ultimate 90	0.9	cup	1	2	0
	all fruit flavors	Light n'Lively Free 50 Cal	6.3	oz.	1	1	0
	all fruit flavors, except banana	Dannon Sprinkl'ins	5.9	oz.	1	4	1
	apple cinnamon	Dannon Fruit on Bottom	0.8	cup	1	4	1
	apple spice or apricot	Colombo	0.9	cup	1	4	1
	banana	Dannon Sprinkl'ins	5.9	oz.	1	4	1
	banana	Tropifruita	6	cup	1	3	0
	banana cream pie	Dannon	0.8	cup	1	2	1
	banana creme strawberry	Dannon Double Delights	6	oz.	1	3	1
	banana strawberry	Colombo Lowfat	1.1	cup	1	4	1
	banana strawberry	Colombo Nonfat	0.9	cup	1	5	0
	Bavarian creme raspberry	Dannon Double Delights	6	oz.	1	3	1

FOOD ITEM	SPECIFICATIONS	BRAND NAME	QUANTITY	SIZE	PROTEIN BLOCKS	CARBOHYDRATE BLOCKS	FAT BLOCKS
	berry, mixed	Breyers	0.9	cup	1	5	1
	berry, mixed	Dannon Fruit on Bottom	0.8	cup	1	4	1
	berry, mixed	Knudsen Free	5.5	oz.	1	4	0
	berry, mixed	Light n' Lively Free	5.5	oz.	1	4	0
	blueberry	Breyers	0.9	cup	1	5	1
	blueberry	Colombo Lowfat	1.1	cup	1	4	1
	blueberry	Colombo Nonfat	0.9	cup	1	4	0
	blueberry	Dannon Danimals	4.9	oz.	1	3	1
	blueberry	Dannon Fruit on the Bottom	0.8	cup	1	4	1
	blueberry	Dannon Nonfat	0.8	cup	1	2	0
	blueberry	Knudsen Cal 70	6	oz.	1	1	0
	blueberry	Light n' Lively Multi	6.3	oz.	1	4	0
	blueberry	Light n' Lively Free	5.5	oz.	1	4	0
	blueberry	Light n' Lively Free 70 Cal	6	oz.	1	1	0
	blueberry and creme	Ultimate 90	0.9	cup	1	1	0
	boysenberry	Dannon Fruit on Bottom	0.8	cup	1	4	1
	cappuccino	Colombo	0.8	cup	1	3	0
	cappuccino	Dannon	0.8	cup	1	2	0
	cappuccino	Ultimate 90	0.9	cup	1	2	0
	cappuccino w/chocolate	Dannon Light'n Crunchy	0.8	cup	1	2	0
	caramel apple	Dannon Light'n Crunchy	0.8	cup	1	2	0
	cheesecake, strawberry/ cherry	Dannon Double Delights	6	oz.	1	3	1
	cherry	Colombo	0.9	cup	1	4	0
	cherry	Dannon Fruit on Bottom	0.8	cup	1	4	1
	cherry, black	Breyers	0.9	cup	1	5	1
	cherry, black	Colombo	1.1	cup	1	4	1
	cherry, black	Knudsen Cal 70	6	oz.	1	1	0
	cherry, black	Light n' Lively Free 70 Cal	6	oz.	1	1	0
	cherry jubilee	Ultimate 90	0.9	cup	1	2	0
	cherry vanilla	Dannon	6.2	oz.	1	2	0
	cherry vanilla	Dannon	0.8	cup	1	2	0

Food	Brand	Amount	Unit			
chocolate, white, and raspberry	Yoplait	6	oz.	1	4	1
coffee	Breyers	0.7	cup	1	3	1
coffee	Dannon	5.7	oz.	1	3	1
coffee	Dannon	0.6	cup	1	3	1
coconut cream pie	Yoplait	6	oz.	1	4	1
cranberry raspberry	Dannon	0.7	cup	1	3	0
cranberry raspberry	Ultimate 90	0.9	cup	1	2	0
cranberry strawberry	Colombo	0.9	cup	1	5	0
creme caramel	Dannon	0.7	cup	1	1	0
French roast	Colombo	0.8	cup	1	3	0
fruit cocktail	Colombo	0.9	cup	1	4	0
guava	Tropifruita	6	oz.	1	3	1
lemon	Colombo	0.7	cup	1	3	0
lemon	Dannon Lowfat	5.7	oz.	1	3	1
lemon	Dannon Lowfat	0.6	cup	1	3	1
lemon	Dannon Nonfat	0.8	cup	1	2	0
lemon	Knudsen Cal 70	6	oz.	1	1	0
lemon	Knudsen Free	5.5	oz.	1	4	0
lemon	Light n' Lively Free	5.5	oz.	1	4	0
lemon	Light n' Lively Free 70 Cal	6	oz.	1	1	0
lemon creamy	Breyers	0.7	cup	1	3	0
lemon ice	Dannon Danimals	4.9	oz.	1	2	0
lemon chiffon	Dannon	6	oz.	1	3	1
lemon chiffon	Ultimate 90	0.9	cup	1	1	0
lemon chiffon w/blueberry	Dannon Light'n Crunchy	0.8	cup	1	2	0
mango	Tropifruita	6	oz.	1	3	0
orange	Dannon Fruit on Bottom	0.8	cup	1	4	0
orange-banana	Dannon Danimals	4.9	oz.	1	3	1
papaya-pineapple	Tropifruita	6	oz.	1	5	0
peach	Breyers	0.9	cup	1	4	1
peach	Colombo	0.9	cup	1	4	1
peach	Dannon Fruit on Bottom	0.8	cup	1	2	1
peach	Dannon Nonfat	0.8	cup	1	1	0
peach	Knudsen Cal 70	6	oz.	1	4	0
peach	Knudsen Free	5.5	oz.	1	4	0

FOOD ITEM	SPECIFICATIONS	BRAND NAME	QUANTITY	SIZE	PROTEIN BLOCKS	CARBOHYDRATE BLOCKS	FAT BLOCKS
	peach	Light n' Lively Multi	6.3	oz.	1	4	0
	peach	Light n' Lively Free	5.5	oz.	1	4	0
	peach	Light n' Lively Free 70 Cal	6.7	oz.	1	1	0
	peach	Ultimate 90	0.9	cup	1	2	0
	peach Melba	Yoplait Tropical	6	oz.	1	4	1
	pear	Colombo Lowfat	1.1	cup	1	4	1
		Dannon Fruit on Bottom	0.8	cup	1	4	1
	pina colada	Tropifruita	6	oz.	1	3	0
	pineapple	Breyers	0.9	cup	1	5	1
	pineapple	Knudsen Cal 70	6	oz.	1	1	0
	pineapple	Light n' Lively Multi	6.3	oz.	1	4	0
	plum	Dannon Fruit on Bottom	0.8	cup	1	4	1
	raspberry	Breyers	0.9	cup	1	5	1
	raspberry	Colombo Lowfat	1.1	cup	1	4	1
	raspberry	Colombo Nonfat	0.9	cup	1	4	0
	raspberry	Dannon Fruit on Bottom	0.8	cup	1	4	1
	raspberry	Dannon Nonfat	0.8	cup	1	2	0
	raspberry	Knudsen Cal 70	6	oz.	1	1	0
	raspberry	Knudsen Free	5.5	oz.	1	3	0
	raspberry	Light n' Lively Multi	6.3	oz.	1	4	0
	raspberry	Light n' Lively Free	5.5	oz.	1	4	0
	raspberry	Light n' Lively Free 70 Cal	6	oz.	1	1	0
	raspberry, creme	Ultimate 90	0.9	cup	1	2	0
	raspberry, w/granola	Dannon Light'n Crunchy	0.7	cup	1	1	1
	raspberry, wild	Dannon Danimals	4.9	oz.	1	2	1
	strawberry	Breyers	0.9	cup	1	5	1
	strawberry	Colombo Lowfat	1.1	cup	1	4	1
	strawberry	Colombo Nonfat	0.9	cup	1	4	0
	strawberry	Dannon Danimals	4.9	oz.	1	3	1
	strawberry	Dannon Nonfat	6.2	oz.	1	2	0
	strawberry	Dannon Nonfat	0.8	cup	1	2	0
	strawberry	Knudsen Cal 70	6	oz.	1	1	0
	strawberry	Knudsen Free	5.5	oz.	1	4	0

Food	Brand	Amount	Unit	Fat	Carbohydrate	Protein
strawberry	Light n' Lively Multi	6.3	oz.	0	4	1
strawberry	Light n' Lively Free	5.5	oz.	0	4	1
strawberry	Light n' Lively Free 70 Cal	6	oz.	0	1	1
strawberry	Tropifruita	6	oz.	0	3	1
strawberry	Ultimate 90	0.9	cup	1	1	1
strawberry	Yoplait	6	oz.	0	4	1
strawberry, fruit basket	Knudsen Cal 70	6	oz.	0	1	1
strawberry, fruit cup	Dannon	0.8	cup	0	2	1
strawberry, fruit cup	Light n' Lively Free	5.5	oz.	0	4	1
strawberry, fruit cup	Light n' Lively Multi	6.3	oz.	0	4	1
strawberry, fruit cup	Light n' Lively Free 70 Cal	6	oz.	0	1	1
strawberry, wild	Light n' Lively Kidpack	6.3	oz.	1	4	1
strawberry-banana	Breyers	0.8	cup	1	5	1
strawberry-banana	Dannon Fruit on Bottom	0.8	cup	0	4	1
strawberry-banana	Dannon Nonfat	0.8	cup	0	2	1
strawberry-banana	Knudsen 70	1	cup	0	1	1
strawberry-banana	Light n' Lively Multi	6.3	oz.	0	4	1
strawberry-banana	Light n' Lively Free 70 Cal	6	oz.	0	1	1
strawberry-banana	Tropifruita	6	oz.	1	3	1
strawberry-banana	Ultimate 90	0.9	cup	0	1	1
strawberry-banana	Yoplait	6	oz.	1	4	1
strawberry-banana	Tropifruita	6	oz.	0	3	1
strawberry-kiwi	Yoplait	6	oz.	0	4	1
strawberry-kiwi	Colombo	0.9	cup	0	4	1
strawberry pineapple, orange	Dannon	0.8	cup	0	2	1
tropical fruit	Dannon Danimals	4.9	oz.	1	3	1
tropical punch	Breyers	0.7	cup	1	3	1
vanilla	Colombo	0.7	cup	0	3	1
vanilla	Dannon Danimals	4.9	oz.	1	3	1
vanilla	Dannon Lowfat	5.7	oz.	1	3	1
vanilla	Dannon Lowfat	0.6	cup	0	2	1
vanilla	Dannon Nonfat	6.2	oz.	0	1	1
vanilla	Dannon Nonfat	0.7	cup	0	1	1
vanilla	Knudsen Cal 70	6	oz.	0	1	1
vanilla	Knudsen Free	5.5	oz.	0	4	1

FOOD ITEM	SPECIFICATIONS	BRAND NAME	QUANTITY	SIZE	PROTEIN BLOCKS	CARBOHYDRATE BLOCKS	FAT BLOCKS
	vanilla	Light n' Lively Free	5.5	oz.	1	4	0
	vanilla	Ultimate 90	0.9	cup	1	2	0
	vanilla, French	Colombo	1	cup	1	3	1
	vanilla, French	Dannon Nonfat	6	oz.	1	3	0
	vanilla, w/chocolate	Dannon Light'n Crunchy	0.8	cup	1	2	0
	vanilla peach apricot or strawberry	Dannon Double Delights	6	oz.	1	3	1
Yogurt, frozen	banana, cream pie	Dannon Light'n Crunchy	0.8	cup	1	5	0
	banana pudding, homestyle	TCBY	1.3	cup	1	5	3
	cappuccino	Ben & Jerry's Nonfat	0.7	cup	1	4	0
	cappuccino	Dannon Light	0.8	cup	1	3	0
	caramel praline crunch	Edy's	0.8	cup	1	3	0
	cherry vanilla, black, swirl	Edy's	0.8	cup	1	3	0
	cherry vanilla, chocolate cherry	Dannon Pure Indulgence	0.8	cup	1	5	2
	cherry vanilla, chocolate chip	Ben & Jerry's Cherry Garcia	1.3	cup	1	8	3
	cherry vanilla, swirl	Dannon Light	1.3	cup	1	5	0
	chocolate	Ben & Jerry's Nonfat	1.3	cup	1	8	0
	chocolate	Dannon Light	0.8	cup	1	3	0
	chocolate	Edy's	1.3	cup	1	5	3
	chocolate	Edy's Nonfat	0.8	cup	1	3	0
	chocolate	Haagen-Dazs	0.5	cup	1	3	1
	chocolate brownie chunk	Edy's	1.3	cup	1	5	3
	chocolate chip cookie dough	Ben & Jerry's	0.7	cup	1	6	1
	chocolate, Dutch	TCBY	1.7	cup	1	7	3
	chocolate nut, chunky	Dannon Pure Indulgence	0.6	cup	1	3	1
	chocolate, triple	Dannon Light'n Crunchy	0.8	cup	1	5	0
	chocolate fudge	Dannon Pure Indulgence Coco-Nut	0.7	cup	1	4	1
	chocolate fudge	Edy's	1.3	cup	1	5	0
	chocolate fudge, brownie	Ben & Jerry's	0.6	cup	1	4	3
	citrus heights	Edy's	1.7	cup	1	7	3
	coffee	Haagen-Dazs	0.5	cup	1	3	1

Food	Brand	Amount	Unit			
coffee fudge	Ben & Jerry's Nonfat	0.8	cup	1	5	0
coffee fudge sundae	Edy's	1.3	cup	1	5	0
cookies 'n cream	Dannon Pure Indulgence	0.7	cup	1	4	1
cookies 'n cream	Edy's	1.3	cup	1	5	3
cookies 'n cream	TCBY	1.3	cup	1	8	3
cone crunch, crispy	TCBY	1.3	cup	1	5	3
espresso, crunchy	Dannon Pure Indulgence	0.7	cup	1	4	1
lemon chiffon	Dannon Light	0.8	cup	1	3	0
marble fudge	Edy's	1.3	cup	1	5	3
marble fudge	Edy's Nonfat	1.3	cup	1	5	0
mocha chocolate chunk	Dannon Light'n Crunchy	0.8	cup	1	5	0
Orange Tango	Haagen-Dazs	0.8	cup	1	5	0
orange vanilla swirl	Edy's	1.3	cup	1	5	3
peach	TCBY	1.3	cup	1	7	0
peach, perfectly	Edy's	1.7	cup	1	3	3
peach, raspberry Melba	Dannon Light	0.8	cup	1	8	0
peanut butter fudge sundae	TCBY	1.3	cup	1	5	3
peanut chocolate	Dannon Light'n Crunchy	0.8	cup	1	8	3
pecan praline crisp	TCBY	1.3	cup	1	8	0
pina colada	Haagen-Dazs	1.3	cup	1	3	3
pine-orange paradise	Edy's	0.8	cup	1	7	0
raspberry	Edy's Nonfat	1.7	cup	1	5	0
raspberry	Ben & Jerry's Nonfat	1.3	cup	1	10	3
raspberry, black	Edy's	1.3	cup	1	5	3
raspberry, vanilla swirl	Haagen-Dazs	1.3	cup	1	5	2
Raspberry Randezvous	Starburst	0.8	cup	1	7	3
raspberry	Edy's	3.3	cup	1	7	3
strawberry	Edy's Nonfat	1.7	cup	1	5	3
strawberry	Dannon Light	1.3	cup	1	3	0
strawberry cheesecake	Edy's	0.8	cup	1	5	0
strawberry, chocolate chip	TCBY	1.3	cup	1	5	3
strawberry, summertime	Haagen-Dazs	1.3	cup	1	8	0
Strawberry Duet	Ben & Jerry's Heath	1.3	cup	1	10	3
toffee crunch	Dannon Pure Indulgence Heath	0.7	cup	1	4	1
toffee crunch	Edy's Heath	0.8	cup	1	3	2

FOOD ITEM	SPECIFICATIONS	BRAND NAME	QUANTITY	SIZE	PROTEIN BLOCKS	CARBOHYDRATE BLOCKS	FAT BLOCKS
	vanilla	Dannon Light	0.8	cup	1	3	0
	vanilla	Edy's	1.3	cup	1	5	3
	vanilla	Edy's Nonfat	0.8	cup	1	3	0
	vanilla	Haagen-Dazs	0.5	cup	1	3	1
	vanilla, classic	TCBY	1.3	cup	1	5	3
	vanilla blueberry swirl	Dannon Light'n Crunchy	0.8	cup	1	5	0
	vanilla chocolate swirl	Edy's	0.8	cup	1	3	0
	vanilla fudge	Ben & Jerry's Nonfat	0.7	cup	1	6	0
	vanilla raspberry truffle	Dannon Pure Indulgence	0.7	cup	1	4	1
Yogurt bar, frozen	all flavors	Starburst	3.3	pc.	1	3	0
	Brownie Nut Blast	Haagen-Dazs Extraas	0.9	pc.	1	3	3
	cherry chocolate chip	Ben & Jerry's Cherry Garcia	1.4	pc.	1	4	7
	cherry chocolate fudge	Haagen-Dazs	1.4	pc.	1	4	6
	chocolate almond	Frozfruit	1.7	pc.	1	5	2
	chocolate fudge	Edy's	1.7	pc.	1	5	8
	peach	Frozfruit	2.5	pc.	1	5	0
	peach	Haagen-Dazs	3.3	pc.	1	7	0
	pina colada	Haagen-Dazs	2.5	pc.	1	5	0
	raspberry and vanilla	Haagen-Dazs	2.5	pc.	1	5	0
	strawberry/strawberry, banana	Frozfruit	2.5	pc.	1	5	0
	Strawberry Cheesecake Craze	Haagen-Dazs Extraas	1	pc.	1	3	3
	strawberry daiquiri	Haagen-Dazs	3.3	pc.	1	7	0
	toffee crunch	Edy's	2.5	pc.	1	8	13
	Tropical Orange Passion	Haagen-Dazs	3.3	pc.	1	7	0
	vanilla almond	Edy's	1.7	pc.	1	5	8

Carbohydrate Table

FOOD ITEM	SPECIFICATIONS	BRAND NAME	QUANTITY	SIZE	PROTEIN BLOCKS	CARBOHYDRATE BLOCKS	FAT BLOCKS
Acerola (fresh)	trimmed		1.5	oz.	0	1	0
	juice		1	cup	0	1	0
Acorn squash	baked, cubed		0.4	cup	0	1	0
	boiled, mashed		0.6	cup	0	1	0
Adzuki beans	Dry	Arrowhead Mills	0.1	cup	1	1	0
	canned	Eden	0.4	cup	1	1	0
	canned	Eden Jars	0.4	cup	0	1	0
Alfalfa sprouts		Arrowhead Mills	4.3	cups	2	1	1
	w/dill or radish sprouts	Jonathan's	10	cups	3	1	2
	w/garlic	Jonathan's	4.3	cups	1	1	1
	w/onion	Jonathan's	4.3	cups	1	1	1
	spiced rings	Jonathan's	10	cups	3	1	2
	hearts	S&W	2.9	rings	1	1	0
Artichoke, globe, frozen			8.2	pkg.	1	1	0
	in brine	Goya	3.8	oz.	0	1	1
	canned	S&W Blended	17.1	pcs.	1	1	0
	frozen, boiled, spears	Green Giant Harvest Fresh	13.3	spears	1	1	1
	frozen, cuts		1.9	cup	1	1	0
Amaranth	whole grain	Arrowhead Mills	0.2	cup	0	1	0
Amaranth flour		Arrowhead Mills	0.1	cup	0	1	0
Amaranth seeds		Arrowhead Mills	0.1	cup	1	1	0
Anasazi beans		Arrowhead Mills	0.1	cup	0	1	0
Apple	w/peel		0.5	2 3/4" apple	0	1	0
	w/peel, sliced		0.8	cup	0	1	0
	peeled		0.6	2 3/4" apple	0	1	0
	peeled, sliced		0.6	cup	0	1	0
	fresh, boiled, peeled, sliced		0.5	cup	0	1	0
Apple, canned	baked, Dutch	Lucky Leaf/Musselman's	0.1	cup	0	1	0
	escalloped	White House	0.1	cup	0	1	0
	fried	Apple Time/Lucky Leaf	0.1	cup	0	1	0
	sliced	Lucky Leaf/Musselman's	0.5	cup	0	1	0
	sliced	Musselman's Home Style	0.1	cup	0	1	0

			Amount	Unit			
Apple, dried	sliced	White House	0.2	cup	0	—	0
	spiced rings	Lucky Leaf/Musselman's	1.1	ring	0	—	0
	spiced rings	White House	0.8	ring	0	—	0
Apple, escalloped	chips	Sonoma	0.5	oz.	0	—	0
	sliced	Smart Snackers	0.8	oz.	0	—	0
	frozen	Del Monte	0.2	cup	0	—	0
Apple butter		Stouffers	1.6	oz.	0	—	0
		Apple Time, Lucky Leaf, Musselman's	1.1	Tbsp.	0	—	0
		Dutch Girl, Mary Ellen, R.W. Knudsen, White House	1	Tbsp.	0	—	0
		Eden	3.3	Tbsp.	0	—	0
		Smucker's, Simply Fruit	0.8	Tbsp.	0	—	0
Apple drink	spread	Apple Time, New Morning	1.4	Tbsp.	0	—	0
		Hi-C Jammin'	2.3	oz.	0	—	0
		Lincoln	2.4	oz.	0	—	0
Apple drink blends	berry, frozen	Dole Burst	2.4	oz.	0	—	0
	black cherry, white grape	Veryfine Quenchers	2.4	oz.	0	—	0
	cranberry	Dole	2.3	oz.	0	—	0
	cranberry	Tree Top	1.8	oz.	0	—	0
	cranberry-tangerine	Veryfine Quenchers	2.4	oz.	0	—	0
	peach-kiwi	Veryfine Quenchers	2.2	oz.	0	—	0
	peach-plum	Veryfine Quenchers	2.2	oz.	0	—	0
	pear-passion fruit	Veryfine Quenchers	2.4	oz.	0	—	0
	punch	Minute Maid	2.2	oz.	0	—	0
	raspberry	Tree Top	1.9	oz.	0	—	0
	raspberry-blackberry	Tropicana Twister	2.2	oz.	0	—	0
	raspberry-cherry	Veryfine Quenchers	2.4	oz.	0	—	0
	raspberry-lime	Veryfine Quenchers	2.4	oz.	0	—	0
	strawberry-banana	Veryfine Quenchers	2.4	oz.	0	—	0
		After the Fall	3.3	oz.	0	—	0
		Apple & Eve	2.8	oz.	0	—	0
		Apple Time/Lincoln/Lucky Leaf/ Speas Farm Regular/Cider	2.4	oz.	0	—	0
Apple juice		Musselman's	2.5	oz.	0	—	0
		Dole	2.3	oz.	0	—	0

FOOD ITEM	SPECIFICATIONS	BRAND NAME	QUANTITY	SIZE	PROTEIN BLOCKS	CARBOHYDRATE BLOCKS	FAT BLOCKS
		Goya/Heinke's Organic/Gravenstein	2.4	oz.	0	1	0
		Minute Maid/Mott's Natural/ Red Cheek/Tree Top	2.5	oz.	0	1	0
		Musselman's Regular/Natural/Cider	2.4	oz.	0	1	0
		Musselman's Premium Natural	2.2	oz.	0	1	0
		R.W. Knudsen Clear	2.6	oz.	0	1	0
		R.W. Knudsen Organic/Gravenstein	2.4	oz.	0	1	0
		S&W/Santa Cruz Organic/ White House	2.4	oz.	0	1	0
		Season's Best	2.6	oz.	0	1	0
		Snapple	2.5	oz.	0	1	0
		Tree Top Fiber Rich	2.4	oz.	0	1	0
		Veryfine	2.1	oz.	0	1	0
		Sparkling Cider Apple Time/ Lucky Leaf/Musselman's	2	oz.	0	1	0
Apple juice, frozen, prepared		Spiced Apple & Eve Cider & Spice	2.8	oz.	0	1	0
		Minute Maid	2.6	oz.	0	1	0
Apple juice blends	all blends except apricot and cherry cider	R.W. Knudsen	2.4	oz.	0	1	0
		Tree Top	2.5	oz.	0	1	0
	apricot	R.W. Knudsen	2.4	oz.	0	1	0
	apricot	After the Fall	3.3	oz.	0	1	0
	apricot	R.W. Knudsen	2.4	oz.	0	1	0
	boysenberry or raspberry	Tree Top Fiber Rich	1.8	oz.	0	1	0
	cherry	Heinke's	2.4	oz.	0	1	0
	cherry cider	After the Fall	3	oz.	0	1	0
	cherry cider	R.W. Knudsen	2.2	oz.	0	1	0
	cranberry	Apple & Eve	2.4	oz.	0	1	0
	cranberry, frozen, prepared	Tree Top	2.2	oz.	0	1	0
	grape	Apple & Eve	2.3	oz.	0	1	0
	grape	Juicy Juice	2.4	oz.	0	1	0

Food		Amount	Unit			
grape	Minute Maid/Tree Top/ Tree Top frozen, prepared	2.2	oz.	0	1	0
orange	Tree Top Fiber Rich	2	oz.	0	1	0
pear	Tree Top	2.5	oz.	0	1	0
raspberry	After the Fall	3.1	oz.	0	1	0
raspberry	Tree Top	2.6	oz.	0	1	0
raspberry frozen, prepared	Tree Top	2.6	oz.	0	1	0
	After the Fall	3	oz.	0	1	0
Apple syrup	R.W. Knudsen	0.1	cup	0	1	0
Applesauce	Apple Time Regular/Granny Smith/ Red Delicious/McIntosh	0.2	cup	0	1	0
	Apple Time/Lucky Leaf/ Musselman's Lite	0.4	cup	0	1	0
	Eden	0.3	cup	0	1	0
	Lincoln/Lucky Leaf Regular/ Chunky/Delicious	0.2	cup	0	1	0
	Lucky Leaf Regular/Cinnamon	2	oz.	0	1	0
	Mott's	0.2	cup	0	1	0
	Mott's Chunky	0.2	cup	0	1	0
	Mott's Cinnamon	0.2	cup	0	1	0
	Musselman's Chunky/Cinnamon/ White House/Cinnamon	0.2	cup	0	1	0
	Musselman's Regular/Cinnamon	1.9	oz.	0	1	0
	Musselman's	2	oz.	0	1	0
	S&W Gravenstein	0.2	cup	0	1	0
	Tree Top Original/Cinnamon	0.2	cup	0	1	0
	White House	0.2	cup	0	1	0
	Apple Time/Lincoln	0.4	cup	0	1	0
Applesauce, unsweetened/natural	Lucky Leaf Regular/Cinn...	0.4	cup	0	1	0
	Musselman's Regular/Cinnamon	0.4	cup	0	1	0
	S&W Gravenstein	0.4	cup	0	1	0
	Tree Top	0.3	cup	0	1	0
	White House	0.4	cup	0	1	0
	Musselman's Fruit 'N Sau...	0.2	cup	0	1	0
Applesauce Blends	w/apricot or cherry					

FOOD ITEM	SPECIFICATIONS	BRAND NAME	QUANTITY	SIZE	PROTEIN BLOCKS	CARBOHYDRATE BLOCKS	FAT BLOCKS
Apricot	w/cherry	Musselman's Fruit 'N Sauce	0.2	cup	0	1	0
	w/peach	Musselman's Fruit 'N Sauce	0.2	cup	0	1	0
	fresh		3	medium	0	1	0
	fresh, pitted, halves		0.7	cup	0	1	0
	canned	Del Monte Lite	0.3	cup	0	1	0
	canned, in juice	Libby's Lite	0.4	cup	0	1	0
	canned, in heavy syrup	Del Monte	0.2	cup	0	1	0
	canned, in heavy syrup	S&W	0.2	cup	0	1	0
	dried	Dole Sun Giant	0.6	oz.	0	1	0
	dried	Sonoma	0.4	oz.	0	1	0
	dried sulfured		0.6	oz.	0	1	0
	sun dried	Del Monte	0.2	cup	0	1	0
	frozen, sweetened		0.2	cup	0	1	0
Apricot nectar		Goya	2.1	fl. oz.	0	1	0
		Libby's/Kern's	2	fl. oz.	0	1	0
		R.W. Knudsen/Santa Cruz	2.4	fl. oz.	0	1	0
		S&W	2.1	fl. oz.	0	1	0
	pineapple	Kern's	1.9	fl. oz.	0	1	0
Arrowroot flour			0.1	cup	0	1	0
Artichoke appetizer, marinated		Contorno Caponata di Carciofi	0.8	cup	1	1	5
Artichoke, globe, fresh	quarters	Progresso	0.6	cup	0	1	8
		S&W	20	pcs.	0	1	7
	boiled	Dole	5	large	1	1	0
	hearts, boiled, drained		13.3	oz.	1	1	0
Artichoke	bottoms	Progresso	1	cup	1	1	0
		S&W	3.3	pcs.	1	1	0
	hearts	S&W	7.5	pcs.	0	1	0
	canned	S&W Colossal	5	pcs.	0	1	0
Asparagus	fresh, raw		12.9	spears	1	1	0
	fresh, boiled		24	spears	1	1	1
	fresh, boiled		30	spears	1	1	1
	fresh, boiled, drained, cuts		2.5	cup	1	1	1

Food	Type	Brand	Amount	Unit	P	C	F
Bacalaitos, mix	canned	Stokely, regular & no salt/Del Monte, all varieties/Green Giant, all varieties	2.5	cup	1	1	0
	imitation	Goya	1.4	Tbsp.	0	1	0
		Durkee	5.7	Tbsp.	0	1	0
		Heluva Good Free	4.4	Tbsp.	0	1	0
Bagel	plain	Awrey's	0.2	pc.	0	1	0
	plain	Thomas'	0.3	pc.	0	1	0
	cinnamon raisin	Awrey's	0.2	pc.	0	1	0
	cinnamon raisin	Thomas'	0.3	pc.	0	1	0
	egg	Thomas'	0.3	pc.	0	1	0
	mini	Awrey's	0.4	pc.	0	1	0
	onion	Thomas'	0.3	pc.	0	1	0
Bagel, frozen	plain	Lender's	0.3	pc.	0	1	0
	plain	Lender's Bagelettes	0.7	pcs.	0	1	0
	plain	Lender's Big'N Crusty	0.2	pc.	0	1	0
	blueberry	Lender's	0.3	pc.	0	1	0
	cinnamon raisin	Lender's	0.2	pc.	0	1	0
	cinnamon raisin	Lender's Big'N Crusty	0.2	pc.	0	1	0
	cinnamon raisin	Sara Lee	0.2	pc.	0	1	0
	egg	Lender's	0.3	pc.	0	1	0
	egg	Lender's Big'N Crusty	0.2	pc.	0	1	0
	garlic	Lender's	0.3	pc.	0	1	0
	oat bran	Lender's	0.3	pc.	0	1	0
	onion	Lender's	0.2	pc.	0	1	0
	onion	Lender's Big'N Crusty	0.3	pc.	0	1	0
	poppy	Lender's	0.3	pc.	0	1	0
	pumpernickel	Lender's	0.3	pc.	0	1	0
	rye	Lender's	0.3	pc.	0	1	0
	sesame	Lender's	0.3	pc.	0	1	0
	soft	Lender's Original	0.3	pc.	0	1	0
Bagel chips	cheese, three	Pepperidge Farm	0.6	oz.	0	1	1
	onion and garlic	Pepperidge Farm	0.3	pc.	0	1	1
	onion multigrain	Pepperidge Farm	0.3	pc.	0	1	0
Baked beans		Allens	0.2	cup	0	1	0
		B&M Brick Oven	0.2	cup	0	1	0
		B&M Extra Hearty	0.2	cup	0	1	0

FOOD ITEM	SPECIFICATIONS	BRAND NAME	QUANTITY	SIZE	PROTEIN BLOCKS	CARBOHYDRATE BLOCKS	FAT BLOCKS
		B&M 99% Fat Free	0.2	cup	0	1	0
		Bush's	0.2	cup	0	1	0
		Campbell's New England Style	0.2	cup	0	1	0
		Campbell's Homestyle	0.2	cup	0	1	0
		Campbell's Old Fashioned	0.2	cup	0	1	0
		Friend's	0.2	cup	0	1	0
		Grandma Brown's	0.2	cup	0	1	0
		Green Giant/Joan of Arc	0.2	cup	0	1	0
		Heartland Iron Kettle	0.2	cup	0	1	0
		S&W Brick Oven	0.2	cup	0	1	0
		Van Camp's Fat Free	0.2	cup	0	1	0
		Van Camp's Premium	0.2	cup	0	1	0
	w/bacon	Grandma Brown's Saucepan	0.2	cup	0	1	0
	bacon/brown sugar	Campbell's/Campbell's Old Fashioned	0.2	cup	0	1	0
	bacon/brown sugar	S&W	0.2	cup	0	1	0
	barbeque	B&M Brick Oven	0.2	cup	0	1	0
	barbeque	Campbell's Old Fashioned/Tangy	0.2	cup	0	1	0
	barbeque	Green Giant/Joan of Arc	0.2	cup	0	1	0
	barbeque	S&W Texas Style	0.3	cup	0	1	0
	brown sugar	Van Camps	0.2	cup	0	1	0
	honey	B&M	0.2	cup	0	1	0
	honey	Health Valley	0.3	cup	0	1	0
	honey bacon	Green Giant/Joan of Arc	0.2	cup	0	1	0
	honey mustard	S&W	0.2	cup	0	1	0
	maple sugar	S&W	0.2	cup	0	1	0
	w/onion	Bush's	0.2	cup	0	1	0
	w/onion	Green Giant/Joan of Arc	0.2	cup	0	1	0
	w/pork	Campbell's	0.3	cup	0	1	0
	w/pork	Crest Top	0.3	cup	0	1	0
	w/pork	Green Giant/Joan of Arc	0.2	cup	0	1	0
	w/pork	Hunt's	0.2	cup	0	1	0
	w/pork	Stokely Sugar	0.2	cup	0	1	0
	w/pork	Stokely Tomato	0.2	cup	0	1	0

Food	Description	Brand	Amount	Unit			
	w/pork	Van Camp's	0.3	cup	0	1	0
	w/pork	Wagon Master/Trappey's	0.3	cup	0	1	0
	w/pork & jalapenos	Trappey's	0.3	cup	0	1	0
	w/pork & peas	East Texas Fair Peas 'n Pork	0.3	cup	0	1	0
	vegetarian	Bush's	0.3	cup	0	1	0
	vegetarian	Campbell's	0.3	cup	0	1	0
	vegetarian	Stokely	0.2	cup	0	1	0
	vegetarian	Van Camp's	0.3	cup	0	1	0
	vegetarian	brown sugar sauce Stokely	0.2	cup	0	1	0
	yellow eye	B&M	0.2	cup	0	1	0
Baking mix	all purpose	Arrowhead Mills	0.1	cup	7	1	4
Balsam pear	leafy tips, raw		25	cup	7	1	0
	leafy tips, boiled, drained		2.5	cup	1	1	1
	pods, raw, 1/2" pcs.		12.5	cup	1	1	0
	pods, boiled, drained, 1/2" pcs.		2.5	cup	1	1	0
Bamboo shoots	fresh, raw slices		1.3	cup	1	1	0
	fresh, boiled, drained, 1/2" slices		5	cup	1	1	0
Banana	canned	La Choy	25	cup	0	0	0
	fresh, whole		0.1	lb.	0	1	0
	fresh		0.4	8 3/4" banana	0	0	0
	fresh, mashed		0.2	cup	0	0	0
	dehydrated		0.1	cup	0	0	0
	dried	Sonoma	0.6	pcs.	0	0	0
Banana drink		After the Fall Casablanca	3.8	fl. oz.	0	0	0
Banana milk drink	chilled, lowfat	Nestle Quick	0.3	cup	1	0	0
	mix	Nestle Quick	0.8	Tbsp.	0	0	0
Banana nectar		Libby's/Kern's	2.2	fl. oz.	0	0	1
	blend	Libby's Quanabana	2.1	fl. oz.	0	0	0
	blend, pineapple	Kern's	2	fl. oz.	0	0	0
Bananaberry shake		Nestle Killer	2	oz.	1	0	0
Barbeque dip		Healthy Choice all varieties	2.9	Tbsp.	0	0	1
		Heluva Good	10	Tbsp.	0	0	0
Barbeque sauce		Heinz Thick & Rich Old Fashioned	1.8	Tbsp.	1	0	9
		Hunt's Light	2.9	Tbsp.	0	0	0

FOOD ITEM	SPECIFICATIONS	BRAND NAME	QUANTITY	SIZE	PROTEIN BLOCKS	CARBOHYDRATE BLOCKS	FAT BLOCKS
		Hunt's Original	2.2	Tbsp.	0	1	0
		Hunt's Original Bold	2	Tbsp.	0	1	0
		KC Masterpiece Original	1.7	Tbsp.	0	1	0
		Kraft Char-Grill	1.5	Tbsp.	0	1	0
		Kraft Original	1.8	Tbsp.	0	1	0
		Kraft Original Extra Rich	1.5	Tbsp.	0	1	0
		Kraft Thick'N Spicy Original	1.5	Tbsp.	0	1	0
		Lea & Perrins Original/Bold & Spicy	1.4	Tbsp.	0	1	0
		Maull's	1.8	Tbsp.	0	1	0
		Mississippi	1.2	Tbsp.	0	1	0
		Open Pit Original	1.7	Tbsp.	0	1	0
		Rice Road	10	Tbsp.	0	1	3
		Woody's Cook-In'	6.7	Tbsp.	0	1	4
	Buffalo wing	Heinz	6.7	Tbsp.	0	1	0
	Cajun	Luzianne	1	Tbsp.	0	1	1
	Dijon, mild	Hunt's	2	Tbsp.	0	1	0
	Dijon and honey	Lawry's	1.5	Tbsp.	0	1	0
	garlic	Kraft	2	Tbsp.	0	1	0
	garlic and herb	Lea & Perrins	2	Tbsp.	0	1	0
	hickory	Hunt's Bold	1.8	Tbsp.	0	1	0
	hickory	Open Pit	1.7	Tbsp.	0	1	0
	hickory	Open Pit Thick and Tangy	1.5	Tbsp.	0	1	0
	hickory and brown sugar	Hunt's	1	Tbsp.	0	1	0
	hickory or honey hickory	Hunt's	2	Tbsp.	0	1	0
	hickory smoke	Kraft	1.8	Tbsp.	0	1	0
	hickory smoke	Kraft Thick'N Spicy	1.5	Tbsp.	0	1	0
	hickory smoke	Open Pit	1.7	Tbsp.	0	1	0
	hickory smoke, hot	Kraft	2	Tbsp.	0	1	0
	hickory smoke, onion bits	Kraft	1.7	Tbsp.	0	1	0
	honey	Heinz Thick & Rich	1.7	Tbsp.	0	1	0
	honey	Kraft	1.4	Tbsp.	0	1	0
	honey	Kraft Thick'N Spicy	1.4	Tbsp.	0	1	0
	honey mustard	Hunt's	1.5	Tbsp.	0	1	0

Food	Brand	Amount			
honey and spice	Open Pit Thick and Tangy	1.7 Tbsp.	0	1	0
honey Dijon	KC Masterpiece	1.8 Tbsp.	0	1	0
hot	Kraft	2 Tbsp.	0	1	0
hot	Open Pit	1.7 Tbsp.	0	1	0
hot and spicy	Hunt's	1.5 Tbsp.	0	1	0
hot and spicy	Master Choice	2.5 Tbsp.	0	1	1
Italian	Porino's	2.5 Tbsp.	0	1	0
Italian, seasonings	Kraft	1.8 Tbsp.	0	1	0
jalapeno	Maull's	1.5 Tbsp.	0	1	0
Kansas City style	Kraft	1.7 Tbsp.	0	1	0
Kansas City style	Kraft Thick'N Spicy	1.4 Tbsp.	0	1	0
Kansas City style	Maull's	1.2 Tbsp.	0	1	0
mesquite	Hunt's	2 Tbsp.	0	1	0
mesquite	Open Pit	1.7 Tbsp.	0	1	0
mesquite smoke	Kraft	2 Tbsp.	0	1	0
mesquite smoke	Kraft Thick'N Spicy	1.5 Tbsp.	0	1	0
mild	Hunt's	1.8 Tbsp.	0	1	0
onion	Open Pit	1.7 Tbsp.	0	1	0
onion	Open Pit Thick and Tangy	1.5 Tbsp.	0	1	0
onion bits	Kraft	1.7 Tbsp.	0	1	0
onion bits	Maull's	2 Tbsp.	0	1	0
Oriental	House of Tsang Hong Kong	10 Tbsp.	0	1	0
Oriental pork	House of Tsang	0.9 Tbsp.	0	1	0
salsa style	Kraft	2 Tbsp.	0	1	0
smoky	Maull's	1.8 Tbsp.	0	1	0
sweet	Maull's Sweet-N-Mild	1.5 Tbsp.	0	1	0
sweet	Maull's Sweet-N-Smokey	1.4 Tbsp.	0	1	0
sweet	Open Pit	1.5 Tbsp.	0	1	0
sweet and sour	Lawry's	0.9 Tbsp.	0	1	0
sweet and sour	Open Pit	1.8 Tbsp.	0	1	0
teriyaki	Hunt's	1.7 Tbsp.	0	1	0
teriyaki	Kraft	1.5 Tbsp.	0	1	0
Barley, pearled, dry	Arrowhead Mills	0.1 cup	0	1	0
dry	Goya	0.1 cup	0	1	0
dry	Quaker Scotch Quick	0.1 cup	0	1	0
dry		0.1 cup	0	1	0

CARBOHYDRATES

FOOD ITEM	SPECIFICATIONS	BRAND NAME	QUANTITY	SIZE	PROTEIN BLOCKS	CARBOHYDRATE BLOCKS	FAT BLOCKS
Barley flakes	dry, medium	Quaker Scotch	0.1	cup	0	1	0
Barley flour	cooked		0.2	cup	0	1	0
		Arrowhead Mills	0.1	cup	0	1	0
Barley malt syrup		Arrowhead Mills	0.1	cup	0	1	0
Barley pilaf mix		Eden	0.6	Tbsp.	0	1	0
Batter, seasoning	prepared	Eden	0.3	cup	0	1	0
Bean dip		House of Tsang Cantonese	1.3	Tbsp.	0	1	0
	black bean	Chi-Chi's Fiesta	6.7	Tbsp.	0	1	2
	black bean	Marie's Fiesta	10	Tbsp.	1	1	24
	black bean, spicy	Old Dutch	5	Tbsp.	0	1	1
	hot	Old El Paso	6.7	Tbsp.	1	1	0
	jalapeno	Tostitos	5	Tbsp.	1	1	0
	pinto, spicy	Guiltless Gourmet	5	Tbsp.	1	1	1
		Frito-Lay's	6.7	Tbsp.	0	1	0
		Frito-Lay's	2.9	Tbsp.	1	1	0
		Guiltless Gourmet	5	Tbsp.	0	1	0
Bean dip mix	black	Knorr	5	Tbsp.	1	1	0
	mexican	Knorr	5	Tbsp.	0	1	0
Bean sauce, brown	spicy	House of Tsang	3.3	tsp.	0	1	0
Beans, mixed	canned	Stokely Chulent	0.3	cup	0	1	0
Bearnaise sauce mix		Knorr	0.5	pkg.	0	1	0
Beef seasoning mix	ground	Durkee Pouch	0.4	pkg.	0	1	0
	marinade	Durkee Pouch	1	pkg.	0	1	0
	marinade	Lawry's	7.5	tsp.	0	1	0
Beef seasoning and coating mix	pot roast	McCormick Bag 'n Season	1.7	Tbsp.	0	1	0
	spare ribs	McCormick Bag 'n Season	1.4	Tbsp.	0	1	0
	Swiss steak	McCormick Bag 'n Season	3.3	tsp.	0	1	0
Beef stew seasoning		Durkee	0.4	pkg.	0	1	0
		Durkee Roasting Bag	0.3	pkg.	0	1	0
		Lawry's	3.3	tsp.	0	1	0
		McCormick	0.4	tsp.	0	1	0
Beer	regular		8	oz.	0	1	0

Food	Description	Brand	Amount	Unit			
Beet	light		24	oz.	0	1	0
	fresh, raw		1.7	medium, 2" diam.	0	1	0
	fresh, raw, trimmed, sliced		1	cup	0	1	0
	fresh, boiled, drained		2.2	medium, 2" diam.	0	1	0
	fresh, boiled, drained, sliced		0.6	cup	0	1	0
	canned, w/liquid		0.6	cup	0	1	0
	canned, whole	Stokely	6.4	oz.	0	1	0
	canned, whole, baby	Green Giant LeSueur	0.7	cup	0	1	0
	canned, whole or sliced	Del Monte	0.7	cup	0	1	0
	canned, whole or sliced	Green Giant	0.7	cup	0	1	0
	canned, whole, sliced, or julienne	S&W	0.7	cup	0	1	0
	canned, sliced	Goya	0.6	cup	0	1	0
	canned, sliced	Green Gian No Salt	0.7	cup	0	1	1
	canned, sliced	Stokely	5	cup	0	1	0
	canned, Harvard w/liquid	Green Giant	0.2	cup	0	1	0
	canned, Harvard w/liquid	Stokely	0.2	cup	0	1	0
	canned, Harvard w/liquid	S&W	0.2	cup	0	1	0
	canned, pickled	Stokely Can	3.3	oz.	0	1	0
	canned, pickled	Stokely Jar	2.5	oz.	0	1	0
	canned, pickled	Del Monte	2.5	oz.	0	1	0
	canned, pickled, crinkle		0.3	oz.	0	1	0
Beet greens	raw, 1" pcs.		50	pc.	3	1	4
	boiled, drained, 1" pcs.		2.5	cup	0	1	1
Berries, mixed, frozen		Big Valley Burst O' Berries	0.5	cup	0	1	0
Berry drink		After the Fall Oregon	2.9	fl. oz.	0	1	0
		Capri Sun Yo Yogi Berry	2.3	fl. oz.	0	1	0
		Hi-C Boppin'	2.2	fl. oz.	0	1	0
		Hi-C Wild	2.4	fl. oz.	0	1	0
		R.W. Knudsen Razzleberry	2.2	fl. oz.	0	1	0
	citrus	Five Alive	2.4	fl. oz.	0	1	0
	nectar	Santa Cruz	2.7	fl. oz.	0	1	0
	punch	Minute Maid	2.2	fl. oz.	0	1	0
	punch	Minute Maid Box	2.2	fl. oz.	0	1	0

FOOD ITEM	SPECIFICATIONS	BRAND NAME	QUANTITY	SIZE	PROTEIN BLOCKS	CARBOHYDRATE BLOCKS	FAT BLOCKS
Berry juice	punch	Tropicana	2.2	fl. oz.	0	1	0
	punch, frozen (prepared)	Minute Maid	2.2	fl. oz.	0	1	0
		Apple & Eve Nothin' But Juice	2.5	fl. oz.	0	1	0
		Heinke's Berry Patch	2.4	fl. oz.	0	1	0
		Juicy Juice	2.4	fl. oz.	0	1	0
		Veryfine Juice-Ups	2.1	fl. oz.	0	1	0
Biscuit		Arnold Old Fashioned	1	pcs.	0	1	1
		Awrey's Country	0.4	pc.	0	1	1
		Awrey's Round	0.9	oz.	0	1	0
Biscuit, refrigerated	plain or buttermilk	Big Country Butter Tastin'	0.7	pc.	0	1	1
	baking powder or buttermilk	Grands! Homestyle	0.4	pc.	0	1	1
	butter	Ballard Extra Lights Ovenready	0.9	pcs.	0	1	0
		1869 Brand	0.8	pc.	0	1	1
	butter or country	Grands!	0.4	pc.	0	1	1
	buttermilk	Pillsbury	0.9	pcs.	0	1	0
	buttermilk	Big Country Butter Tastin'	0.6	pc.	0	1	1
	buttermilk	Grands!	0.4	pc.	0	1	1
	buttermilk	Pillsbury	0.9	pcs.	0	1	0
		Pillsbury Tender Layer	1	pcs.	0	1	1
	cinnamon raisin	Grands!	0.3	pc.	0	1	1
	flaky	Grands!	0.4	pc.	0	1	1
	flaky	Hungry Jack	0.8	pcs.	0	1	1
	flaky	Hungry Jack Butter Tastin'	0.8	pcs.	0	1	1
	flaky	Hungry Jack Honey Tastin'	0.7	pcs.	0	1	0
	fluffy	Hungry Jack	0.8	pc.	0	1	1
	Southern style	Big Country	0.6	pc.	0	1	1
		Grands!	0.4	pc.	0	1	1
	Southern style, flaky	Hungry Jack	0.8	pc.	0	1	1
Biscuit, frozen	garlic and cheese	Pepperidge Farm	0.4	pc.	0	1	1
Biscuit mix		Arrowhead Mills	0.1	cup	0	1	0
		Bisquick	0.1	cup	0	1	1
Black bean mix		Fantastic	0.2	cup, prepared	0	1	1
Black bean garlic sauce		Lee Kum Kee	3.3	Tbsp.	0	1	1

Food	Description	Brand	Amount	Unit	P	C	F
Black beans	dried	Frieda's	3.3	oz.	0	1	1
	dried	Goya	0.3	cup	0	1	1
	dried, boiled		0.4	cup	0	1	1
	canned	Eden Organic	0.4	cup	0	1	1
	canned	Goya	0.4	cup	0	1	0
	canned	Green Giant/Joan of Arc	0.4	cup	0	1	1
	canned	Old El Paso	0.5	cup	0	1	1
	canned	Progresso	0.5	cup	0	1	0
	canned	S&W	0.4	cup	0	1	0
	canned	Stokely	0.3	cup	0	1	0
	canned	Sun-Vista	0.4	cup	0	1	1
	canned, seasoned	Allens/Trappey's	0.4	cup	0	1	1
	turtle soup, dried		0.1	cup	0	1	0
	turtle soup, dried	Arrowhead Mills	0.1	cup	0	1	1
	turtle soup, dried, boiled		0.1	cup	0	1	0
	fresh trimmed		0.8	cup	0	1	1
Blackberry	canned	Allens/Wolco	1.7	cup	1	1	0
	canned, heavy syrup		0.2	cup	0	1	0
	frozen	Stilwell	0.6	cup	0	1	0
	frozen, unsweetened		0.6	cup	0	1	0
Blackberry syrup		Knott's Berry Farm	0.6	Tbsp.	0	1	1
Black-eyed peas	canned, fresh shell	Allens/East Texas Fair/Homefolks	0.3	cup	0	1	0
	canned, fresh shell	Goya Cowpeas	0.3	cup	0	1	0
	canned, fresh shell	Green Giant/Joan of Arc	0.4	cup	0	1	0
	canned, fresh shell	Stokely	0.3	cup	0	1	1
	canned, fresh shell	Sun-Vista	0.4	cup	0	1	0
	canned, fresh shell w/ jalapeno	Homefolks	0.3	cup	0	1	0
	canned, fresh shell w/snaps	Allens/East Texas Fair/Homefolks	0.3	cup	0	1	1
	canned, dry	Allens/East Texas Fair	0.3	cup	0	1	0
	canned, dry w/bacon	Allens	0.3	cup	0	1	0
	canned, dry w/bacon	Trappey's	0.3	cup	0	1	0
	canned, dry w/bacon and jalapeno	Trappey's	0.3	cup	0	1	0
Blintz, frozen	frozen	Stilwell	0.3	cup	0	1	0
	apple	Empire Kosher	0.6	pcs.	1	1	0

FOOD ITEM	SPECIFICATIONS	BRAND NAME	QUANTITY	SIZE	PROTEIN BLOCKS	CARBOHYDRATE BLOCKS	FAT BLOCKS
	blueberry	Empire Kosher	0.5	pcs.	0	1	0
	cheese	Empire Kosher	0.7	pcs.	0	1	1
	cherry	Empire Kosher	0.5	pcs.	0	1	0
	potato	Empire Kosher	0.6	pcs.	0	1	1
Bloody Mary mixer	rich and spicy	Mr. & Mrs. "T"	8.9	fl. oz.	0	1	0
		V-8	9.6	fl. oz.	0	1	0
		Mr. & Mrs. "T"	7.3	fl. oz.	0	1	0
Blueberry	fresh		0.6	cup	0	1	0
	canned, heavy syrup	Lucky Leaf/Musselman's	0.2	cup	0	1	0
	canned, heavy syrup	S&W Wild Maine	0.3	cup	0	1	0
	dried	Sonoma	0.1	cup	0	1	0
	frozen	Cascadian Farm Organic	0.9	cup	0	1	0
	frozen	Stilwell	0.6	cup	0	1	0
	frozen sweetened		0.2	cup	0	1	0
Blueberry juice		After the fall	2.9	fl. oz.	0	1	0
Blueberry syrup		Knott's Berry Farm	0.6	Tbsp.	0	1	0
		R.W. Knudsen	0.1	cup	0	1	0
		S&W Reduced Cal	0.1	cup	0	1	0
Bouillabaisse seasoning mix		Knorr Recipe	3.3	Tbsp.	0	1	1
Bouillon	beef	Herb-Ox	10	tsp. or cube	0	1	0
	beef	Herb-Ox Instant	10	tsp. or cube	0	1	0
	beef	Knorr	10	tsp. or cube	1	1	5
	beef	MBT/Wyler's Instant	5	pkt.	1	1	0
	beef	MBT/Wyler's Low Sodium	3.3	pkt.	1	1	0
	beef or chicken	Wyler's/Steero	10	tsp. or cube	0	1	0
	beef or chicken	Wyler's/Steero Reduced Sodium	10	tsp. or cube	0	1	0
	chicken	Herb-Ox	10	tsp. or cube	0	1	0
	chicken	Knorr	10	tsp. or cube	1	1	5
	chicken	MBT/Wyler's Instant	5	pkt.	1	1	0
	chicken	MBT/Wyler's Low Sodium	3.3	pkt.	0	1	0
	onion	MBT Instant	3.3	pkt.	0	1	0
	vegetable	MBT Instant	5	pkt.	0	1	0

Food	Type	Brand	Amount	Unit			
Bowtie dishes mix	vegetable	Wyler's	10	tsp. or cube	0	1	0
	vegetable, vegetarian	Knorr	5	cube	3	1	1
	Bourguignonne seasoning and beans with herb sauce	Knorr	1.4	Tbsp.	0	1	0
	Italian cheese	Knorr	0.1	cup	0	1	0
		Lipton Pasta & Sauce	0.1	pkg.	0	1	0
Boysenberries	canned, heavy syrup	Farmer's Market	0.2	cup	0	1	0
	frozen, unsweetened	Heinke's	0.8	cup	0	1	0
Boysenberry drink	cider	Knott's Berry Farm	2.4	fl. oz.	0	1	0
Boysenberry syrup		Knott's Berry Farm	2.4	fl. oz.	0	1	0
Bread	apple honey wheat	Arnold Bran'nola Country	0.6	Tbsp.	0	1	0
	apple walnut	Arnold/Brownberry Bran'nola Original	0.6	slice	1	1	0
	bran, honey	Brownberry	0.6	slice	0	1	0
	bran, light	Pepperidge Farm	0.8	slice	0	1	0
	bran, whole	Pepperidge Farm	0.7	slice	0	1	0
	buttermilk	August Bros./Brownberry Bakery Country	0.6	slice	0	1	0
	cinnamon	Brownberry	1.1	slices	0	1	1
	cinnamon	Arnold	0.9	slice	0	1	0
	cranberry	Brownberry	0.5	slice	0	1	0
	date nut	Pepperidge Farm	0.6	slice	0	1	0
	French	Arnold	0.8	slice	0	1	0
	French	Thomas'	0.7	slice	0	1	0
	French, twin	Arnold Francisco	0.6	oz.	0	1	0
	golden, light	Pepperidge Farm	0.6	oz.	0	1	0
	golden, swirl	Pepperidge Farm Sliced	0.04	loaf	0	1	0
	Italian	Brownberry Francisco Intl.	0.04	loaf	0	1	0
	Italian	Brownberry Bakery	0.5	slice	0	1	0
	Italian, brown and serve	Pepperidge Farm Vermont Maple	1.2	slices	0	1	0
	Italian, light	Arnold Francisco	0.6	slice	0	1	0
	Italian, stick	Arnold Savoni's	0.8	slice	0	1	0
	Italian, stick, sliced	Pepperidge Farm	0.7	slice	0	1	0
		Arnold/Brownberry Bakery	0.04	loaf	0	1	0
		Arnold Francisco 10 oz.	1.1	slices	0	1	0
		Arnold Francisco 1 lb.	0.7	oz.	0	1	0
			0.6	slice	0	1	0

FOOD ITEM	SPECIFICATIONS	BRAND NAME	QUANTITY	SIZE	PROTEIN BLOCKS	CARBOHYDRATE BLOCKS	FAT BLOCKS
	Italian, thick	Brownberry Francisco Intl.	0.8	slice	0	1	0
	kamut, sprout	Shiloh Farms Egyptian	0.6	slice	0	1	0
	mixed/multigrain	Brownberry Hearth	0.6	slice	0	1	0
	mixed/multigrain	Roman Meal Round Top	0.8	slice	0	1	0
	mixed/multigrain	Roman Meal Sun	0.8	slice	0	1	0
	mixed/multigrain, 5 sprouted	Shiloh Farms	0.6	slice	0	1	0
	mixed/multigrain, 5 sprouted	Shiloh Farms No Salt	0.6	slice	0	1	0
	mixed/multigrain, 7	Roman Meal	0.6	slice	0	1	0
	mixed/multigrain, 7, hearty	Pepperidge Farm	0.6	slice	0	1	0
	mixed/multigrain, 7, light	Pepperidge Farm	1.2	slices	0	1	0
	mixed/multigrain, 7, light	Roman Meal	1.3	slices	0	1	0
	mixed/multigrain, 7 sprouted	Breads for Life/Shiloh Farms	0.6	slice	0	1	0
	mixed/multigrain, 7 white	Arnold/Brownberry Bran'nola	0.6	slice	0	1	0
	mixed/multigrain, 9	Pepperidge Farm	0.6	slice	0	1	0
	mixed/multigrain, 12	Arnold Bran'nola	0.6	slice	0	1	0
	mixed/multigrain, 12	Brownberry	1	slice	0	1	0
	mixed/multigrain, 12	Roman Meal	0.8	slice	0	1	0
	mixed/multigrain, crunchy	Pepperidge Farm	0.7	slice	0	1	0
	mixed/multigrain w/oat bran	Roman Meal	0.8	slice	0	1	0
	mixed/multigrain, nutty	Arnold Bran'nola	0.6	slice	0	1	0
	mixed/multigrain, nutty	Brownberry Bran'nola	0.6	slice	0	1	0
	mixed/multigrain, sprouted	Shiloh Farms Sandwich	0.6	slice	0	1	0
	mixed/multigrain, whole	Pepperidge Farm 100%	0.7	slice	0	1	0
	nut	Brownberry Natural Health	0.8	slice	0	1	0
	oat	Brownberry Bran'nola	0.6	slice	0	1	0
	oat	Roman Meal	0.8	slice	0	1	0
	oat, crunchy, hearty	Pepperidge Farm	0.6	slice	0	1	0
	oat bran, honey	Roman Meal	0.8	slice	0	1	0
	oat bran, honey nut	Roman Meal	0.8	slice	0	1	0
	oat bran, light	Roman Meal	1.3	slices	0	1	0
	oatmeal	Brownberry Natural	0.8	slice	0	1	0
	oatmeal	Pepperidge Farm	0.6	slice	0	1	0
	oatmeal, light	Arnold/Brownberry Bakery	1.1	slices	0	1	0

CARBOHYDRATES

Food	Brand	P	C	F	Amount	Unit
oatmeal, light	Pepperidge Farm	0	1	0	1.3	slices
oatmeal, soft	Brownberry	0	1	0	0.7	slice
oatmeal, soft	Pepperidge Farm	0	1	0	0.8	slice
oatmeal, thin	Pepperidge Farm	0	1	0	0.9	slice
orange raisin	Brownberry	0	1	0	0.6	slice
pita/pocket	Arnold	0	1	0	0.3	2 oz. pc.
pita/pocket	Arnold	0	1	0	0.2	3 oz. pc.
pita/pocket	Pepperidge Farm	0	1	0	0.3	pc
pita/pocket	Pepperidge Farm Mini	0	1	0	0.6	1 oz. pc.
pita/pocket	Thomas' Sahara	0	1	0	0.3	2 oz. pc.
pita/pocket	Thomas' Sahara	0	1	0	0.2	3 oz. pc.
pita/pocket garlic	Thomas' Sahara Mini	0	1	0	0.6	1 oz. pc.
pita/pocket oat bran	Arnold	0	1	0	0.3	pc.
pita/pocket onion	Thomas' Sahara	0	1	0	0.3	pc.
pita/pocket onion	Arnold	0	1	0	0.3	pc.
pita/pocket salsa	Thomas' Sahara	0	1	0	0.3	pc.
pita/pocket sourdough	Thomas' Sahara	0	1	0	0.3	pc.
pita/pocket wheat	Thomas' Sahara	0	1	0	0.3	pc.
pita/pocket wheat	Arnold 4	0	1	0	0.8	oz.
pita/pocket wheat	Arnold	0	1	0	0.7	oz.
pita/pocket wheat	Thomas' Sahara	0	1	0	0.8	oz.
pita/pocket white	Thomas' Sahara Mini	0	1	0	0.8	oz.
poppy seed, hazelnut	Arnold 4	0	1	0	0.6	oz.
potato	Roman Meal	0	1	0	0.6	pc.
potato, hearty	Arnold Country	0	1	0	0.5	slice
potato	Pepperidge Farm Russet	0	1	0	0.6	slice
pumpernickel	Arnold	0	1	0	0.6	slice
pumpernickel	Arnold August Bros. 1 Lb.	0	1	0	0.6	slice
pumpernickel	Arnold August Bros. 24 oz.	0	1	0	0.5	slice
pumpernickel	Arnold Levy's	0	1	0	0.6	slice
pumpernickel, dark	Pepperidge Farm	0	1	0	0.6	slice
pumpernickel, party	Pepperidge Farm	0	1	0	4	slices
pumpernickel, rye	Brownberry	0	1	0	0.7	slice
raisin	Arnold Sunmaid	0	1	0	0.6	slice
raisin, cinnamon	Arnold	0	1	0	0.6	slice
raisin, cinnamon	Brownberry	0	1	0	0.6	slice

FOOD ITEM	SPECIFICATIONS	BRAND NAME	QUANTITY	SIZE	PROTEIN BLOCKS	CARBOHYDRATE BLOCKS	FAT BLOCKS
	raisin, cinnamon	Pepperidge Farm	0.7	slice	0	1	0
	raisin, walnut	Brownberry	0.8	slice	0	1	1
	raisin, whole wheat	Shiloh Farms	0.7	slice	0	1	1
	rye	Arnold Deli	0.6	slice	0	1	0
	rye	Brownberry Hearth	0.6	slice	0	1	0
	rye, Dijon	Arnold Real Jewish	0.6	slice	0	1	0
	rye, Dijon, thin	Pepperidge Farm	1.1	slices	0	1	0
	rye, dill	Arnold	0.6	slice	0	1	0
	rye, dill	Brownberry	0.6	slice	0	1	0
	rye, onion	Arnold August Bros.	0.6	slice	0	1	0
	rye, onion, w/ seeds	Arnold August Bros.	0.5	slice	0	1	0
	rye, onion	Pepperidge Farm	0.6	slice	0	1	0
	rye, party	Pepperidge Farm	3.8	slices	0	1	0
	rye, seeded	Arnold August Bros. 1 lb.	0.6	slice	0	1	0
	rye, seeded	Arnold/Levy's Real Jewish	0.6	slice	0	1	0
	rye, seeded	Brownberry Natural	0.6	slice	0	1	0
	rye, seeded or unseeded	Arnold August Bros. 24 oz.	0.5	slice	0	1	0
	rye, seeded or unseeded	Pepperidge Farm	0.6	slice	0	1	0
	rye, soft	Arnold Country	0.7	slice	0	1	0
	rye, soft, light	Arnold/Brownberry Bakery	1.1	slices	0	1	0
	rye, soft, seeded	Arnold Bakery	0.6	slice	0	1	0
	rye, soft, unseeded	Arnold Bakery	0.6	slice	0	1	0
	rye, thin	Arnold Levy's Melba	1.1	slices	0	1	0
	rye, unseeded	Arnold August Bros. 1 lb.	0.6	slice	0	1	0
	rye, unseeded	Arnold Real Jewish 1 lb.	0.6	slice	0	1	0
	rye, unseeded	Arnold Real Jewish 2 lb.	0.6	slice	0	1	0
	rye, unseeded	Arnold Levy's Real Jewish	0.6	slice	0	1	0
	rye, unseeded	Brownberry Natural	0.6	slice	0	1	0
	rye, unseeded, thin	Arnold August Bros.	1	slice	0	1	0
	rye, unseeded, thin	Brownberry	1	slice	0	1	0
	rye and pump	Arnold August Bros.	0.5	slice	0	1	0
	sourdough	Arnold August Bros.	0.4	slice	0	1	0
	sourdough	Arnold Francisco	0.5	slice	0	1	0

		Amount	Unit	P	C	F
sourdough, brown and serve	Arnold Francisco	0.7	oz.	0	1	0
sourdough, light	Arnold	1.1	slices	0	1	0
sourdough, light	Pepperidge Farm	1.2	slices	0	1	0
sourdough, thick	Brownberry Francisco Intl.	0.5	slice	0	1	0
sourdough, whole grain	Roman Meal	0.8	slice	0	1	0
spelt	Shiloh Farms	0.5	slice	0	1	0
stick, sliced	Arnold August Bros.	0.9	slice	0	1	0
stick, sliced	Brownberry Francisco	0.5	slice	0	1	0
toast, Texas	Arnold August Bros.	0.3	slice	0	1	0
Vienna, light	Pepperidge Farm	1.2	slices	0	1	0
Vienna, thick	Pepperidge Farm	0.8	slice	1	1	0
wheat	Arnold Brick Oven	0.8	slice	0	1	0
wheat	Arnold Brick Oven 8 oz.	1.1	slices	1	1	0
wheat	Arnold Brick Oven 1 lb.	1	slice	0	1	0
wheat	Arnold Sunny Valley	1	slice	0	1	0
wheat	Arnold/Brownberry Country	0.5	slice	0	1	0
wheat	Brownberry Hearth	0.6	slice	0	1	0
wheat	Brownberry Natural	0.6	slice	0	1	0
wheat	Pepperidge Farm	0.6	slice	0	1	0
wheat	Pepperidge Farm Family	0.8	slice	0	1	0
wheat	Pepperidge Farm Natural	0.6	slice	0	1	0
wheat	Roman Meal Natural	0.9	slice	0	1	0
wheat	Shiloh Farms Homestyle	0.3	1/2" slice	0	1	0
wheat, cracked, thin	Pepperidge Farm	0.8	slice	1	1	0
wheat, dark	Arnold/Brownberry Bran'nola	0.7	slice	1	1	0
wheat, hearty	Arnold/Brownberry Bran'nola	0.7	slice	0	1	0
wheat, light	Pepperidge Farm	1.2	slices	0	1	0
wheat, light	Roman Meal	1.2	slices	0	1	0
wheat, light, golden	Arnold	1.2	slices	0	1	0
wheat, light, hearty	Roman Meal Light	1.3	slices	1	1	0
wheat, sesame, hearty	Pepperidge Farm	0.6	slice	0	1	0
wheat, soft	Brownberry	0.7	slice	0	1	0
wheat, soft	Brownberry 16 oz.	1	slice	0	1	0
wheat, very thin	Pepperidge Farm	1.5	slices	0	1	0
wheat, whole	Arnold Stoneground 1 lb. 4 oz.	0.9	slice	0	1	0
wheat, whole	Arnold Stoneground 2 lb.	1.1	slices	0	1	0

FOOD ITEM	SPECIFICATIONS	BRAND NAME	QUANTITY	SIZE	PROTEIN BLOCKS	CARBOHYDRATE BLOCKS	FAT BLOCKS
	wheat, whole	Roman Meal	0.8	slice	0	1	0
	wheat, whole	Shiloh Farms	0.8	slice	0	1	0
	wheat, whole	Shiloh Farms No Salt	0.8	slice	0	1	0
	wheat, whole, light	Roman Meal	1.4	slices	0	1	0
	wheat, whole, soft	Pepperidge Farm	1.4	slices	0	1	0
	wheat, whole, thin	Pepperidge Farm	0.8	slice	0	1	0
	wheatberry, honey	Arnold	0.7	slice	0	1	0
	wheatberry, honey	Arnold Bran'nola	0.6	slice	0	1	0
	wheatberry, honey	Roman Meal	0.8	slice	0	1	0
	wheatberry, honey	Pepperidge Farm	0.6	slice	0	1	0
	wheatberry, honey, hearty	Roman Meal	1.8	slices	0	1	0
	wheatberry, honey, light						
	white	Arnold Brick Oven	0.6	slice	0	1	0
	white	Arnold Brick Oven 8 oz.	0.8	slice	0	1	0
	white	Arnold Brick Oven 1 lb.	0.8	slice	0	1	0
	white	Arnold Country	0.5	slice	0	1	0
	white	Arnold Sunny Valley	0.9	slice	0	1	0
	white	Brownberry Country	0.5	slice	0	1	0
	white	Brownberry Natural	0.8	slice	0	1	0
	white, hearty	Pepperidge Farm	0.5	slice	0	1	0
	white, hearty	Pepperidge Farm Country	0.5	slice	0	1	0
	white, light	Arnold/Brownberry Bakery	1.1	slices	0	1	0
	white, light	Roman Meal	1.2	slices	0	1	0
	white, sandwich	Pepperidge Farm	0.8	slice	0	1	0
	white, sandwich	Roman Meal	1	slice	0	1	3
	white, soft	Arnold Country	0.6	slice	0	1	0
	white, soft	Brownberry	0.7	slice	0	1	0
	white, soft	Brownberry 16 oz.	0.9	slice	0	1	0
	white, toasting	Pepperidge Farm	0.6	slice	0	1	0
	white, thin	Pepperidge Farm	0.7	slice	0	1	1
	white, thin	Pepperidge Farm Large Family	0.6	slice	0	1	0
	white, very thin	Pepperidge Farm	1.3	slices	0	1	0
Brown bread, canned		B&M/Friend's	0.3	1/2" slice	0	1	0
		S&W	0.5	1/2" slice	0	1	0

Category	Food	Brand	Amount	Unit	P	C	F
Bread, frozen	raisin	B&M/Friend's	0.3	1/2" slice	0	1	0
	cheddar, two	Pepperidge Farm	0.1	loaf	0	1	2
	garlic	Pepperidge Farm	0.1	loaf	0	1	2
	garlic mozzarella	Pepperidge Farm	0.1	loaf	0	1	2
	garlic Parmesan	Pepperidge Farm	0.1	loaf	0	1	1
	garlic sourdough	Pepperidge Farm	0.1	loaf	0	1	2
	Monterey Jack/ jalapeno cheese	Pepperidge Farm	0.1	loaf	0	1	1
Bread, refrigerated	corn bread twists	Pillsbury Pipin' Hot	0.1	loaf	0	1	0
	French	Pillsbury	0.5	twist	0	1	1
	French	Pillsbury	0.1	loaf	0	1	0
Bread, stuffed	broccoli and cheese	Stuffed Breads	1.2	oz.	0	1	1
	pepperoni and cheese	Stuffed Breads	1.4	oz.	1	1	3
Bread crumbs	Italian	Contadina	0.2	cup	0	1	0
	Italian	Devonsheer/Old London	0.1	cup	0	1	0
		Progresso	0.1	cup	0	1	0
		Devonsheer	0.1	cup	0	1	0
	Lemon herb	Progresso	0.1	cup	0	1	0
	seasoned	Progresso	0.1	cup	0	1	0
	tomato basil	Old London	0.1	cup	0	1	0
		Progresso	0.1	cup	0	1	0
Bread mix, dry	beer	Buckeye	0.02	pkg.	0	1	0
	beer, whole wheat	Buckeye	0.03	pkg.	0	1	0
	cheddar cheese	Dromedary	0.04	pkg.	0	1	0
	corn bread	Arrowhead Mills	0.1	cup	0	1	1
	corn bread	Aunt Jemima Easy Mix	0.2	cup	0	1	0
	corn bread	Ballard	0.02	pkg.	0	1	0
	corn bread	Buckeye	0.02	pkg.	0	1	0
	corn bread	Dromedary	0.04	pkg.	0	1	0
	herb, Italian	Dromedary	0.04	pkg.	0	1	0
	Kamut	Arrowhead Mills	0.1	cup	0	1	0
	multigrain	Arrowhead Mills	0.1	cup	0	1	0
	oatmeal, honey	Dromedary	0.04	pkg.	0	1	0
	rye	Arrowhead Mills	0.1	pkg.	0	1	0
	sourdough	Buckeye	0.02	cup	0	1	0
	sourdough	Dromedary	0.04	pkg.	0	1	0

FOOD ITEM	SPECIFICATIONS	BRAND NAME	QUANTITY	SIZE	PROTEIN BLOCKS	CARBOHYDRATE BLOCKS	FAT BLOCKS
	spelt	Arrowhead Mills	0.1	cup	0	1	0
	wheat, cracked	Pillsbury Bread Machine	0.03	loaf, prepared	0	1	0
	wheat, stoneground	Dromedary	0.04	pkg.	0	1	0
	wheat, whole	Arrowhead Mills	0.1	cup	0	1	0
	white	Arrowhead Mills	0.1	cup	0	1	0
	white, country	Dromedary	0.04	pkg.	0	1	0
	white, crusty	Pillsbury Bread Machine	0.03	loaf, prepared	0	1	0
Bread mix, sweet (dry except as noted)	apple cinnamon	Buckeye	0.02	pkg.	0	1	0
	apple cinnamon	Dromedary	0.04	pkg.	0	1	0
	apple cinnamon	Pillsbury	0.03	pkg.	0	1	1
	banana	Pillsbury	0.03	loaf, prepared	0	1	0
	banana	Pillsbury	0.03	pkg.	0	1	1
	blueberry	Pillsbury	0.03	loaf, prepared	0	1	0
	blueberry	Pillsbury	0.03	pkg.	0	1	1
	carrot	Pillsbury	0.03	loaf, prepared	0	1	0
	carrot	Pillsbury	0.03	pkg.	0	1	1
	cranberry	Pillsbury	0.04	loaf, prepared	0	1	0
	cranberry	Pillsbury	0.03	pkg.	0	1	1
	date	Pillsbury	0.02	loaf, prepared	0	1	0
	date	Pillsbury	0.02	pkg.	0	1	1
	date nut	Dromedary	0.1	pkg.	0	1	2
	gingerbread	Dromedary	0.03	pkg.	0	1	0
	gingerbread	Pillsbury Bread Machine	0.03	loaf, prepared	0	1	0
	nut	Pillsbury	0.03	pkg.	0	1	1
	nut	Pillsbury	0.03	loaf, prepared	0	1	0
	pumpkin	Pillsbury	0.03	pkg.	0	1	1
	pumpkin	Pillsbury	0.03	loaf, prepared	0	1	1
Bread snack	crisps, swirl, cinnamon raisin	Pepperidge Farm	0.6	oz.	0	1	1
	crisps, swirl, garlic butter	Pepperidge Farm	0.6	oz.	0	1	2
	sticks, three cheese	Pepperidge Farm	4.1	pcs.	0	1	0
	sticks, pretzel	Pepperidge Farm	3.5	pcs.	0	1	0
	sticks, pumpernickel/sesame	Pepperidge Farm	4.3	pcs.	0	1	1

Food	Description	Brand	Amount	Unit	Protein	Carbohydrate	Fat
Breadfruit			0.2	cup	0	1	0
			0.1	small	0	1	0
Breadfruit nuts		Goya Pana de Pepita	6.7	nuts	0	1	0
Breadsticks		Pepperidge Farm Brown and Serve	0.3	stick	0	1	0
		Pillsbury	0.5	stick	0	1	0
		Stella D'Oro	1.3	sticks	0	1	0
		Stella D'Oro Fat Free Original	3.8	sticks	0	1	0
		Stella D'Oro Fat Free Traditional	1.3	sticks	0	1	0
		Stella D'Oro No Sodium	1.3	sticks	0	1	0
	cheddar, thin	Pepperidge Farm	5.8	stick	1	1	1
	w/cheese	Handi-Snacks	0.8	stick	2	1	1
	garlic	Stella D'Oro	1.3	sticks	0	1	0
	garlic	Stella D'Oro Fat Free	1.4	sticks	0	1	0
	garlic	Stella D'Oro Fat Free Deli	3.8	sticks	0	1	0
	onion	Stella D'Oro	1.4	sticks	0	1	0
	onion, thin	Pepperidge Farms	5.8	sticks	1	1	1
	sesame	Stella D'Oro	1.3	sticks	0	1	0
	sesame	Stella D'Oro Low Fat	1.4	sticks	0	1	0
	sesame	Stella D'Oro No Sodium	1.3	sticks	0	1	0
	sesame, thin	Pepperidge Farm	5.8	sticks	1	1	1
	wheat	Stella D'Oro	1.7	sticks	0	1	0
Broad beans	raw		1	cup	1	1	0
	boiled, drained		3.6	oz.	0	1	0
Broad beans, mature	dried	Goya	0.1	cup	0	1	0
	boiled		0.4	cup	0	1	0
	canned	Progresso Fava Beans	0.3	cup	0	1	0
Broccoli, fresh	raw		2.5	8.7-oz. stalk	0	1	0
	raw, chopped		5	cup	1	1	0
	raw	Dole	10	stalk	1	1	0
	raw, florets	Dole	30	oz.	3	1	0
	boiled, drained		2.5	stalk	2	1	0
	boiled, drained, chopped		2.5	cup	1	1	0
Broccoli, frozen	spears	Green Giant	14.3	pkg.	1	1	0
	spears	Green Giant Harvest Fresh	15	oz.	0	1	0
	spears	Green Giant	17.5	oz.	0	1	0
	florets	Green Giant	6.7	cup	0	1	0

CARBOHYDRATES

FOOD ITEM	SPECIFICATIONS	BRAND NAME	QUANTITY	SIZE	PROTEIN BLOCKS	CARBOHYDRATE BLOCKS	FAT BLOCKS
	florets	Stilwell	20	florets	1	1	0
	cut	Green Giant	5	cup	1	1	0
	cut	Green Giant Harvest Fresh	3.3	cup	1	1	0
	cut	Stilwell	2.5	cup	1	1	0
	chopped		16.7	oz.	1	1	1
	chopped	Green Giant	3.8	cup	1	1	0
	chopped	Seabrook	3.8	cup	1	1	0
	butter sauce, spears	Green Giant	6.7	oz.	1	1	1
	cheese sauce	Green Giant	1	cup	0	1	1
Broccoli combinations, frozen	and cauliflower	Stilwell	2.5	cup	1	1	0
	cauliflower/carrots	Green Giant Harvest Fresh	5	cup	1	1	0
	cauliflower/carrots, cheese sauce	Green Giant	0.7	cup	0	1	0
	cauliflower/carrots, w/corn and peas, butter sauce	Green Giant	1.1	cup	0	1	1
	pasta, peas, corn, and peppers, butter sauce	Green Giant	0.8	cup	0	1	1
	stir-fry	Bird's Eye	3.3	cup	1	1	0
	stir-fry	Green Giant Create-A-Meal	1.8	cup	0	1	1
Broth concentrate	beef flavor	Knorr	20	tsp.	2	1	0
	chicken flavor	Knorr	20	tsp.	1	1	0
	vegetable flavor	Knorr	5	tsp.	0	1	0
Brown gravy	w/onions	Franco-American	0.6	cup	1	1	1
	savory	Heinz	0.8	cup	0	1	1
	mix, prepared	Durkee/French's	0.8	cup	0	1	1
	mix, prepared	Knorr Classic	0.8	cup	0	1	1
	mix, prepared	Loma Linda Gravy Quick	0.6	cup	0	1	0
	mix, prepared	McCormick	0.8	cup	0	1	0
	mix, prepared	Pillsbury	0.8	cup	0	1	0
	mix, prepared	Tone's Cook Up	1.3	cup	0	1	0
	mix, prepared, herb	Durkee/French's	0.8	cup	0	1	1
Brown gravy sauce		La Choy	0	cup	0	1	0
Brownie		Hostess Light	0.3	pcs.	0	1	0

Food	Type	Source	P	C	F	Amount	Unit
	chocolate	Awrey's Decadent	0	1	1	0.3	pc.
	chocolate	Little Debbie Low Fat	0	1	0	0.2	pc.
	chocolate, Bavarian	Awrey's	0	1	2	0.3	pc.
	chocolate, peanut	Awrey's Sensation	0	1	1	0.3	pc.
	fudge	Entenmann's Fat Free	0	1	0	0.03	strip
	fudge	Little Debbie	0	1	1	0.2	pc.
	fudge, w/out nuts	Awrey's	0	1	1	0.3	pc.
	fudge nut	Awrey's	0	1	1	0.4	pc.
	fudge nut	Drake's Reduced Fat	0	1	0	0.3	pc.
	fudge nut, chewy	Awrey's	0	1	1	0.3	pc.
	fudge walnut	Tastycake	0	1	1	0.2	pc.
	mini	Hostess Bites	0	1	1	1.5	pc.
	mini, walnut	Hostess Bites	0	1	2	0.3	pc.
Brownie, refrigerated	fudge	Pillsbury	0	1	1	0.02	pkg.
Brownie mix	chocolate	Arrowhead Mills	0	1	0	0.4	pc., prepared
		Arrowhead Mills Fat Free	0	1	0	0.3	pc., prepared
		Arrowhead Mills Wheat Free	0	1	0	0.4	pc., prepared
	chocolate	Pillsbury	0	1	1	0.3	pc., prepared
	fudge	Betty Crocker	0	1	0	0.02	pkg.
	fudge	Betty Crocker Light	0	1	0	0.02	pkg.
	fudge	Pillsbury, 15 oz.	0	1	1	0.4	pc., prepared
	fudge	Pillsbury, 21.5 oz.	0	1	1	0.4	pc., prepared
	fudge	Pillsbury Lovin' Lites	0	1	1	0.3	pc., prepared
	fudge, hot	Pillsbury	0	1	1	0.4	pc., prepared
	cream cheese swirl	Pillsbury Deluxe	0	1	1	0.4	pc., prepared
	walnut	Betty Crocker Supreme	0	1	1	0.02	pkg.
	walnut	Pillsbury	0	1	2	0.4	pc., prepared
Browning sauce		Gravy Master	0	1	0	1.3	tsp.
Brussels sprouts	fresh, raw		1	1	0	2.5	cup
	fresh, boiled		1	1	0	10	.7 oz. sprout
	frozen, boiled, drained		2	1	0	0.8	cup
	frozen, boiled, drained	Stilwell	0	1	0	30	sprouts
Buckwheat	whole grain		0	1	0	0.5	oz.
	whole grain		0	1	0	0.1	cup
Buckwheat flour	whole grain		0	1	0	1	oz.
	whole grain		0	1	0	0.1	cup

FOOD ITEM	SPECIFICATIONS	BRAND NAME	QUANTITY	SIZE	PROTEIN BLOCKS	CARBOHYDRATE BLOCKS	FAT BLOCKS
Buckwheat groats	brown	Arrowhead Mills	0.1	cup	0	1	0
Bulgur	dry	Arrowhead Mills	0.1	cup	0	1	0
	dry		0.6	oz.	0	1	0
	dry	Arrowhead Mills	0.1	cup	0	1	0
Bulgur pilaf mix	cooked		0.4	cup	0	1	0
Bun, sweet	apple	Casbah	0.5	oz.	0	1	0
	cheese, blueberry	Entenmann's Fat Free	0.3	bun	0	1	0
	cheese, pineapple	Entenmann's Fat Free	0.3	bun	0	1	0
	cheese, raspberry	Entenmann's Fat Free	0.3	bun	0	1	0
	cinnamon	Entenmann's	0.3	bun	0	1	1
	cinnamon, raisin	Entenmann's Fat Free	0.3	bun	0	1	0
	cinnamon roll	Hostess	0.2	bun	0	1	0
	cinnamon roll	Hostess Home Baked	0.4	bun	0	1	1
	cinnamon roll	Weight Watchers	0.3	bun	0	1	1
	honey	Aunt Fanny's	0.7	oz.	0	1	2
	honey	Aunt Fanny's	0.7	oz.	0	1	2
	honey	Grandma's	0.2	bun	0	1	1
	honey	Little Debbie	0.8	oz.	0	1	2
	honey	Morton	0.6	oz.	0	1	1
	honey	Morton Mini	0.7	oz.	0	1	1
	honey, applesauce filled	Aunt Fanny's	0.2	bun	0	1	1
	honey, banana, chocolate or valilla creme filled	Aunt Fanny's	0.3	bun	0	1	2
	honey, glazed	Hostess	0.3	bun	0	1	2
	honey, glazed or iced	Tastykake	0.2	bun	0	1	1
	honey, iced	Aunt Fanny's	0.3	bun	0	1	2
	honey, iced	Hostess	0.2	bun	0	1	1
	honey, raspberry filled	Aunt Fanny's	0.2	bun	0	1	1
	honey, frozen	Rich's	0.3	bun	0	1	1
	pecan roll	Little Debbie Spinwheels	0.3	bun	0	1	1
Bun, sweet, frozen or refrigerated	apple cinnamon, iced	Pillsbury	0.4	pc.	0	1	1

Food	Description	Brand	Amount	Unit	P	C	F
	carmel	Pillsbury	0.4	pc.	0	1	1
	cinnamon	Pepperidge Farm	0.3	pc.	0	1	1
	cinnamon, iced	Pillsbury	0.4	pc.	0	1	1
	cinnamon, raisin, iced	Pillsbury	0.3	pc.	0	1	1
	orange, iced	Pillsbury	0.4	pc.	0	1	1
Burdock root	raw		1.1	7.3-oz. pc.	0	1	0
	raw, pieces		0.6	cup	0	1	0
	boiled, 1 pc.		0.4	cup	0	1	0
Burrito sauce		Hunt's Manwich	0.6	cup	0	1	0
Burrito seasoning mix		Durkee Pouch	0.3	pkg.	0	1	0
		Lawry's	1.4	Tbsp.	0	1	1
		Old El Paso	10	tsp.	1	1	0
Butternut squash	fresh, raw, cubed		0.6	cup	0	1	0
	fresh, baked, cubed		0.6	cup	0	1	0
	frozen		2.4	pkg.	0	1	0
	frozen, boiled, drained, mashed		0.4	cup	0	1	0
Butterscotch chips	baking	Nestle Morsels	0.9	Tbsp.	0	1	1
Butterscotch topping		Kraft	0.6	tsp.	0	1	0
	carmel	Smucker's Sundae	0.7	tsp.	0	1	0
	carmel	Smucker's Nonfat	0.6	tsp.	0	1	0
	raw	Smucker's Special Recipe	0.3	tsp.	0	1	0
Cabbage	raw, shredded		5	cup (5 3/4 head, 2 1/2 lbs)	1	1	0
	boiled, drained, shredded		5	cup	1	1	1
Cabbage, Chinese	Bok choy, raw, whole		2	lb.	1	1	1
	pe-tsai, raw, whole		1	lb.	1	1	0
	pe-tsai, raw, shredded		5	cup	1	1	0
	pe-tsai, boiled, drained, shredded		12.5	cup	2	1	2
Cabbage, napa	raw	Frieda's	10	oz.	0	1	0
	raw, shredded	Dole	150	oz.	3	1	2
Cabbage, red, fresh	raw, whole		0.6	lb.	0	1	0
	raw, shredded		2.5	cup	1	1	0
	boiled, drained, shredded		2.5	cup	1	1	1

FOOD ITEM	SPECIFICATIONS	BRAND NAME	QUANTITY	SIZE	PROTEIN BLOCKS	CARBOHYDRATE BLOCKS	FAT BLOCKS
Cabbage, red, sweet and sour, in jars		Greenwood	0.2	cup	0	1	0
Cabbage, savoy		S&W	6.7	Tbsp.	0	1	0
	raw, whole		0.8	lb.	1	1	1
	raw, shredded		5	cup	1	1	1
	boiled, drained, shredded		1.3	cup	0	1	0
Cactus leaves		Frieda's	2.5	cup	0	1	0
Cake	angel food ring	Hostess	0.1	cake	0	1	0
	apple-spice crumb	Entenmann's Fat Free	0.04	cake	0	1	0
	banana	Awrey's Sheet	0.01	cake	0	1	2
	banana	Entenmann's Fat Free	0.03	cake	0	1	0
	banana, chocolate chip	Awrey's Marquise	0.01	cake	0	1	1
	banana crunch	Entenmann's	0.03	cake	0	1	1
	banana crunch	Entenmann's Fat Free	0.04	cake	0	1	0
	Black Forest torte	Awrey's	0.03	cake	0	1	2
	blueberry crunch	Entenmann's Fat Free	0.04	cake	0	1	0
	Boston creme	Awrey's	0.02	cake	0	1	1
	butter, French crumb	Entenmann's	0.04	cake	0	1	1
	butter	Entenmann's	0.05	loaf	0	1	1
	carrot	Entenmann's	0.03	cake	0	1	1
	carrot	Entenmann's Fat Free	0.03	cake	0	1	0
	carrot, cream cheese iced	Awrey's	0.01	cake	0	1	2
	carrot, supreme	Awrey's Sheet	0.01	cake	0	1	2
	cherries cordial	Awrey's Marquise	0.02	cake	0	1	1
	chocolate, crunch	Entenmann's Fat Free	0.04	cake	0	1	0
	chocolate, fudge	Entenmann's	0.03	cake	0	1	1
	chocolate, fudge iced	Entenmann's Fat Free	0.03	cake	0	1	0
	chocolate, German	Awrey's Sheet	0.01	cake	0	1	1
	chocolate, German, layer	Awrey's	0.01	cake	0	1	0
	chocolate, loaf	Entenmann's Fat Free	0.04	cake	0	1	1
	chocolate, mocha iced	Entenmann's Fat Free	0.03	cake	0	1	0
	chocolate, peanut	Awrey's Marquise	0.01	cake	0	1	2
	chocolate, tropical	Awrey's Marquise	0.02	cake	0	1	1

Item	Brand		Unit			
chocolate, white iced, layer	Awrey's	0.02	cake	0	1	1
chocolate, double	Awrey's	0.01	cake	0	1	1
chocolate, double	Awrey's Sheet	0.01	cake	0	1	1
chocolate, double, 3 layer	Awrey's	0.01	cake	0	1	1
chocolate, double, 2 layer	Awrey's	0.02	cake	0	1	1
coconut buttercream	Awrey's Sheet	0.01	cake	0	1	2
coconut buttercream, layer	Awrey's	0.01	cake	0	1	2
coffee	Awrey's Long John	0.04	cake	0	1	2
coffee, cheese	Entenmann's	0.04	cake	0	1	1
coffee, cheese, crumb	Entenmann's	0.04	cake	0	1	1
coffee, cinnamon apple	Entenmann's Fat Free	0.04	cake	0	1	0
coffee, crumb	Entenmann's	0.03	cake	0	1	1
crunch, Louisiana	Entenmann's	0.02	cake	0	1	1
crunch, Louisiana	Entenmann's Fat Free	0.03	cake	0	1	1
danish cake, Black Forest	Entenmann's Fat Free	0.03	cake	0	1	0
danish cake, raspberry cheese	Entenmann's Fat Free	0.03	cake	0	1	0
danish ring, cinnamon filbert	Entenmann's	0.1	ring	0	1	2
danish ring, pecan	Entenmann's	0.1	cake	0	1	2
danish ring, walnut	Entenmann's	0.1	cake	0	1	2
danish twist, apricot	Entenmann's Fat Free	0.03	cake	0	1	0
danish twist, cinnamon apple	Entenmann's Fat Free	0.03	cake	0	1	0
danish twist, lemon	Entenmann's Fat Free	0.04	cake	0	1	0
danish twist, raspberry	Entenmann's	0.04	cake	0	1	1
danish twist, raspberry	Entenmann's Fat Free	0.04	cake	0	1	0
devil's food, marshmallow iced	Entenmann's	0.03	cake	0	1	1
espresso, French	Awrey's Marquise	0.02	cake	0	1	2
fruit cake	Hostess 2 lb.	0.02	cake	0	1	0
fruit cake	Hostess 3 lbs.	0.01	cake	0	1	0
golden, crumb, French	Entenmann's Fat Free	0.03	cake	0	1	0
golden, fudge, thick	Entenmann's	0.03	cake	0	1	1
golden, fudge, iced	Entenmann's	0.03	cake	0	1	0
golden loaf	Entenmann's Fat Free	0.04	cake	0	1	0
golden loaf, chocolatey chip	Entenmann's Fat Free	0.04	cake	0	1	0
lemon layer	Awrey's	0.01	cake	0	1	2
marble loaf	Entenmann's	0.04	cake	0	1	1
marble loaf	Entenmann's Fat Free	0.04	cake	0	1	0

FOOD ITEM	SPECIFICATIONS	BRAND NAME	QUANTITY	SIZE	PROTEIN BLOCKS	CARBOHYDRATE BLOCKS	FAT BLOCKS
	Neapolitan	Awrey's	0.02	cake	0	1	2
	orange, frosty	Awrey's Sheet	0.01	cake	0	1	1
	orange, frosty, layer	Awrey's	0.01	cake	0	1	1
	peach, Georgia	Awrey's Marquise	0.02	cake	0	1	1
	pound	Hostess	0.04	cake	0	1	1
	pound, golden	Awrey's	0.04	cake	0	1	1
	raisin loaf	Entenmann's	0.03	cake	0	1	0
	raisin loaf	Entenmann's Fat Free	0.03	cake	0	1	1
	raspberry and cream	Awrey's Marquise	0.02	cake	0	1	1
	raspberry nut	Awrey's Marquise	0.01	cake	0	1	1
	sour cream chip-nut loaf	Entenmann's	0.04	cake	0	1	2
	sponge, uniced	Awrey's	0.01	cake	0	1	1
	strawberry supreme	Awrey's Marquise	0.02	cake	0	1	1
	strawberry supreme torte	Awrey's	0.02	cake	0	1	2
	yellow, lemon iced, 2 layer	Awrey's	0.02	cake	0	1	1
	yellow, white iced	Awrey's Sheet	0.01	cake	0	1	1
	Boston creme	Mrs. Smith's	0.04	cake	0	1	1
	Boston creme	Pepperidge Farm	0.03	cake	0	1	1
	carrot	Pepperidge Farm Deluxe	0.03	cake	0	1	1
Cake, frozen	cheesecake, strawberry	Amy's	1	oz.	0	1	1
	cheesecake, strawberry, French	Sara Lee	0.04	cake	0	1	1
	chocolate, double layer	Sara Lee	0.04	cake	0	1	1
	chocolate, fudge	Amy's	0.5	oz.	0	1	0
	chocolate, fudge, layer	Pepperidge Farm	0.04	cake	0	1	1
	chocolate, fudge stripe, layer	Pepperidge Farm	0.04	cake	0	1	1
	chocolate, German, layer	Pepperidge Farm	0.04	cake	0	1	1
	chocolate, mousse	Pepperidge Farm	0.03	cake	0	1	1
	coconut layer	Pepperidge Farm	0.04	cake	0	1	1
	coffee cake	Sara Lee	0.03	cake	0	1	1
	devil's food layer	Pepperidge Farm	0.04	cake	0	1	1
	golden layer	Pepperidge Farm	0.04	cake	0	1	1
	lemon mousse	Pepperidge Farm	0.03	cake	0	1	1

Cake, mix

Food	Brand	Amount	Unit			
pineapple cream	Pepperidge Farm	0.03	cake	0	—	—
pound	Goya	0.1	cake	0	—	—
pound, butter	Pepperidge Farm	0.05	cake	0	—	—
strawberry cream	Pepperidge Farm	0.03	cake	0	—	—
strawberry stripe layer	Pepperidge Farm	0.03	cake	0	—	—
vanilla layer	Pepperidge Farm	0.04	cake	0	—	—
angel food, prepared	Betty Crocker	0.02	pkg.	0	—	0
angel food, prepared	Pillsbury Moist Supreme	0.1	pkg.	0	—	0
angel food, prepared	Pillsbury Plus	0.03	cake	0	—	0
banana	Pillsbury Moist Supreme	0.02	pkg.	0	—	0
banana, prepared	Pillsbury Moist Supreme	0.02	pkg.	0	—	—
banana	Pillsbury Plus	0.02	pkg.	0	—	0
banana, prepared	Pillsbury Plus	0.02	pkg.	0	—	—
butter pecan	Betty Crocker SuperMoist	0.02	pkg.	0	—	0
butter recipe	Pillsbury Moist Supreme	0.02	pkg.	0	—	0
butter recipe, prepared	Pillsbury Moist Supreme	0.02	pkg.	0	—	—
butter recipe	Pillsbury Plus	0.02	pkg.	0	—	0
butter recipe, prepared	Pillsbury Plus	0.02	pkg.	0	—	—
butter recipe, chocolate	Pillsbury Moist Supreme	0.02	pkg.	0	—	0
butter recipe, chocolate, prepared	Pillsbury Moist Supreme	0.02	pkg.	0	—	—
butter recipe, chocolate	Pillsbury Plus	0.02	pkg.	0	—	0
butter recipe, chocolate, prepared	Pillsbury Plus	0.02	pkg.	0	—	—
carrot	Betty Crocker SuperMoist	0.02	pkg.	0	—	0
carrot	Pillsbury Moist Supreme	0.02	pkg.	0	—	—
carrot, prepared	Pillsbury Moist Supreme	0.02	pkg.	0	—	0
carrot	Pillsbury Plus	0.02	pkg.	0	—	0
carrot, prepared	Pillsbury Plus	0.02	pkg.	0	—	—
cheesecake, prepared	Jell-O Homestyle	0.03	cake	0	—	4
cheesecake, prepared	Jell-O Real	0.03	cake	0	—	—
cheesecake, blueberry, prepared	Jell-O	0.03	cake	0	—	—
cheesecake, cherry, prepared	Jell-O	0.03	cake	0	—	—
cheesecake, strawberry, prepared	Jell-O	0.03	cake	0	—	—

FOOD ITEM	SPECIFICATIONS	BRAND NAME	QUANTITY	SIZE	PROTEIN BLOCKS	CARBOHYDRATE BLOCKS	FAT BLOCKS
	chocolate	Betty Crocker SuperMoist	0.05	cake	0	1	0
	chocolate	Pillsbury Moist Supreme	0.04	cake	0	1	0
	chocolate, prepared	Pillsbury Moist Supreme	0.04	cake	0	1	1
	chocolate	Pillsbury Plus	0.04	cake	0	1	0
	chocolate, prepared	Pillsbury Plus	0.04	cake	0	1	1
	chocolate caramel nut	Pillsbury Bundt	0.02	cake	0	1	1
	chocolate chip	Pillsbury Moist Supreme/Plus	0.04	cake	0	1	0
	chocolate chip, prepared	Pillsbury Moist Supreme/Plus	0.04	cake	0	1	1
	chocolate, dark	Pillsbury Moist Supreme	0.05	cake	0	1	0
	chocolate, dark, prepared	Pillsbury Moist Supreme	0.05	cake	0	1	1
	chocolate, dark	Pillsbury Plus	0.05	cake	0	1	0
	chocolate, dark, prepared	Pillsbury Plus	0.05	cake	0	1	1
	chocolate, German	Betty Crocker SuperMoist	0.04	cake	0	1	0
	chocolate, German	Pillsbury Moist Supreme/Plus	0.04	cake	0	1	0
	chocolate, German, prepared	Pillsbury Moist Supreme	0.04	cake	0	1	1
	chocolate, German, prepared	Pillsbury Plus	0.04	cake	0	1	1
	cinnamon streusel	Pillsbury Streusel Swirl	0.01	pkg.	0	1	0
	cinnamon streusel, prepared	Pillsbury Streusel Swirl	0.01	cake	0	1	1
	coffee	Aunt Jemima Easy Mix	0.3	cup	0	1	1
	date nut roll	Dromedary	0.1	pk.	0	1	0
	devil's food	Betty Crocker SuperMoist	0.04	cake	0	1	0
	devil's food	Pillsbury Moist Supreme/Plus	0.05	cake	0	1	0
	devil's food, prepared	Pillsbury Moist Supreme/Plus	0.05	cake	0	1	1
	devil's food	Pillsbury Moist Supreme/ Plus Lovin' Lites	0.02	pkg.	0	1	0
	devil's food, prepared	Pillsbury Moist Supreme/ Plus Lovin' Lites	0.02	cake	0	1	0
	fudge, double hot	Pillsbury Bundt	0.02	cake	0	1	0
	fudge swirl	Pillsbury Moist Supreme	0.04	cake	0	1	1
	fudge swirl, prepared	Pillsbury Moist Supreme	0.04	cake	0	1	1
	fudge swirl	Pillsbury Plus	0.04	cake	0	1	0
	fudge swirl, prepared	Pillsbury Plus	0.04	cake	0	1	1
	lemon	Pillsbury Moist Supreme	0.02	pkg.	0	1	0

Food	Brand	Amount	Unit			
lemon, prepared	Pillsbury Moist Supreme	0.02	pkg.	0	—	1
lemon	Pillsbury Plus	0.02	pkg.	0	—	0
lemon, prepared	Pillsbury Plus	0.02	pkg.	0	—	1
lemon	Pillsbury Moist Supreme/Plus Funfetti	0.03	pkg.	0	—	0
lemon, prepared	Pillsbury Moist Supreme/Plus Funfetti	0.03	pkg.	0	—	1
pound	Betty Crocker	0.03	pkg.	0	—	1
pound	Dromedary	0.03	pkg.	0	—	0
strawberry	Pillsbury Plus	0.04	cake	0	—	1
strawberry, prepared	Pillsbury Plus	0.04	cake	0	—	0
strawberry, cream cheese	Pillsbury Bundt	0.02	cake	0	—	0
strawberry, swirl	Betty Crocker SuperMoist	0.02	pkg.	0	—	0
vanilla, French	Betty Crocker SuperMoist	0.04	cake	0	—	0
vanilla, French	Pillsbury Moist Supreme	0.02	pkg.	0	—	1
vanilla, French, prepared	Pillsbury Moist Supreme	0.02	pkg.	0	—	0
vanilla, French	Pillsbury Plus	0.02	pkg.	0	—	1
vanilla, French, prepared	Pillsbury Plus	0.02	pkg.	0	—	0
vanilla, sunshine	Pillsbury Moist Supreme/Plus	0.04	cake	0	—	1
vanilla, sunshine, prepared	Pillsbury Moist Supreme/Plus	0.04	cake	0	—	0
white	Betty Crocker SuperMoist	0.04	cake	0	—	0
white	Pillsbury Moist Supreme/Plus	0.02	pkg.	0	—	1
white, prepared	Pillsbury Moist Supreme/Plus	0.02	cake	0	—	0
white	Pillsbury Moist Supreme/ Plus Lovin' Lites	0.02	pkg.	0	—	0
white, prepared	Pillsbury Moist Supreme/ Plus Lovin' Lites	0.02	cake	0	—	0
white 'n fudge swirl	Pillsbury Moist Supreme	0.04	cake	0	—	0
white 'n fudge swirl, prepared	Pillsbury Moist Supreme	0.04	cake	0	—	1
white 'n fudge swirl	Pillsbury Plus	0.04	cake	0	—	0
white 'n fudge swirl, prepared	Pillsbury Plus	0.04	cake	0	—	1
yellow	Betty Crocker SuperMoist	0.04	cake	0	—	0
yellow	Pillsbury Moist Supreme	0.04	cake	0	—	0
yellow, prepared	Pillsbury Moist Supreme	0.04	cake	0	—	1
yellow	Pillsbury Plus	0.04	cake	0	—	0
yellow, prepared	Pillsbury Plus	0.04	cake	0	—	1
yellow	Pillsbury Moist Supreme/ Plus Lovin' Lites	0.02	pkg.	0	—	0

FOOD ITEM	SPECIFICATIONS	BRAND NAME	QUANTITY	SIZE	PROTEIN BLOCKS	CARBOHYDRATE BLOCKS	FAT BLOCKS
	yellow, prepared	Pillsbury Moist Supreme/ Plus Lovin' Lites	0.02	cake	0	1	0
	yellow, butter recipe	Betty Crocker SuperMoist	0.04	cake	0	1	0
Cake, snack		Tastykake Koffee Kake	0.5	oz.	0	1	1
	all varieties	Tastykake Kreme Krimpies	0.5	pc.	0	1	1
	almond swirl	Health Valley Healthy Tarts	0.3	pc.	0	1	0
	apple bar	Aunt Fanny's	0.6	pc.	0	1	1
	apple filled	Health Valley	0.3	pc.	0	1	0
	apricot bar	Tastykake Krimpets Low Fat	0.5	pc.	0	1	0
		Health Valley	0.3	pc.	0	1	0
	banana	Little Debbie Twins	0.2	pc.	0	1	1
	banana	Suzy Q's	0.3	pc.	0	1	1
	banana	Tastykake Creamies	0.3	pc.	0	1	1
	banana	Twinkies	0.4	pc.	0	1	1
	Boston Creme	Drake's	0.4	pc.	0	1	1
	brownie, fudge filled	Health Valley	0.4	pc.	0	1	0
	butterscotch iced	Tastykake Krimpets	0.5	pc.	0	1	0
	cheesecake	Boar's Head New York	0.4	pc.	0	1	4
	cheesecake, bar all varieties	Health Valley	0.3	pc.	0	1	0
	chocolate	Devil Dogs	0.6	oz.	0	1	1
	chocolate	Ding Dongs	0.6	oz.	0	1	1
	chocolate	Funny Bones	0.5	pc.	0	1	1
	chocolate	Ho-Hos	0.5	pc.	0	1	1
	chocolate	Hostess Choco-Diles	0.3	pc.	0	1	1
	chocolate	Hostess Choco Licious	0.3	pc.	0	1	1
	chocolate	Ring Dings	0.5	pc.	0	1	1
	chocolate	Suzy Q's	0.3	pc.	0	1	1
	chocolate	Tastykake Creamies	0.3	pc.	0	1	1
	chocolate	Tastykake Juniors	0.2	pc.	0	1	1
	chocolate	Tastykake Kandy Kakes	0.8	pc.	0	1	1
	chocolate	Yodels	0.5	pc.	0	1	1
	chocolate, fingers	Aunt Fanny's	0.4	pc.	0	1	1
	chocolate chip	Little Debbie	0.3	pc.	0	1	1

Food	Brand	Amount	Unit			
cinnamon twirl	Aunt Fanny's	0.1	pc.	0	—	0
coconut covered	Sno Balls	0.3	pc.	0	—	1
coconut covered	Tastykake Juniors	0.2	pc.	0	—	0
coconut covered	Tastykake Kandy Kakes	0.8	pc.	0	—	1
coconut twirl	Aunt Fanny's	0.6	pc.	0	—	1
coffee cake	Drake's	0.5	pc.	0	—	1
coffee cake	Drake's Low Fat	0.5	pc.	0	—	0
coffee cake	Little Debbie	0.2	pc.	0	—	1
crumb	Hostess	0.6	pc.	0	—	0
crumb	Hostess Lites	0.5	pc.	0	—	1
cupcake	Tastykake Kreme Kup	0.6	pc.	0	—	0
cupcake	Yankee Doodles	0.6	pc.	0	—	1
cupcake, apple filled	Tastykake Koffee Kake Low Fat	0.5	pc.	0	—	1
cupcake, buttercreme iced	Tastykake	0.5	pc.	0	—	1
cupcake, buttercreme iced, mini	Tastykake	1.1	pcs.	0	—	0
cupcake, creme	Tastykake Koffee Kake	0.5	pc.	0	—	1
cupcake, creme, mini	Tastykake Koffee Kake	1.1	pcs.	0	—	1
cupcake, lemon filled	Tastykake Koffee Kake, Low Fat	0.5	pc.	0	—	0
cupcake, raspberry filled	Tastykake Koffee Kake, Low Fat	0.5	pc.	0	—	0
cupcake, chocolate	Aunt Fanny's	0.4	pc.	0	—	1
cupcake, chocolate	Hostess	0.6	pc.	0	—	1
cupcake, chocolate	Hostess, Light	0.7	pc.	0	—	0
cupcake, chocolate	Tastykake	0.5	pc.	0	—	0
cupcake, chocolate	Tastykake	0.5	pc.	0	—	0
cupcake, chocolate, creme	Tastykake, Low Fat	0.4	pc.	0	—	0
cupcake, chocolate, iced, creme	Tastykake	0.5	pc.	0	—	1
cupcake, chocolate, iced, creme, mini	Tastykake	1.1	pcs.	0	—	1
cupcake, chocolate, iced, creme, vanilla, mini	Tastykake	1.1	pcs.	0	—	1
cupcake, orange	Aunt Fanny's	0.4	pc.	0	—	1
cupcake, orange	Hostess	0.3	pc.	0	—	1
cupcake, vanilla, creme	Tastycake Low Fat	0.4	pc.	0	—	0
date bar	Health Valley	0.3	pc.	0	—	0

FOOD ITEM	SPECIFICATIONS	BRAND NAME	QUANTITY	SIZE	PROTEIN BLOCKS	CARBOHYDRATE BLOCKS	FAT BLOCKS
	devil's food	Little Debbie Devil Cremes	0.2	pc.	0	1	1
	devil's food	Twinkies	0.4	pc.	0	1	1
	frosty	Tastykake Kandy Kakes	0.7	pc.	0	1	1
	fruit loaf	Hostess	0.1	1 pc.	0	1	0
	fudge, frosted	Little Debbie	0.3	pc.	0	1	1
	fudge, rounds	Little Debbie	0.2	pc.	0	1	1
	golden, creme filled	Hostess Dessert Cup	0.5	pc.	0	1	0
	golden, creme filled	Hostess Lil Angels	0.5	pc.	0	1	1
	golden, creme filled	Hostess Tiger Tails	0.3	pc.	0	1	1
	golden, creme filled	Little Debbie Golden Cremes	0.2	pc.	0	1	1
	golden, creme filled	Sunny Doodles	0.6	pcs.	0	1	1
	golden, creme filled	Sunny Doodles Reduced Fat	0.6	pcs.	0	1	0
	golden, creme filled	Twinkies	0.5	oz.	0	1	0
	golden, creme filled	Twinkies Light	0.5	oz.	0	1	0
	jelly filled	Tastykake Krimpets	0.5	pc.	0	1	0
	jelly filled	Tastykake Krimpets Low Fat	0.5	pc.	0	1	0
	lemon filled	Tastykake Krimpets Low Fat	0.5	pc.	0	1	0
	peanut butter	Tastykake Kandy Kakes	0.3	pc.	0	1	1
	pecan twirl	Aunt Fanny's	0.6	pc.	0	1	1
	pound	Aunt Fanny's	0.3	pc.	0	1	1
	pound	Tastykake	0.2	pc.	0	1	1
	raisin bar	Health Valley Fat Free	0.3	pc.	0	1	0
	raspberry fingers	Aunt Fanny's	0.4	pc.	0	1	1
	sprinkled	Tastycake Creamies	0.4	pc.	0	1	1
	stick, dunking	Aunt Fanny's	0.6	oz.	0	1	2
	stick, dunking	Aunt Fanny's	0.6	oz.	0	1	2
	stick, dunking	Little Debbie	0.3	pc.	0	1	2
	stick, dunking	Tastykake Stix	0.2	pc.	0	1	1
	stick, dunking, cherry	Aunt Fanny's	0.5	pc.	0	1	2
	stick, dunking, chocolate	Aunt Fanny's	0.5	pc.	0	1	2
	stick, dunking, twin sticks	Awrey's	0.8	oz.	0	1	2
	strawberry	Twinkies Fruit 'n Creme	0.3	pc.	0	1	0
	strawberry, iced	Tastykake Krimpets	0.2	pc.	0	1	0

Item	Brand	Amount	Unit	Protein	Carbohydrate	Fat
strawberry shortcake	Little Debbie	0.2	pc.	0	1	1
Swiss roll	Little Debbie	0.2	pc.	0	1	1
vanilla	Little Debbie	0.2	pc.	0	1	1
vanilla	Tastykake Creamies	0.3	pc.	0	1	1
vanilla, fingers	Aunt Fanny's	0.4	pc.	0	1	0
yellow	Hostess Baseball	0.3	pc.	0	1	0
zebra	Little Debbie	0.2	pc.	0	1	1
Cake mix, dry						
apple cinnamon	Betty Crocker Easy Layer Bar	0.03	pkg.	0	1	0
apple streusel bar	Sweet Rewards	0.03	pkg.	0	1	1
apple streusel bar, prepared	Pillsbury	0.02	pkg.	0	1	0
banana	Pillsbury	0.4	bar	0	1	0
chocolate bar	Sweet Rewards	0.03	pkg.	0	1	1
chocolate bar, chip	Sweet Rewards	0.03	pkg.	0	1	0
chocolate bar, chip, prepared	Pillsbury Chips Ahoy!	0.02	pkg.	0	1	1
chocolate bar, chunk	Pillsbury Chips Ahoy!	0.3	bar	0	1	1
chocolate bar, peanut butter	Betty Crocker	0.02	pkg.	0	1	1
chocolate cookie bar	Betty Crocker	0.02	pkg.	0	1	1
chocolate cookie bar, prepared	Pillsbury Oreo	0.02	pkg.	0	1	1
chocolate cookie bar, prepared	Pillsbury Oreo	0.4	bar	0	1	1
date bar, prepared	Betty Crocker	0.03	pkg.	0	1	1
fudge swirl cookie	Pillsbury	0.02	pkg.	0	1	0
fudge swirl cookie, prepared	Pillsbury	0.4	bar	0	1	0
gingerbread	Betty Crocker	0.03	pkg.	0	1	1
lemon bar	Sweet Rewards	0.03	pkg.	0	1	2
lemon bar	Betty Crocker Sunkist	0.02	pkg.	0	1	1
lemon cheesecake bar	Pillsbury	0.02	pkg.	0	1	1
lemon cheesecake bar, prepared	Pillsbury	0.5	bar	0	1	0
peanut butter bar	Pillsbury Nutter Butter	0.02	pkg.	0	1	1
peanut butter bar, prepared	Pillsbury Nutter Butter	0.3	bar	0	1	0
raspberry	Betty Crocker	0.02	pkg.	0	1	0
Cake decoration						
confetti or nonpareils	Dec-A-Cake Dec-A-Cone	3.3	tsp.	0	1	0
hearts, bats, or pumpkins	Dec-A-Cake	3.3	tsp.	0	1	0
party imperials or fruit cocktail	Dec-A-Cake	2.5	tsp.	0	1	0
party imperials or fruit cocktail	Dec-A-Cake	22.5	pcs.	0	1	0

FOOD ITEM	SPECIFICATIONS	BRAND NAME	QUANTITY	SIZE	PROTEIN BLOCKS	CARBOHYDRATE BLOCKS	FAT BLOCKS
	rainbow	Dec-A-Cake	2.5	tsp.	0	1	1
	sprinkles	Hershey's Cookies 'n Mint	0.8	tsp.	0	1	2
	sprinkles, chocolate, milk	Hershey's	0.8	Tbsp.	0	1	1
	sprinkles, fun	Dec-A-Cake	2.5	tsp.	0	1	0
	sprinkles, holiday	Dec-A-Cake	3.3	tsp.	0	1	1
	sprinkles, peanut butter	Reese's	1.1	Tbsp.	0	1	2
	sugar crystals	Dec-A-Cake	3.3	tsp.	0	1	0
	trims, chocolate	Dec-A-Cake	5	tsp.	0	1	1
	trims, chocolate, mint	Dec-A-Cake	3.3	tsp.	0	1	1
Canary beans	dry	Goya	0.1	cup	1	1	0
Candy		Baby Ruth	0.3	2.1-oz. bar	0	1	1
		Baby Ruth Fun Size	0.7	bar	0	1	1
		Bar None	0.6	oz.	0	1	2
		Buncha Crunch	3.9	oz.	0	1	1
	butter rum	Lifesavers	3.3	pcs.	0	1	0
	butter rum	Pearson Nips	1.5	pcs.	0	1	0
	buttercrunch/almond	Almond Roca	1.4	pcs.	0	1	2
		Butterfinger	0.2	2.1-oz. bar	0	1	1
		Butterfinger, Fun Size	0.6	bars	0	1	1
		Butterfinger BB's	0.3	1.7-oz. bag	0	1	1
	butterscotch	Brach's Disks	0.5	pc.	0	1	0
	candy corn	Heide/Heide Indian	1.3	oz.	0	1	0
	caramel	Kraft	1.4	pcs.	0	1	0
	caramel	Pearson Nips	1.5	pcs.	0	1	0
	caramel, chocolate	Milk Duds	0.4	oz.	0	1	1
	caramel, chocolate	Pom Poms	0.4	oz.	0	1	1
	caramel, chocolate	Rolo	0.5	oz.	0	1	1
	caramel, w/cookies	Twix	0.5	pc.	0	1	1
	caramel, w/cookies	Twix, Fun Size	0.9	pc.	0	1	1
	caramel, w/cookies	Twix Single	0.5	pc.	0	1	1
	cherry, chocolate coated	Perugina	0.4	oz.	0	1	1
	chocolate, w/hazelnuts	Ferraro Rocher	1.7	pcs.	0	1	3
	chocolate parfait	Pearson Nips	1.7	pcs.	0	1	1

chocolate, candy coated	M&M's	0.5 oz.	0	1	1
chocolate, candy coated w/almonds	M&M's	0.6 oz.	0	1	2
chocolate, candy coated, peanut butter	M&M's	0.6 oz.	0	1	2
chocolate, candy coated w/peanuts	M&M's	0.6 oz.	0	1	1
chocolate, dark	Dove	0.1 of 6-oz. bar	0	1	2
chocolate, dark	Dove Mini	2.6 pcs.	0	1	2
chocolate, dark	Dove Single	0.6 oz.	0	1	2
chocolate, dark	Ghirardelli	0.5 oz.	0	1	2
chocolate, dark	Ghirardelli	0.4 1 1/4-oz. bar	0	1	2
chocolate, dark	Hershey's Special Dark	0.4 1.45-oz. bar	0	1	2
chocolate, dark w/almonds	Ghirardelli	0.4 1 1/2-oz. bar	0	1	2
chocolate, dark bittersweet	Toblerone	0.6 of 3 1/2-oz. bar	0	1	2
chocolate, dark w/raspberries	Ghirardelli	1.4 pcs.	0	1	1
chocolate, milk	Cadbury's Dairy Milk	0.5 oz.	0	1	2
chocolate, milk	Dove	0.1 of 6-oz. bar	0	1	2
chocolate, milk	Dove Mini	2.6 pcs.	0	1	2
chocolate, milk	Dove Single	0.4 1.3-oz. bar	0	1	2
chocolate, milk	Ghirardelli	0.5 oz.	0	1	2
chocolate, milk	Ghirardelli	0.5 oz.	0	1	2
chocolate, milk	Hershey's	0.7 oz.	0	1	2
chocolate, milk	Hershey's Hugs	3.3 pcs.	0	1	2
chocolate, milk	Hershey's Nuggets	1.7 pcs.	0	1	2
chocolate, milk	Hershey's Kisses	3.3 pcs.	0	1	2
chocolate, milk	Nestle	0.4 1.45-oz. bar	0	1	2
chocolate, milk	Symphony	0.6 oz.	0	1	2
chocolate, milk, w/almonds	Cadbury	0.6 oz.	0	1	2
chocolate, milk, w/almonds	Ghirardelli	0.5 1 1/4-oz. bar	0	1	2
chocolate, milk, w/almonds	Ghirardelli	0.7 oz.	0	1	2
chocolate, milk, w/almonds	Ghirardelli	0.3 2.1-oz. bar	0	1	2
chocolate, milk, w/almonds	Hershey's	0.7 oz.	0	1	2
chocolate, milk, w/almonds	Hershey Nuggets	1.9 pcs.	0	1	2
chocolate, milk, w/almonds	Hershey's Kisses	4 pcs.	0	1	2
chocolate, milk, w/almonds, toffee	Symphony	0.7 oz.	0	1	2

FOOD ITEM	SPECIFICATIONS	BRAND NAME	QUANTITY	SIZE	PROTEIN BLOCKS	CARBOHYDRATE BLOCKS	FAT BLOCKS
	chocolate, milk, w/caramel	Caramello	0.3	1.6-oz. bar	0	1	1
	chocolate, milk, cookies and cream	Ghirardelli	0.5	oz.	0	1	2
	chocolate, milk, cookies and cream	Hershey's Nuggets	1.7	pcs.	0	1	2
	chocolate, milk, w/crisps	Crunch	0.3	1.55-oz. bar	0	1	1
	chocolate, milk, w/crisps	Crunch Fun Size	1.5	bars	0	1	1
	chocolate, milk, w/crisps	Ghirardelli	0.4	1 1/4-oz. bar	0	1	1
	chocolate, milk, w/crisps	Ghirardelli	0.2	2.1-oz. bar	0	1	1
	chocolate, milk, w/crisps	Ghirardelli	0.2	2 1/2-oz. bar	0	1	1
	chocolate, milk, w/crisps	Krackel	0.2	2.6-oz. bar	0	1	1
	chocolate, milk w/ fruit and nuts	Chunky	0.5	1.4-oz. bar	0	1	2
	chocolate, milk w/hazelnuts	Mon Cheri	1.4	pcs.	0	1	3
	chocolate, milk w/ honey and nougat	Toblerone	0.2	of 3 1/2-oz. bar	0	1	2
	chocolate, milk w/ macadamias	Ghirardelli	0.5	1 1/4-oz. bar	0	1	2
	chocolate, milk w/peanuts	Mr. Goodbar	0.4	1 3/4-oz. bar	0	1	2
	chocolate, milk w/pecans	Ghirardelli	0.4	1 3/4-oz. bar	0	1	2
	chocolate, milk w/ raisins and almonds	Cadbury Fruit and Nut	0.5	oz.	0	1	1
	chocolate, milk, thins	Lindt Swiss	6.3	pcs.	0	1	2
	chocolate, milk w/toffee	Ghirardelli	1.4	pcs.	0	1	1
	chocolate, milk wafers	Ghirardelli	3.4	pcs.	0	1	1
	chocolate mint	Ghirardelli	0.5	oz.	0	1	2
	chocolate mint	Ghirardelli	0.2	bar	0	1	2
	chocolate mint	Pearson Nips	1.7	pcs.	0	1	0
	chocolate mint, cookies and	Hershey's	0.3	1.55-oz. bar	0	1	1
	chocolate mint, cookies and	Hershey's Nuggets	1.5	pcs.	0	1	1
	chocolate mint, candy coated	M&M's	0.5	oz.	0	1	1
	chocolate mint, wafers	Ghirardelli	3.7	pcs.	0	1	1
	chocolate, white, raspberry cream	Ghirardelli	1.7	pcs.	0	1	2

Food	Description	Amount	Unit	Protein	Carbohydrate	Fat
coconut, w/chocolate	Mounds	0.3	1.9-oz. bar	0	1	—
coconut, w/chocolate, w/almonds	Almond Joy	0.3	1.76-oz. bar	0	1	—
coffee	Pearson Nips	1.5	pcs.	0	1	○
fruit flavor	Skittles Original	0.4	oz.	0	1	○
fruit flavor	Skittles Singles Original	0.4	oz.	0	1	○
fruit flavor, chews	Starburst	2.2	pcs.	0	1	○
fruit flavor, tropical or wild berry	Skittles	0.4	oz.	0	1	○
fruit flavor, tropical or wild berry	Skittles, Single	0.2	oz.	0	1	○
fruit flavor, gummed	Amazin' Fruit	0.4	oz.	0	1	○
fruit flavor, gummed	Brach's Fruit Bunch	0.7	pc.	0	1	○
fruit flavor, gummed	Gummi Savers	0.4	oz.	0	1	○
fudge	Kraft Fudgies	1.4	pcs.	0	1	○
gum, chewing, all flavors	Beech-Nut	5	pcs.	0	1	○
gum, chewing, all flavors	Big Red	5	pcs.	0	1	○
gum, chewing, all flavors	Care*Free	5	pcs.	0	1	○
gum, chewing, all flavors	Doublemint/Winterfresh/ Wrigley's Spearmint	5	pcs.	0	1	○
gum, chewing, all flavors	Extra/Winterfresh Sugarfree	5	pcs.	0	1	○
gum, chewing, all flavors	Freedent	5	pcs.	0	1	○
gum, chewing, all flavors	Fruit Stripe	5	pcs.	0	1	○
gum, chewing, all flavors	Juicy Fruit	5	pcs.	0	1	○
gum, bubble	Bubble Yum	1.4	pcs.	0	1	○
gum, bubble	Bubble Yum, Sugarless	3.3	pcs.	0	1	○
gum, bubble	Care*Free	5	pcs.	0	1	○
gum, bubble, stick	Care*Free	5	pcs.	0	1	○
hard, all flavors	Brach's Sparklers	1.6	pcs.	0	1	○
hard, all flavors	Lifesavers	3.3	pcs.	0	1	○
hard, all flavors	Pez	1	.3-oz. roll	0	1	○
hard, all flavors	Pez Sugar Free	1.1	.3-oz. roll	0	1	—
hard, all flavors, chocolate dipped	Bogdon's Reception Sticks	3.3	pcs	0	1	○
honey	Bit-O-Honey	0.4	oz.	0	1	○
jelly/jellied	Jujubes	0.4	oz.	0	1	○

FOOD ITEM	SPECIFICATIONS	BRAND NAME	QUANTITY	SIZE	PROTEIN BLOCKS	CARBOHYDRATE BLOCKS	FAT BLOCKS
	jelly/jellied	Jujyfruits	0.4	oz.	0	1	0
	jelly/jellied, spearmint leaves	Brach's	1.3	pcs.	0	1	0
	licorice	Pearson Nips	1.5	pcs.	0	1	0
	licorice	Twizzler Nibs	0.4	oz.	0	1	0
	licorice	Twizzlers	1.1	pcs.	0	1	0
	licorice, cherry	Twizzler Pull-n-Peel	0.4	pcs.	0	1	0
	licorice, cherry	Twizzler Nibs	0.4	pkg.	0	1	0
	licorice, strawberry	Twizzlers	1.1	pcs.	0	1	0
	licorice, candy coated	Good & Fruity	0.3	1.8-oz. box	0	1	0
	licorice, candy coated	Good & Plenty	0.4	oz.	0	1	0
	lollipop, all flavors	Astro Pops	0.3	pop	0	1	0
	lollipop, all flavors	Dum-Dums	0.5	pop	0	1	0
	lollipop, all flavors	Lifesavers	0.8	pop	0	1	0
	lollipop, all flavors	Save-A-Sucker/Suck An Egg	0.3	oz.	0	1	0
	lollipop, all flavors	Save-A-Sucker	0.3	oz.	0	1	0
	malted milk balls	Whoppers	0.4	oz.	0	1	1
		Mars	0.3	1.76-oz. bar	0	1	1
	marshmallow	Mars Fun Size	0.8	bar	0	1	0
	marshmallow	Funmallows	1.4	pcs.	0	1	0
	marshmallow, mini	Kraft Jet-Puffed	1.7	pcs.	0	1	0
	marshmallow, mini	Funmallows	0.2	cup	0	1	0
	marshmallow, peanut	Kraft	0.2	cup	0	1	0
		Spangler	1.3	pcs.	0	1	0
		Milky Way	0.2	2.15-oz. bar	0	1	1
		Milky Way Fun Size	0.6	bar	0	1	1
		Milky Way Dark	0.3	1.76-oz. bar	0	1	1
		Milky Way Fun Size Dark	0.6	.7-oz. bar	0	1	1
	mint	Lifesavers Cryst-O-Mint	3.3	pcs.	0	1	0
	mint	Pez Peppermint	15	pcs.	0	1	0
	mint, all flavors	Lifesavers	5	pcs.	0	1	0
	mint, all flavors except iced and vanilla	Breath Savers	5	pcs.	0	1	0
	mint, butter	Kraft	4.4	pcs.	0	1	0

Description	Brand	Amount	Unit			
mint, chocolate coated	After Eight	1.5	pcs.	0	1	1
mint, chocolate coated	Junior Mint	0.2	1.6-oz. bar	0	1	0
mint, chocolate coated	York Peppermint Pattie	0.3	1 1/2-oz. pc.	0	1	0
mint, chocolate coated	York Peppermint Pattie, Mini	0.8	pc.	0	1	0
mint, iced/vanilla	Breath Savers	5	pcs.	0	1	0
mint, party	Kraft	4.4	pcs.	0	1	0
	Nestle Turtles	1	pc.	0	1	1
nonpareils	Ghirardelli	0.4	oz.	0	1	1
nonpareils	Sno-Caps	0.5	oz.	0	1	1
nougat	Brach's	1	pc.	0	1	0
nougat bar, chocolate coated, chocolate	Charleston Chew	0.2	1.9-oz. bar	0	1	0
nougat bar, chocolate coated, strawberry	Charleston Chew	0.2	1.9-oz. bar	0	1	0
nougat bar, chocolate coated, vanilla	Charleston Chew	0.2	1.9-oz. bar	0	1	1
peanut	Oh Henry!	0.3	1.8-oz. bar	0	1	1
	100 Grand	0.5	1 1/2-oz. bar	0	1	1
	Pay Day	0.3	1.85-oz. bar	0	1	2
	Planters	0.5	1.6-oz. bar	0	1	2
peanut, chocolate coated	Goobers	0.7	oz.	0	1	1
peanut brittle	Kraft	0.4	oz.	0	1	1
peanut butter, chocolate	5th Avenue	0.2	2-oz. bar	0	1	1
peanut butter, chocolate, candy coated	Reese's Pieces	0.5	oz.	0	1	2
peanut butter, chocolate, w/cookie	Twix	0.7	oz.	0	1	2
peanut butter cup	Reese's	0.6	oz.	0	1	2
peanut butter cup	Reese's	1	pc.	0	1	2
peanut butter cup	Reese's Mini	2.2	pcs.	0	1	2
peanut butter parfait	Pearson Nips	1.7	pcs.	0	1	1
raisins, chocolate coated	Raisinets	0.5	oz.	0	1	1
raisins, yogurt coated, strawberry or vanilla	Del Monte	0.4	oz.	0	1	0
raisins, yogurt coated, vanilla	Del Monte	0.4	oz.	0	1	0
rock	Brach's	0.3	oz.	0	1	0

FOOD ITEM	SPECIFICATIONS	BRAND NAME	QUANTITY	SIZE	PROTEIN BLOCKS	CARBOHYDRATE BLOCKS	FAT BLOCKS
		Snickers	0.3	2.07-oz. bar	0	1	1
		Snickers Fun Size	0.8	bars	0	1	1
		Snickers Mini	1.7	pcs.	0	1	1
		Snickers Peanut Butter	0.3	2-oz. bar	0	1	2
		Snickers Munch	0.8	oz.	0	1	3
		3 Musketeers	0.2	2.13-oz. bar	0	1	1
		3 Musketeers Fun Size	0.7	bars	0	1	0
	toffee	Brach's Treasures	1.2	pcs.	0	1	0
	toffee bar	Heath	0.5	oz.	0	1	2
	toffee bar	Skor	0.5	oz.	0	1	2
		Tootsie Roll Midgets	1.4	pcs.	0	1	0
	wafer, chocolate coated	Kit Kat	0.3	1 1/2-oz. bar	0	1	1
		Whatchamacallit	0.3	1.7-oz. bar	0	1	1
Cane syrup			0.7	Tbsp.	0	1	0
Cantaloupe	pulp, cubed		0.7	cup	0	1	0
			0.2	of 5" melon	0	1	0
Cantaloupe cocktail		Snapple	2.2	fl. oz.	0	1	0
Cappuccino	iced	Jamaican Gold	3.4	fl. oz.	0	1	0
	iced, coffee	Maxwell House	3	fl. oz.	0	1	0
	iced, mocha	Maxwell House	2.7	fl. oz.	0	1	0
	iced, vanilla	Maxwell House	2.7	fl. oz.	0	1	0
Cappuccino bar	frozen	Frozfruit	0.5	bar	0	1	1
Caramel Dip		Marie's	0.8	Tbsp.	0	1	1
		Marie's Low Fat	0.6	Tbsp.	0	1	0
Caramel topping		Kraft	0.6	Tbsp.	0	1	0
		Smucker's Sundae	0.7	Tbsp.	0	1	0
	hot	Smucker's	0.6	Tbsp.	0	1	0
Caraway seed			8.3	tsp.	0	1	1
Carbonara sauce mix		Knorr	3.3	Tbsp.	1	1	2
Cardamom	ground	McCormick	12.5	tsp.	0	1	0
	seed	Tone's	10	tsp.	0	1	0
		Spice Island	10	tsp.	0	1	0
Cardoon	raw, shredded		1.7	cup	0	1	0

Food	Brand	Amount	Unit	P	C	F
Carob drink mix, powder		2.5	tsp.	0	1	0
Carob flour		0.2	cup	0	1	0
Carrot, fresh, raw, whole		1.7	7 1/2" long, 2.8 oz.	0	1	0
raw, shredded	Dole	1.3	cup	0	1	0
raw, shredded		3.3	oz.	0	1	0
raw, baby		10	medium	0	1	0
raw, mini	Frieda's	3.3	oz.	0	1	0
raw, mini, peeled	Dole	3.3	oz.	0	1	0
boiled, drained, sliced		0.8	cup	0	1	0
Carrot, canned, all varieties	S&W	1.3	cup	0	1	0
baby, whole	Green Giant LeSueur	0.8	cup	0	1	0
whole or sliced	Stokely	15	oz.	0	1	0
sliced, w/liquid		0.8	cup	0	1	0
sliced, drained		1.7	cup	0	1	0
sliced	Allens/Crest Top	0.8	cup	0	1	0
sliced	Del Monte	0.8	cup	0	1	0
sliced	Goya	1.3	cup	0	1	0
sliced	Green Giant	1.3	cup	0	1	0
sliced	Stokely No Salt	1.7	cup	0	1	0
Carrot, frozen, boiled, drained, sliced		1.3	cup	0	1	0
baby, whole	Stilwell	1.7	cup	0	1	0
baby cut	Green Giant	1.9	cup	0	1	0
baby cut	Green Giant Harvest Fresh	2.2	cup	0	1	0
crinkle	Stilwell	1.7	cup	0	1	0
Carrot juice, canned		3.5	fl. oz.	0	1	0
Casaba		0.1	of 7 3/4" melon	0	1	0
pulp, cubed		1	cup	0	1	0
Cassava, see also Yuca		1.3	oz.	0	1	0
Cauliflower, fresh, raw		15	florets	1	1	1
raw		5	cup, 1" pcs.	1	1	1
raw, florets	Dole	150	oz.	10	1	10
boiled, drained		5	cup, 1" pcs.	1	1	1
green, raw		0.7	head	1	1	1
green, raw	Dole	0.3	head	1	1	1
green, raw		2.5	cup, 1" pcs.	1	8	1

FOOD ITEM	SPECIFICATIONS	BRAND NAME	QUANTITY	SIZE	PROTEIN BLOCKS	CARBOHYDRATE BLOCKS	FAT BLOCKS
Cauliflower, frozen	green, boiled, drained		2.5	cup, 1" pcs.	1	1	1
	boiled, drained		2.5	cup, 1" pcs.	1	1	1
	florets	Stilwell	10	cup	2	1	0
	in cheese sauce	Green Giant	5	cup	1	1	0
Cauliflower, pickled	sweet	Vlasic	0.7	cup	0	1	1
Cactus	marinated	Goya Napolitos	1	oz.	0	1	0
Cavatelli	frozen	Celentano	30	pcs.	1	1	0
Celeriac	trimmed		0.4	oz.	0	1	0
	trimmed		3.6	oz.	0	1	0
	raw		0.8	cup	0	1	0
Celery	raw		10	7 1/2"-stalk / 1.6 oz.	0	1	0
	raw, diced		5	cup	1	1	0
	boiled, drained, diced		2.5	cup	1	1	0
Celery, dried	flakes or seeds	Tone's	10	tsp.	0	1	2
Cereal, ready-to-eat	amaranth flakes	Arrowhead Mills	0.5	cup	0	1	0
	bran (see also oat bran below)	Kellogg's All-Bran	0.4	cup	1	1	0
	bran	Kellogg's All-Bran Extra Fiber	0.6	cup	0	1	0
	bran	Kellogg's Bran Buds	0.2	cup	0	1	0
	bran	Kellogg's Frosted Bran	0.3	cup	0	1	0
	bran	Kellogg's Fruitful Bran	0.3	cup	0	1	0
	bran	Post Bran'nola	0.1	cup	0	1	0
	bran	Nabisco 100% Bran	0.2	cup	0	1	0
	bran	Quaker Crunchy	0.4	cup	0	1	0
	bran flakes	Arrowhead Mills	0.5	cup	0	1	0
	bran flakes	Kellogg's Complete	0.3	cup	0	1	0
	bran flakes	Malt-O-Meal	0.4	cup	0	1	0
	bran flakes	New Morning Multi-Bran	0.6	cup	0	1	0
	bran flakes	Post	0.4	cup	0	1	0
	bran, raisin	Kellogg's	0.3	cup	0	1	0
	bran, raisin	Malt-O-Meal	0.3	cup	0	1	0
	bran, raisin	New Morning Multi-Bran	0.6	cup	0	1	0
	bran, raisin	Post	0.2	cup	0	1	0

Food		Amount	Unit			
bran, raisin	Post Bran'nola	0.1	cup	0	1	0
corn	Arrowhead Mills Maple Corns	0.2	cup	0	1	0
corn	Barbara's Frosted Funnies	0.4	cup	0	1	0
corn	Barbara's Puffins	0.4	cup	0	1	0
corn	Cocoa Comets	0.3	cup	0	1	0
corn	Corn Bursts	0.3	cup	0	1	0
corn	Kellogg's Corn Pops	0.3	cup	0	1	0
corn	Nut & Honey Crunch	0.3	cup	0	1	0
corn	Perky's Nutty Rice	0.2	cup	0	1	0
corn	Post Toasties	0.4	cup	0	1	0
corn, almond raisin	New Morning Crunchy	0.4	cup	0	1	0
corn, flakes	Arrowhead Mills	0.3	cup	0	1	0
corn, flakes	Barbara's	0.4	cup	0	1	0
corn, flakes	Kellogg's Corn Flakes	0.4	cup	0	1	0
corn, flakes	Kellogg's Frosted Flakes	0.2	cup	0	1	0
corn, flakes	Malt-O-Meal	0.4	cup	0	1	0
corn, flakes	Malt-O-Meal Frosted	0.3	cup	0	1	0
corn, flakes	New Morning	0.4	cup	0	1	0
corn, flakes	New Morning	0.2	cup	0	1	0
corn, flakes, honey	Kellogg's Temptations	0.4	cup	0	1	0
corn, honey roasted pecan	Arrowhead Mills	0.6	cup	0	1	0
corn, puffed	Health Valley	0.5	cup	0	1	0
corn, puffed, honey	Kellogg's Mini Buns	0.3	cup	0	1	0
corn and oat, cinnamon	Kellogg's Temptations	0.3	cup	0	1	0
corn and oat, vanilla almond	Kellogg's Crispix	0.4	cup	0	1	0
corn and rice	Kellogg's Double Dip Crunch	0.3	cup	0	1	0
corn and rice	C.W. Post Hearty	0.1	cup	0	1	0
granola	Heartland	0.1	cup	1	1	0
granola	Heartland Lowfat	0.1	cup	1	1	0
granola	Kellogg's Lowfat	0.1	cup	0	1	0
granola	New Morning Oatiola	0.2	cup	0	1	0
granola, almond	Sun Country	0.1	cup	1	1	0
granola, blueberries, milk	Mountain House	0.2	cup	1	1	0
granola, carob cashew	Roman Meal	0.1	cup	0	1	0
granola, figs and filberts	Roman Meal	0.1	cup	0	1	0
granola, honey nut	Roman Meal	0.1	cup	0	1	0

FOOD ITEM	SPECIFICATIONS	BRAND NAME	QUANTITY	SIZE	PROTEIN BLOCKS	CARBOHYDRATE BLOCKS	FAT BLOCKS
	granola, raisin	Heartland	0.1	cup	0	1	1
	granola, raisin	Kellogg's Low Fat	0.2	cup	0	1	0
	granola, raisin and date	Sun Country	0.1	cup	0	1	1
	granola, raisin nut	Roman Meal	0.1	cup	0	1	0
	kamut	New Morning Kamutios	0.4	cup	0	1	0
	kamut, flakes	Arrowhead Mills	0.4	cup	0	1	0
	kamut, puffed	Arrowhead Mills	0.5	cup	0	1	0
	millet, puffed	Arrowhead Mills	0.5	cup	0	1	0
	mixed/multigrain	Apple Jacks	0.3	cup	0	1	0
	mixed/multigrain	Arrowhead Mills Crispy Puffs	0.6	cup	0	1	0
	mixed/multigrain	Barbara's Shredded Spoonsfuls	0.4	cup	0	1	0
	mixed/multigrain	Barbara's High 5	0.4	cup	0	1	0
	mixed/multigrain	Froot Loops	0.4	cup	0	1	0
	mixed/multigrain	Fruiteo's	0.4	cup	0	1	0
	mixed/multigrain	Grape-Nuts	0.1	cup	0	1	0
	mixed/multigrain	Grape-Nuts Flakes	0.3	cup	0	1	0
	mixed/multigrain	Just Right Crunchy Nuggets	0.2	cup	0	1	0
	mixed/multigrain	Kellogg's Mueslix Crispy	0.2	cup	0	1	0
	mixed/multigrain	Kellogg's Mueslix Golden Cru ch	0.2	cup	0	1	0
	mixed/multigrain	Product 19	0.4	cup	0	1	0
	mixed/multigrain	Team Flakes	0.2	cup	0	1	0
	mixed/multigrain	Tootie Fruities	0.3	cup	0	1	0
	mixed/multigrain, all varieties	Granola O's	0.3	cup	0	1	0
	mixed/multigrain, all varieties	Health Valley Honey Clusters & Flakes	0.3	cup	0	1	0
	mixed/multigrain, brown sugar cinnamon	Pop Tarts Crunch	0.3	cup	0	1	0
	mixed/multigrain, cocoa	Startoons	0.4	cup	0	1	0
	mixed/multigrain, dates, raisins, walnuts	Fruit & Fibre	0.2	cup	0	1	0
	mixed/multigrain, honey	Startoons	0.4	cup	0	1	0
	mixed/multigrain, flakes	Arrowhead Mills	0.3	cup	0	1	0
	mixed/multigrain, flakes	Healthy Choice	0.4	cup	0	1	0
	mixed/multigrain, fruit nut	Just Right	0.2	cup	0	1	0

mixed/multigrain, peaches, raisins, almonds	Fruit & Fibre	0.2	cup	0	1	0
mixed/multigrain, pecan	Great Grains	0.2	cup	0	1	1
mixed/multigrain, raisin, dates, pecans	Great Grains	0.2	cup	0	1	0
mixed/multigrain, raisins, oats, almonds	Healthy Choice	0.2	cup	0	1	0
mixed/multigrain, squares	Healthy Choice	0.3	cup	0	1	0
mixed/multigrain, strawberry	Pop Tarts Crunch	0.3	cup	0	1	0
oat	Alpha-Bits	0.3	cup	0	1	0
oat	Arrowhead Mills Nature O's	0.4	cup	0	1	0
oat	Barbara's Breakfast O's	0.5	cup	0	1	0
oat	Cheerios	0.5	cup	0	1	0
oat	Honey Bunches of Oats	0.3	cup	0	1	0
oat	Kellogg's Nut & Honey Crunch	0.3	cup	0	1	0
oat	New Morning Oatios Original	0.5	cup	0	1	0
oat	Quaker Squares	0.2	cup	0	1	0
oat	Toasty O's	0.5	cup	0	1	0
oat, almonds	Honey Bunches of Oats	0.3	cup	0	1	0
oat, apple cinnamon	New Morning Oatios	0.6	cup	0	1	0
oat, apple cinnamon	Toasty O's	0.3	cup	0	1	0
oat, blueberry	New Morning Oatiola	0.2	cup	0	1	0
oat, cinnamon	Quaker Life	0.3	cup	0	1	0
oat, cocoa	New Morning Oatios	0.3	cup	0	1	0
oat and honey	Quaker 100% Natural	0.3	cup	0	1	1
oat, honey almond	New Morning Oatios	0.5	cup	0	1	0
oat, honey graham	Quaker Ohls	0.4	cup	0	1	0
oat, honey nut	Toasty O's	0.4	cup	0	1	0
oat, honey, raisins	Quaker 100% Natural	0.3	cup	0	1	1
oat, marshmallow	Alpha-Bits	0.4	cup	0	1	0
oat, marshmallow	Mateys	0.4	cup	0	1	0
oat bran	Common Sense	0.4	cup	0	1	0
oat bran	Cracklin' Oat Bran	0.2	cup	0	1	1
oat bran	New Morning Ultimate Oat Bran	0.6	cup	0	1	0
oat bran	Quaker	0.3	cup	0	1	0
oat bran, flakes	Arrowhead Mills	0.5	cup	0	1	0

FOOD ITEM	SPECIFICATIONS	BRAND NAME	QUANTITY	SIZE	PROTEIN BLOCKS	CARBOHYDRATE BLOCKS	FAT BLOCKS
	rice	Apple Cinnamon Rice Krispies	0.3	cup	0	1	0
	rice	Cocoa Krispies	0.3	cup	0	1	0
	rice	Frosted Krispies	0.3	cup	0	1	0
	rice	Fruity Marshmallow Krispies	0.3	cup	0	1	0
	rice	Perky's Nutty Rice	0.2	cup	0	1	0
	rice	Rice Krispies	0.4	cup	0	1	0
	rice	Rice Krispies Treats	0.3	cup	0	1	0
	rice	Special K	0.5	cup	0	1	0
	rice, crispy	Malt-O-Meal	0.3	cup	0	1	0
	rice, puffed	Arrowhead Mills	0.5	cup	0	1	0
	rice, puffed	Malt-O-Meal	0.7	cup	0	1	0
	rice, brown, crisp	Barbara's	0.4	cup	0	1	0
	rice, brown, crisp	Health Valley	0.3	cup	0	1	0
	rice, brown, crisp	New Morning	0.4	cup	0	1	0
	rice, brown, crisp, frosted	New Morning	0.2	cup	0	1	0
	rice and corn, almond raisin	Nutri-Grain	0.3	cup	0	1	0
	rice and rye	Kellogg's Apple Raisin Crisp	0.2	cup	0	1	0
	spelt flakes	Arrowhead Mills	0.5	cup	0	1	0
	wheat	Golden Puffs	0.3	cup	0	1	0
	wheat	Kellogg's Apple Cinnamon/ Blueberry Squares	0.2	cup	0	1	0
	wheat	Kellogg's Frosted Mini-Wheats	0.2	cup	0	1	0
	wheat	Kellogg's Raisin Squares	0.2	cup	0	1	0
	wheat	Kellogg's Smacks	0.3	cup	0	1	0
	wheat	Kellogg's Strawberry Squares	0.2	cup	0	1	0
	wheat	Nabisco Frosted Wheat Bites	0.2	cup	0	1	0
	wheat	Nutri-Grain Golden	0.3	cup	0	1	0
	wheat, blueberry or strawberry	Nabisco Wheat Bites	0.2	cup	0	1	0
	wheat, honey grahams	New Morning	0.8	pcs.	0	1	0
	wheat, puffed	Arrowhead Mills	0.5	cup	0	1	0
	wheat, puffed	Malt-O-Meal	0.9	cup	0	1	0
	wheat, raisin	Nutri-Grain Golden	0.3	cup	0	1	0

Food	Brand	Amount	Unit			
wheat, raspberry	Nabisco Wheat Bites	0.2	cup	0	1	0
wheat, shredded	Barbara's	0.7	pcs.	0	1	0
wheat, shredded	Nabisco	0.5	pcs.	0	1	0
wheat, shredded	Nabisco Shredded Wheat 'n Bran	0.2	cups	0	1	0
wheat, shredded	Nabisco Spoon Size	0.3	cup	0	1	0
wheat, shredded	Quaker	0.6	pcs.	0	1	0
wheat and barley	Perky's Nutty Wheat & Barley	0.2	cup	0	1	0
barley	Arrowhead Mills Bits O Barley	0.4	cup	0	1	0
mixed/multigrain	Mothers	0.2	cup	0	1	0
	Pritkin	0.3	pkt.	0	1	0
Cereal, cooking, hot						
4 Grain, w/flax	Roman Meal	0.5	pkt.	0	1	0
7 grain	Roman Meal Instant	0.5	pkt.	0	1	0
7 grain	Arrowhead Mills	0.1	cup	0	1	0
apple cinnamon	Arrowhead Mills	0.2	cup	0	1	0
apple cinnamon	Arrowhead Mills Wheat Free	0.1	cup	0	1	0
raisin date-nut	Roman Meal	0.5	pkt.	0	1	0
raisin date-nut	Roman Meal Instant	0.4	pkt.	0	1	0
oat bran	Roman Meal	0.4	pkt.	0	1	0
oat bran	Roman Meal Instant	0.4	pkt.	0	1	0
oat flakes, raisin and spice	Mothers	0.3	cup	0	1	0
oatmeal, instant	Quaker	0.3	cup	0	1	0
oatmeal, instant	H-O Instant	0.3	pkt.	1	1	0
oatmeal, instant	Arrowhead Mills	0.5	pkt.	1	1	0
oatmeal, instant	H-O	0.2	cup	0	1	0
oatmeal, instant	Maypo	0.1	cup	0	1	0
oatmeal, instant	Mothers	0.2	cup	0	1	0
oatmeal, instant	Quaker	0.5	pkt.	0	1	0
oatmeal, instant	Roman Meal Premium	0.3	pkt.	0	1	0
oatmeal, instant w/ apples and cinnamon	Quaker	0.4	pkt.	0	1	0
oatmeal, instant apple, raisin, and walnut	Quaker	0.4	pkt.	0	1	0
oatmeal, instant cinnamon, raisin, almond	Arrowhead Mills	0.4	pkt.	0	1	0
oatmeal, instant cinnamon spice	Quaker	0.3	pkt.	0	1	0

FOOD ITEM	SPECIFICATIONS	BRAND NAME	QUANTITY	SIZE	PROTEIN BLOCKS	CARBOHYDRATE BLOCKS	FAT BLOCKS
	oatmeal, instant cinnamon toast	Quaker	0.4	pkt.	0	1	0
	oatmeal, instant fruit and cream	Quaker	0.4	pkt.	0	1	0
	oatmeal, instant honey nut	Quaker	0.4	pkt.	0	1	0
	oatmeal, instant maple	Maypo	0.1	cup	0	1	0
	oatmeal, instant maple, apple, spice	Arrowhead Mills	0.4	pkt.	0	1	0
	oatmeal, instant maple, brown sugar	Quaker	0.3	pkt.	0	1	0
	oatmeal, instant peaches and cream	Quaker	0.4	pkt.	0	1	0
	oatmeal, instant raisin, date, walnut	Quaker	0.4	pkt.	0	1	0
	oatmeal, instant raisin spice	Quaker	0.3	pkt.	0	1	0
	oatmeal, instant raspberry	Quaker	0.3	pkt.	0	1	0
	oatmeal, instant strawberries and cream	Quaker	0.4	pkt.	0	1	0
	oatmeal, instant strawberries 'n stuff	Quaker	0.3	pkt.	0	1	0
	oats	H-O Quick	0.2	cup	0	1	0
	oats	H-O Quick Oats 'n Fiber	0.6	pkt.	0	1	0
	oats, cinnamon graham	Quaker Instant	0.3	pkt.	0	1	0
	oats, rolled	H-O Instant	0.6	pkt.	0	1	0
	oats, rolled	H-O Sweet & Mellow Instant	0.3	pkt.	0	1	0
	oats, rolled	Quaker Quick/Old Fashioned	0.2	cup	0	1	0
	oats, rolled, banana creme	H-O Explo Instant	0.3	pkt.	0	1	0
	oats, rolled, almond raisin	H-O Explo Instant	0.3	pkt.	0	1	0
	oats, rolled, apple and cinnamon	H-O Instant	0.4	pkt.	0	1	0
	oats, rolled, apple maple spice	H-O Explo Instant	0.3	pkt.	0	1	0
	oats, rolled, apricot honey	H-O Explo Instant	0.3	pkt.	0	1	0
	oats, rolled, maple and brown sugar	H-O Instant	0.3	pkt.	0	1	0

CARBOHYDRATES

Food	Brand	Amount	Unit	Protein	Carb	Fat
oats, toasted	H-O Old Fashioned	0.1	cup	0	1	0
rice	Lundberg Amber	0.2	pkt.	0	1	0
rice	Lundberg Organic Hot 'n Creamy	0.1	cup	0	1	0
rice	Arrowhead Mills Rice and Shine	0.1	cup	0	1	0
rice, almond, sweet	Lundberg Hot 'n Creamy	0.1	cup	0	1	0
rice, cinnamon raisin	Lundberg Hot 'n Creamy	0.1	cup	0	1	0
rye, cream of	Roman Meal	0.5	pkt.	0	1	0
rye, cream of	Roman Meal Instant	0.5	pkt.	0	1	0
wheat	Arrowhead Mills Bear Mush	0.1	cup	0	1	0
wheat	Malt-O-Meal Quick	1.1	Tbsp.	0	1	0
wheat	Mothers	0.2	cup	0	1	0
wheat	Wheatena	0.1	cup	0	1	0
wheat, all varieties	Malt-O-Meal	1	Tbsp.	0	1	0
wheat 'n berries	Fantastic Cup	0.4	oz.	0	1	0
wheat, cracked	Arrowhead Mills	0.1	cup	0	1	0
wheat, farina	H-O	1.1	Tbsp.	0	1	0
wheat free, apple cinnamon	Fantastic Cup	0.4	oz.	0	1	0
wheat free, banana nut	Fantastic Cup	0.5	oz.	0	1	0
wheat free, cranberry orange	Fantastic Cup	0.4	oz.	0	1	0
Chayote — raw		2	medium	0	1	0
raw		2.5	cup, 1" pcs.	0	1	0
raw	Frieda's	4.4	oz.	0	1	0
boiled, drained		1	cup, 1" pcs.	0	1	0
Cheese pastry — see Danish						
Cheese stick		5	3/4-oz. slice	2	1	2
Cherry — w/cornmeal coating	Goya Surullitos	1.5	pcs.	1	1	1
fresh, sour, red w/pits		0.8	cup	0	1	0
fresh, sour, red pitted		0.6	cup	0	1	0
fresh, sweet, w/pits		0.5	cup	0	1	0
fresh, sweet		9.1	medium	0	1	0
canned, sour, pitted, red, water	Lucky Leaf/Musselman's	0.4	cup	0	1	0
canned, sour, pitted, heavy syrup		0.2	cup	0	1	0
canned, sweet, pitted, heavy syrup		0.2	cup	0	1	0
canned, sweet, pitted, dark	Del Monte	0.2	cup	0	1	0

FOOD ITEM	SPECIFICATIONS	BRAND NAME	QUANTITY	SIZE	PROTEIN BLOCKS	CARBOHYDRATE BLOCKS	FAT BLOCKS
	canned, sweet, pitted, dark	S&W	0.1	cup	0	1	0
	canned, sweet, pitted, light	S&W Royal Anne	0.1	cup	0	1	0
	dried, pitted	Sonoma	0.1	cup	0	1	0
	frozen, unsweetened, dark, sweet	Big Valley	0.4	cup	0	1	0
	frozen, unsweetened, tart, red	Stilwell	0.8	cup	0	1	0
Cherry, candied	frozen, sweetened	Paradise/White Swan	1.5	oz.	0	1	0
	green or red	S&W Glace	2.5	.2-oz. pcs.	0	1	0
	green or red	Paradise/White Swan	2.3	pcs.	0	1	0
	green or red, and pineapple mix w/liquid	Paradise/White Swan	0.6	Tbsp.	0	1	0
Cherry, maraschino	green or red	Haddon House	1.1	oz.	0	1	0
	green or red	S&W	5	pcs.	0	1	0
Cherry drink		After the Fall Very Cherry	3.3	pcs.	0	1	0
		Farmer's Market	2.8	fl. oz.	0	1	0
		Hi-C	2.4	fl. oz.	0	1	0
		Tree Top Not Plain Cherry	2.1	fl. oz.	0	1	0
	blend	Capri Sun	2.4	fl. oz.	0	1	0
	wild	Hi-C	1.6	fl. oz.	0	1	0
Cherry drink mix, prepared		Kool-Aid	2.8	fl. oz.	0	1	0
Cherry juice		Juicy Juice	2.9	fl. oz.	0	1	0
	black	Heinke's	2.2	fl. oz.	0	1	0
	black	R.W. Knudsen	1.7	fl. oz.	0	1	0
Cherry juice blends		Apple & Eve Nothin' But Juice	1.7	fl. oz.	0	1	0
		Dole Mountain	2.5	fl. oz.	0	1	0
		Verfine Juice-Ups	2.4	fl. oz.	0	1	0
		R.W. Knudsen Concentrate	2.2	fl. oz.	0	1	0
	black	Heinke's	3.1	fl. oz.	0	1	0
	cider	R.W. Knudsen	2.6	fl. oz.	0	1	0
Cherry nectar	cider	Santa Cruz	2.2	fl. oz.	0	1	0
			2.8	fl. oz.	0	1	0

Food	Description	Brand	Amount	Unit	Protein	Fat	Carbohydrate
Cherry pastry	dumpling, frozen	Pepperidge Farm	0.2	pc.	0	1	1
Cherry pastry	pocket	Tastykake	1.7	fl. oz.	0	1	1
Cherry syrup	black	Fox's No Cal	0.9	Tbsp.	0	0	1
Cherries julibee		Lucky Leaf/Musselman's	0.1	cup	0	0	1
Chestnut, Chinese	shelled, dried		0.4	oz.	0	0	1
	shelled, boiled or steamed		0.9	oz.	0	0	1
	shelled, roasted		0.6	oz.	0	0	1
Chestnut, European	raw, in shell		0.1	lb.	0	0	1
	raw, shelled, w/peel		0.2	cup	0	0	1
	dried, peeled		0.4	oz.	0	0	1
	boiled		1.1	oz.	0	0	1
	roasted, peeled		0.8	cup	0	0	1
Chestnut, Japanese	roasted, peeled		0.2	oz.	0	0	1
	dried		0.4	oz.	0	0	1
	boiled or steamed		2.5	oz.	0	0	2
	roasted		0.7	oz.	0	0	1
Chicken gravy	cream of	Franco-American	0.8	cup	0	1	1
	giblet	Heinz Home Style	0.8	cup	1	1	1
	golden, with chicken	Pepperidge Farm	0.8	cup	1	1	1
		Franco-American	0.8	cup	1	1	1
	rotisserie	Pepperidge Farm Rotissore	0.8	cup	1	1	1
Chicken Gravy mix		Durkee	0.6	cup, prepared	0	0	1
		French's	0.6	cup, prepared	0	0	1
		McCormick	0.6	cup, prepared	0	0	1
		Pillsbury w/Water	0.8	cup, prepared	0	0	1
		Pillsbury w/Water and Skim Milk	0.6	cup, prepared	1	1	1
		Weight Watchers	2.5	cup, prepared	0	0	1
	roasted	Knorr	0.8	cup, prepared	1	0	1
Chicken sauce	vegetarian	Loma Linda Gravy Quick	0.8	cup, prepared	0	0	1
	barbeque flavor	Hunt's Chicken Sensations	3.3	Tbsp.	0	0	1
	Caesar	Lawry's	3.3	Tbsp.	0	0	1
	lemon herb	Hunt's Chicken Sensations	5	Tbsp.	0	0	1
	sherried	Lawry's	1.7	Tbsp.	0	0	1
	Southwestern	Hunt's Chicken Sensations	10	Tbsp.	0	0	1
	Thai; satay	Lawry's	2.5	Tbsp.	0	0	1

FOOD ITEM	SPECIFICATIONS	BRAND NAME	QUANTITY	SIZE	PROTEIN BLOCKS	CARBOHYDRATE BLOCKS	FAT BLOCKS
	wing, hot	Nance's	6.7	Tbsp.	0	1	0
	wing, mild	Nance's	6.7	Tbsp.	0	1	0
Chicken seasoning and coating mix		Durkee/French's Roasting Bag	0.4	pkg.	0	1	0
		McCormick Bag 'n Season	2.5	Tbsp.	0	1	0
	barbeque	Shake'n Bake Original	0.2	pkg.	0	1	0
	barbeque glaze	Durkee Roasting Bag	0.2	pkg.	0	1	0
	Buffalo wing, cajun	Shake 'n Bake	0.1	pkg.	0	1	0
	Buffalo wing, garlic and herb	Durkee	0.4	pkg.	0	1	0
	Buffalo wing, hot or screaming hot	Durkee	0.4	pkg.	0	1	0
	Buffalo wing, mild	Durkee	0.4	pkg.	0	1	1
	caccaitore	Durkee Easy	0.4	pkg.	0	1	1
	coq au vin	Knorr Recipe	0.3	pkg.	0	1	0
	country	Durkee Roasting Bag	1.7	Tbsp.	0	1	1
	country	McCormick Bag 'n Season	0.3	pkg.	0	1	1
	Dijonne	Knorr Recipe	6.7	tsp.	0	1	1
	extra crispy	Oven Fry	0.3	pkg.	0	1	1
	homestyle flour	Oven Fry	0.1	pkg.	0	1	0
	hot and spicy	Shake 'n Bake	0.2	pkg.	0	1	0
	hot, spicy	McCormick Bag 'n Season	0.2	pkg.	0	1	0
	Mexican salsa	Durkee Easy	1.7	Tbsp.	0	1	0
	mushroon	Durkee Easy	0.3	pkg.	0	1	0
	Southwest, marinade	Lawry's	0.7	pkg.	0	1	0
	sweet and sour	Durkee Easy	10	tsp.	0	1	0
Chickpea flour		Durkee Easy	0.2	pkg.	0	1	0
Chickpeas	dry	Arrowhead Mills	0.1	cup	0	1	0
	dry, boiled	Arrowhead Mills	0.2	cup	0	1	0
	canned, w/liquid		0.2	cup	0	1	0
	canned	Allens/East Texas	0.2	cup	0	1	0
	canned	Eden Organic	0.4	cup	0	1	1
	canned	Eden Organic Jars	0.4	cup	0	1	0
	canned	Goya	0.3	cup	0	1	0
			0.4	cup	0	1	1

Food	Variety	Brand	Amount	Unit			
Chicory greens	canned	Green Giant/Joan of Ark	0.4	cup	0	1	0
	canned	Old El Paso	0.4	cup	1	1	0
	canned	Progresso	0.4	cup	1	1	0
	canned	Stokely	0.4	cup	0	1	1
	canned, in tomato sauce	Goya Guisados	0.4	cup	0	1	0
Chicory, witloof	trimmed		50	oz.	2	1	3
			10	5-7" head 2.1 oz.	1	1	2
	chopped, 1/2 cup		5	cup	0	1	1
			12.5	cup	0	1	1
Chili, mix	all varieties	Health Valley Chili in a Cup	0.2	cup	0	1	0
	4 bean	Knorr Cup	0.2	pkg.	0	1	0
	3 bean	Spice Island Quick Meal	0.4	pkg.	0	1	0
	vegetarian	Spice Island Quick Meal	0.4	pkg.	0	1	0
Chili base, canned		Hunt's Homestyle Fixings	0.4	cup	0	1	1
	black bean	S&W Chili Makin's	0.3	cup	1	1	0
	homestyle	S&W Chili Makin's	0.4	cup	0	1	0
	Santa Fe	S&W Chili Makin's	0.4	cup	0	1	1
		S&W Chili Makin's	0.4	cup	0	1	0
Chili beans, canned		Gebhardt	0.2	cup	0	1	0
		Hunt's	0.4	cup	0	1	1
		S&W	0.3	cup	0	1	0
		Stokely	0.3	cup	0	1	0
		Sun-Vista	0.3	cup	0	1	1
	hot	Van Camp's Mexican	0.4	cup	1	1	0
	spicy	S&W Chipotle	0.3	cup	0	1	0
	zesty	Green Giant/Joan of Arc	0.3	cup	0	1	1
		Campbell's	0.3	cup	1	1	0
Chili dip	green	La Victoria	10	Tbsp.	0	1	0
	caliente	Knorr	5	tsp.	0	1	0
Chili dip mix			5	Tbsp.	0	1	1
Chili Powder			10	tsp.	2	1	0
Chili sauce		Del Monte	1.7	Tbsp.	1	1	0
		Las Palmas	2.5	cup	0	1	0
		Nance's	3.3	Tbsp.	2	1	0
		S&W Steakhouse	2.5	Tbsp.	0	1	0
	hot dog	Gebhardt	0.6	cup	0	1	1

FOOD ITEM	SPECIFICATIONS	BRAND NAME	QUANTITY	SIZE	PROTEIN BLOCKS	CARBOHYDRATE BLOCKS	FAT BLOCKS
	hot dog	Just Rite	6.7	oz.	1	1	3
	hot dog	Wolf	5	Tbsp.	1	1	2
	hot dog, w/beef	Stenger	0.4	cup	0	1	2
Chili seasoning mix		Durkee	0.3	pkg.	0	1	0
		Durkee Pot-O	0.2	pkg.	0	1	0
		Gebhardt Chili Quick	3.3	Tbsp.	0	1	0
		Lawry's	1.7	Tbsp.	0	1	0
		Lawry's Tex-Mex	3.3	Tbsp.	0	1	1
		McCormick	13.3	tsp. approx.	0	1	0
		Mick Fowler's 2-Alarm Kit	2.7	Tbsp.	0	1	0
		Mick Fowler's 2-Alarm Family	2	Tbsp.	0	1	1
		Old El Paso	3.3	Tbsp.	0	1	1
	mild	Durkee	0.3	pkg.	0	1	0
	Texas red	Durkee	1.7	pkg.	1	1	2
Chives	fresh		33.3	oz.	3	1	2
	canned, fudge, mocha or raspberry truffle	Sweet Success	2.8	fl. oz.	0	1	2
	canned, regular or malt	Sego	2	fl. oz.	0	1	0
	canned, regular or Dutch	Sego Lite	4.3	fl. oz.	1	1	0
	canned, rich almond or creamy milk	Sweet Success	2.8	fl. oz.	0	1	0
	refrigerated, creamy milk or almond	Sweet Success	2.8	fl. oz.	0	1	0
	refrigerated, fudge	Sweet Success	2.8	fl. oz.	0	1	0
Chocolate, baking		Choco Bake	2.5	oz.	1	1	14
Chocolate, baking bar	bittersweet	Ghirardelli	1.2	squares	0	1	2
	milk	Ghirardelli	1.1	squares	0	1	2
	milk	Ghirardelli	0.5	oz.	0	1	1
	semisweet	Baker's	0.5	oz.	0	1	2
	semisweet	Ghirardelli	1.1	squares	0	1	2
	semisweet	Nestle	0.6	oz.	0	1	2
	sweet	Baker's German	0.6	oz.	0	1	2
	sweet, dark	Ghirardelli	1	squares	0	1	2

Food	Description	Brand	Amount	Unit	Protein	Carbohydrate	Fat
Chocolate, chips or morsels	unsweetened	Baker's	1.7	oz.	1	1	8
	unsweetened	Ghirardelli	2.5	squares	0	1	6
	unsweetened	Nestle	2.5	oz.	1	1	12
	white	Baker's	0.5	oz.	0	1	2
	white	Ghirardelli	1.1	squares	0	1	2
	white	Ghirardelli Flickettes	0.6	oz.	0	1	2
	milk	Baker's	0.5	oz.	0	1	1
	milk	Ghirardelli	3	squares	0	1	1
	milk	Hershey's Bake Shoppe	2.7	squares	1	1	1
	milk	M&M's	3	squares	0	1	2
	milk	Nestle	2.7	squares	0	1	1
	mint	Nestle	2.7	squares	0	1	1
	raspberry	Hershey's Bake Shoppe	3.8	squares	0	1	2
	semisweet	Ghirardelli	2.7	squares	0	1	1
	semisweet	Hershey's Bake Shoppe	2.7	squares	0	1	1
	white	Ghirardelli	2.7	squares	0	1	1
	white	Hershey's Bake Shoppe	3	squares	0	1	1
Chocolate, semisweet		Baker's Real	0.5	oz.	0	1	1
		M&M's	0.6	oz.	1	1	1
	flavor	Baker's	0.5	oz.	0	1	2
	plain or mint	Nestle	0.6	oz.	0	1	0
Chocolate drink	bottled	Yoo-Hoo	2.4	fl. oz.	0	1	0
Chocolate flavor drink	canned	Yoo-Hoo	2.5	fl. oz.	0	1	0
	canned	Sego Lite	4.3	fl. oz.	1	1	0
	canned, creamy milk	Nestle Instant Breakfast	2.5	fl. oz.	0	1	0
Chocolate flavor drink mix	canned, creamy milk	Nestle Quick	1	Tbsp.	0	1	0
	almond, creamy milk, fudge, or mocha	Nestle Quick No Sugar	3.3	Tbsp.	0	1	0
	chocolate chip	Pillsbury Instant Breakfast	0.3	pkt.	0	1	1
	creamy milk	Sweet Success	0.7	pkt.	1	1	0
	creamy milk or malt	Sweet Success	0.7	pkt.	0	1	0
	malt, classic	Sweet Success	0.3	pkt.	0	1	0
		Carnation Instant Breakfast No Sugar	0.8	pkt.	1	1	1
		Carnation Instant Breakfast	0.3	pkt.	0	1	0

FOOD ITEM	SPECIFICATIONS	BRAND NAME	QUANTITY	SIZE	PROTEIN BLOCKS	CARBOHYDRATE BLOCKS	FAT BLOCKS
	raspberry truffle	Sweet Success	0.7	pkt.	1	1	0
	shake	Weight Watchers	0.9	pkt.	1	1	0
Chocolate milk	lowfat	Nestle Quick	0.3	cup	0	1	1
	lowfat	Hershey's	0.3	cup	0	1	0
	lowfat	Nestle Quick	0.3	cup	0	1	1
		Nestle Quick	2.4	fl. oz.	0	1	1
Chocolate pastry	dark	Pepperidge Farm Clouds	0.4	pcs.	0	1	2
	milk	Pepperidge Farm Clouds	0.4	pcs.	0	1	2
Chocolate shake		Nestle Killer	2.1	oz.	0	1	1
		Nestle Quick	2.2	oz.	0	1	1
Chocolate syrup		Fox's U-Bet	0.6	Tbsp.	0	1	0
		Hershey's	0.7	Tbsp.	0	1	0
		Smucker's Sundae	0.7	Tbsp.	0	1	0
		Yoo-Hoo	0.7	Tbsp.	0	1	0
	malt	Hershey's	0.7	Tbsp.	0	1	0
		Kraft	0.7	Tbsp.	0	1	0
Chocolate topping	all varieties	Smucker's Magic Shell	1.1	Tbsp.	0	1	3
	caramel	Hershey's	0.7	Tbsp.	0	1	0
	cherry Melba	Dickinson's Black Forest	0.7	Tbsp.	0	1	0
	double	Hershey's	0.7	Tbsp.	0	1	0
	fudge, chocolate	Smucker's	0.7	Tbsp.	0	1	0
	fudge, double	Hershey's	0.7	Tbsp.	0	1	0
	fudge, hot	Hershey's	0.9	Tbsp.	0	1	0
	fudge, hot, fat free	Hershey's	0.8	Tbsp.	0	1	1
	fudge, hot	Kraft	0.7	Tbsp.	0	1	0
	fudge, hot	Smucker's	0.8	Tbsp.	0	1	0
	fudge, hot	Smucker's Special Recipe	0.8	Tbsp.	0	1	1
	fudge, hot, light	Smucker's	0.9	Tbsp.	0	1	1
	mint	Hershey's	0.7	Tbsp.	0	1	0
Churro	cinnamon	Tio Pete's	0.8	oz.	0	1	0
Chutney	mango	Patak's Major Grey's	0.8	Tbsp.	0	1	1
	tomato, dried	Sonoma	1	Tbsp.	0	1	0
	tropical fruit and nut	Patak's	0.8	Tbsp.	0	1	0

Food	Description	Brand	Amount	Unit			
Cinnamon	ground		10	tsp.	○	—	○
Citron	candied	S&W	16.3	pcs.	○	—	○
Citrus juice blend	diced	Paradise/White Swan	1	Tbsp.	○	—	○
Citrus drink		Pet/Season's Best Medley	2.4	fl. oz.	○	—	○
	punch	Five Alive	2.4	fl. oz.	○	—	○
	punch	Goya	2.4	fl. oz.	○	—	○
	punch	Minute Maid	2.2	fl. oz.	○	—	○
	tropical	Tropicana	2	fl. oz.	○	—	○
	frozen, prepared	Five Alive	2.5	fl. oz.	○	—	○
	frozen, prepared, punch	Minute Maid	2.4	fl. oz.	○	—	○
	frozen, prepared, tropical	Minute Maid	2.4	fl. oz.	○	—	○
		Five Alive	2.5	fl. oz.	○	—	2
Clam juice		Bookbinder's	10.5	oz.	○	—	○
	peach	Stilwell	0.03	pkg.	—	—	○
	peach	Stilwell Lite	0.1	pkg.	—	—	○
	peach, crumb	Pet-Ritz	0.04	pkg.	—	—	○
	strawberry	Pet-Ritz	0.04	pkg.	—	—	○
	strawberry	Stilwell	0.03	pkg.	—	—	○
Cobbler, frozen	apple	Marie Callender's	0.9	oz.	—	—	○
	apple	Pet-Ritz	0.04	pkg.	—	—	○
	apple	Stilwell	0.03	pkg.	—	—	○
	apple	Stilwell Lite	0.1	pkg.	—	—	○
	apple crumb	Pet-Ritz	0.03	pkg.	—	—	○
	apricot	Stilwell	0.03	pkg.	—	—	○
	berry	Marie Callender's	1	oz.	—	—	○
	berry	Stilwell	0.03	pkg.	—	—	○
	berry	Stilwell Lite	0.1	pkg.	—	—	○
	blackberry	Pet-Ritz	0.04	pkg.	—	—	○
	blackberry	Stilwell	0.03	pkg.	—	—	○
	blackberry	Stilwell Lite	0.1	pkg.	—	—	○
	blackberry, crumb	Pet-Ritz	0.03	pkg.	—	—	○
	blueberry	Marie Callender's	0.9	oz.	—	—	○
	blueberry	Pet-Ritz	0.04	pkg.	—	—	○
	cherry	Marie Callender's	0.8	oz.	—	—	○
	cherry	Pet-Ritz	0.03	pkg.	—	—	○
	cherry	Stilwell	0.03	pkg.	—	—	○

FOOD ITEM	SPECIFICATIONS	BRAND NAME	QUANTITY	SIZE	PROTEIN BLOCKS	CARBOHYDRATE BLOCKS	FAT BLOCKS
	cherry	Stilwell Lite	0.1	pkg.	0	1	1
	cherry, crumb	Pet-Ritz	0.03	pkg.	0	1	0
	peach	Marie Callender's	0.8	oz.	0	1	1
	peach	Pet-Ritz	0.04	pkg.	0	1	1
Cobbler, freeze dried	apple-blueberry	AlpineAire	0.1	cup	0	1	0
Cocoa, baking	unsweetened	Hershey's	5	Tbsp.	1	1	1
	unsweetened	Ghirardelli	5	Tbsp.	1	1	5
	unsweetened	Nestle Baking	10	Tbsp.	0	1	3
	sweetened	Ghirardelli	0.7	Tbsp.	1	1	0
Cocoa mix, hot		Carnation Fat Free	3.3	pkt.	1	1	0
		Carnation No Sugar	1.1	pkt.	0	1	0
		Carnation 70	0.6	pkt.	0	1	0
		Swiss Miss	0.3	pkt.	0	1	0
		Swiss Miss Diet	2.5	pkt.	1	1	0
		Swiss Miss Fat Free	1	pkt.	0	1	0
		Swiss Miss Lite	0.6	pkt.	0	1	0
		Swiss Miss Sugar Free	0.2	cup	0	1	0
		Weight Watchers	1	pkt.	0	1	0
	almond mocha	Swiss Miss Premiere	0.3	pkt.	0	1	0
	chocolate	Land O Lakes	0.4	pkt.	0	1	1
	chocolate	Swiss Miss Sensations	0.4	pkt.	0	1	0
	chocolate, cinnamon or raspberry	Land O Lakes	0.4	pkt.	0	1	1
	chocolate, double	Ghirardelli	0.5	pkt.	0	1	0
	chocolate, hazelnut	Ghirardelli	0.5	pkt.	0	1	0
	chocolate, Irish cream	Nestle	1.7	Tbsp.	0	1	0
	chocolate, milk	Carnation	1.1	pkt.	0	1	0
	chocolate, milk	Swiss Miss	0.4	pkt.	0	1	0
	chocolate, milk	Swiss Miss Sugar Free	0.9	pkt.	0	1	0
	chocolate, mint	Land O Lakes	0.4	pkt.	0	1	1
	chocolate, mocha	Ghirardelli	0.5	pkt.	0	1	0
	chocolate, raspberry truffle	Swiss Miss Premiere	0.3	pkt.	0	1	0
	chocolate, rich	Carnation	1.1	Tbsp.	0	1	0

Food	Brand	Amount	Unit	Protein Blocks	Carbohydrate Blocks	Fat Blocks
chocolate, rich	Swiss Miss	0.4	pkt.	0	1	0
chocolate, rich, w/marshmallow	Carnation	1.1	Tbsp.	0	1	0
chocolate, rich, w/ or w/out marshmallow	Nestle	0.4	pkt.	0	1	0
chocolate, Suisse truffle	Swiss Miss Premiere	0.3	pkt.	0	1	0
chocolate, Suisse truffle	Nestle	1.6	Tbsp.	0	1	0
chocolate, toffee, English	Swiss Miss Premiere	0.3	pkt.	0	1	0
chocolate, white	Ghirardelli	0.8	Tbsp.	0	1	0
chocolate, white	Swiss Miss	0.4	pkt.	0	1	0
and cream	Swiss Miss	0.4	pkt.	0	1	1
mini-marshmallow	Swiss Miss	0.4	pkt.	0	1	0
mini-marshmallow	Swiss Miss No Sugar	0.8	pkt.	0	1	0
Coconut						
fresh, shelled		5	oz.	1	1	16
fresh, shelled, shredded or grated		1.7	cup, not packed	1	1	15
canned, flaked, sweetened	Angel Flake	0.3	cup	0	1	3
canned, flaked	Durkee	2.9	Tbsp.	0	1	2
canned, flaked		5	Tbsp.	0	1	5
dried toasted		0.8	oz.	0	1	3
packaged, flaked, sweetened	Angel Flake	0.3	cup	0	1	2
packaged, flaked, sweetened	Mounds	2.9	Tbsp.	0	1	2
packaged, flaked, sweetened	Baker's Premium	2.5	Tbsp.	0	1	2
shredded	Coco Casa	3.3	Tbsp.	0	1	2
	Coco Goya	0.8	Tbsp.	0	1	0
	Coco Lopez	0.4	Tbsp.	0	1	1
	Coco Lopez	0.8	Tbsp.	0	1	0
Coffee						
instant, regular		10	rounded tsp, prepared	0	1	0
Coffee, flavored						
café Francais	General Foods International	10	fl. oz., prepared	0	1	2
café Vienna	General Foods International	6.7	fl. oz., prepared	0	1	1
cappuccino	Nestle Instant	0.6	pkt.	0	1	0
cappuccino, cinnamon	Maxwell House	4.4	fl. oz., prepared	0	1	0
cappuccino, coffee	Maxwell House	4	fl. oz., prepared	0	1	0
cappuccino, Italian	General Foods International	7.3	fl. oz., prepared	0	1	0
cappuccino, mocha	Maxwell House	4.2	fl. oz., prepared	0	1	0

FOOD ITEM	SPECIFICATIONS	BRAND NAME	QUANTITY	SIZE	PROTEIN BLOCKS	CARBOHYDRATE BLOCKS	FAT BLOCKS
	cappuccino, mocha	Nestle	0.4	pkt.	0	1	0
	cappuccino, orange	General Foods International	6.7	fl. oz., prepared	0	1	1
	cappuccino, vanilla	Maxwell House	3.8	fl. oz., prepared	0	1	0
	chocolate, Viennese	General Foods International	7.3	fl. oz., prepared	0	1	1
	hazelnut, Belgian	General Foods International	6.2	fl. oz., prepared	0	1	1
	Kahlua Café	General Foods International	7.3	fl. oz., prepared	0	1	1
	mocha, café	Carnation Instant Breakfast	2.6	fl. oz., prepared	0	1	0
	mocha, Suisse	General Foods International	8.9	fl. oz., prepared	0	1	1
	vanilla, French	General Foods International	7.3	fl. oz., prepared	0	1	1
Coffee, iced	canned	Jamaican Gold	3.4	oz.	0	1	0
	canned, latte	Jamaican Gold	3.7	oz.	0	1	0
Coffee substitute	cereal grain	Kaffree Roma	5	tsp.	0	1	0
	cereal grain	Postum Instant	5	tsp.	0	1	0
	cereal grain, regular or coffee flavor		3.3	tsp.	0	1	0
Coleslaw	salad blend mix	Dole	11.7	oz.	0	1	1
Collard greens	fresh, raw		10	oz.	0	1	0
	fresh, raw, chopped		5	cup	0	1	0
	fresh, boiled, drained, chopped		1.7	cup	0	1	0
	canned	Allens/Sunshine	2.5	cup	1	1	1
	frozen, chopped, boiled, drained		0.7	cup	0	1	0
Cookie	almond	Archway Crescents	1.1	pcs.	0	1	1
	almond	Stella D'Oro Breakfast Treats	0.6	.8-oz. pc.	0	1	1
	almond	Stella D'Oro Chinese Dessert	0.4	1.2-oz. pc.	0	1	0
	almond	Sunshine Crescents	1.7	pcs.	0	1	1
	almond, toast	Stella D'Oro Mandel	0.9	pc.	0	1	1
	amaretti di Saronno, chocolate dipped	Lazzaroni	1.7	pcs.	0	1	1
	animal	Barnum's Animals	0.5	oz.	0	1	1
	animal	Sunshine	0.4	oz.	0	1	0
	animal, vanilla	Barbara's	3.8	pcs.	0	1	1

Food	Brand	Amount	Unit			
anisette	Stella D'Oro Sponge	1	pc.	0	—	0
anisette	Stella D'Oro Toast	1	pc.	0	—	0
anisette	Stella D'Oro Toast Jumbo	0.4	pcs.	0	—	0
apple	Newton's Fat Free	0.8	pcs.	0	—	0
apple	Sunshine Golden Fruit	0.6	pcs.	0	—	0
apple, bar	Archway Nonfat	0.6	pc.	0	—	0
apple, bran	Archway	0.4	pc.	0	—	0
apple, cinnamon bar	Tastykake	0.3	pc.	0	—	1
apple, pastry	Stella D'Oro Low Sodium	0.7	pc.	0	—	1
apple and raisin	Archway	0.5	pc.	0	—	1
apple, raisin	Health Valley Fat Free Jumbo	0.6	pc.	0	—	0
apple raisin bar	Smart Snackers	0.8	pc.	0	—	1
apple spice	Health Valley Fat Free	0.4	pc.	0	—	0
apricot filled	Archway	0.5	pc.	0	—	1
apricot filled, raspberry	Pepperidge Farm	1.3	pcs.	0	—	1
apricot or date	Health Valley Non Fat	1.3	pcs.	0	—	1
apricot or date	Archway Bells and Stars	1.4	pcs.	0	—	0
	Archway Old Fashion Windmill	0.6	pc.	0	—	1
	Archway Party Treats	0.5	pc.	0	—	1
arrowroot	National	3.3	pc.	0	—	1
banana bran	Archway Low Fat	0.4	pc.	0	—	1
biscotti, all varieties	Health Valley	0.9	pc.	0	—	0
biscotti, almond	Pepperidge Farm Caruso	0.8	pc.	0	—	0
biscotti, anise	Pepperidge Farm La Scala	0.6	pc.	0	—	1
biscotti, chocolate dipped	Pepperidge Farm Figaro	0.7	pc.	0	—	1
biscotti, cranberry pistachio	Pepperidge Farm Tosca	0.7	pc.	0	—	1
biscottini cashews	Stella D'Oro	0.7	pc.	0	—	1
blueberry	Archway	0.5	pc.	0	—	1
blueberry	Fruitastic Bar	0.8	pc.	0	—	0
brown edge wafer	Nabisco	2.2	pcs.	0	—	1
butter, see also shortbread below	Master Choice Southern Classics	4.2	pcs.	0	—	1
butter	Peak Freans Petit Beurre	1.7	pcs.	0	—	1
butter	Pepperidge Farm Medaillon au Beurre	1.4	pcs.	0	—	1
butter	Pepperidge Farm Chessman	1.5	pcs.	0	—	1
butter	Sunshine	2.2	pcs.	0	—	1

FOOD ITEM	SPECIFICATIONS	BRAND NAME	QUANTITY	SIZE	PROTEIN BLOCKS	CARBOHYDRATE BLOCKS	FAT BLOCKS
	butter, assorted	Pepperidge Farm Toy Chest	0.5	pc.	0	1	1
	butter, sandwich w/fudge	E.L. Fudge	1.1	pcs.	0	1	1
	butter pecan bites	Barbara's Small Indulgences	3.3	pcs.	0	1	2
	caramel, apple	Barbara's Fat Free Mini	2.5	pcs.	0	1	0
	caramel, pecan	Pepperidge Farm	0.6	pc.	0	1	1
	carrot cake	Archway	0.5	pc.	0	1	1
	cherry, cobbler	Pepperidge Farm	0.8	pc.	0	1	1
	cherry, filled	Archway	0.5	pc.	0	1	1
	cherry nougat	Archway	1.5	pcs.	0	1	2
	chocolate	Archway Fat Free	0.5	pc.	0	1	0
	chocolate	Pepperidge Farm Goldfish	0.5	oz.	0	1	1
	chocolate	Stella D'Oro Castelets	1	pcs.	0	1	1
	chocolate	Stella D'Oro Margherite	1.1	pcs.	0	1	1
	chocolate bits	Grandma's	3.5	pcs.	0	1	1
	chocolate brownie	Entenmann's Fat Free	1	pc.	0	1	0
	chocolate brownie nut	Pepperidge Farm	1.7	pcs.	0	1	2
	chocolate, caramel or fudge center	Health Valley Fat Free	1.3	pcs.	0	1	0
	chocolate, covered	Ritz	1.7	pcs.	0	1	2
	chocolate, dark	Pepperidge Farm Espirits Noir	0.9	pc.	0	1	2
	chocolate, double	Barbara's Fat Free Mini	2.7	pcs.	0	1	0
	chocolate, fudge	Dare	0.7	pc.	0	1	1
	chocolate, fudge, iced	Tastykake	0.4	pc.	0	1	1
	chocolate, fudge mint	Grasshopper	1.8	pcs.	0	1	1
	chocolate, laced	Pepperidge Farm Pirouette	2.3	pcs.	0	1	2
	chocolate, milk, peanut butter	Pepperidge Farm Chocolate Heaven	1.2	pcs.	0	1	1
	chocolate, milk, w/nuts	Pepperidge Farm Geneve	1.5	pcs.	0	1	2
	chocolate, orange	Pepperidge Farm Chocolate a l'Orange	0.8	pc.	0	1	1
	chocolate, snaps	Nabisco	2.9	pcs.	0	1	1
	chocolate, wafer	Nabisco Famous	1.9	pcs.	0	1	1
	chocolate, wafer, light	Keebler	2.9	pc.	0	1	0
	chocolate chip/chunk	Archway	0.5	pc.	0	1	1
	chocolate chip/chunk	Archway Bag	1.6	pcs.	0	1	1

chocolate chip/chunk	Archway Ice Box	0.5	pc.	0	1	1
chocolate chip/chunk	Barbara's	0.8	pc.	0	1	1
chocolate chip/chunk	Chip-A-Roos	1.3	pcs.	0	1	1
chocolate chip/chunk	Chips Ahoy! Chewy	1.2	pcs.	0	1	1
chocolate chip/chunk	Chips Ahoy! Mini	6.1	pcs.	0	1	1
chocolate chip/chunk	Chips Ahoy! Real Chocolate	1.4	pcs.	0	1	1
chocolate chip/chunk	Chips Ahoy! Reduced Fat	1.3	pcs.	0	1	2
chocolate chip/chunk	Chips Deluxe	1	pc.	0	1	1
chocolate chip/chunk	Chips Deluxe Chocolate Lovers	0.8	pc.	0	1	1
chocolate chip/chunk	Chips Deluxe Light	0.8	pc.	0	1	1
chocolate chip/chunk	Dare	1	pc.	0	1	1
chocolate chip/chunk	Dare Breaktime	2	pcs.	0	1	2
chocolate chip/chunk	Entenmann's	1.4	pcs.	0	1	1
chocolate chip/chunk	Grandma's Big	0.4	pc.	0	1	1
chocolate chip/chunk	Little Debbie	0.8	pc.	0	1	1
chocolate chip/chunk	Pepperidge Farm Old Fashioned	1.5	pcs.	0	1	1
chocolate chip/chunk	Pepperidge Farm Chesapeake	0.6	pc.	0	1	1
chocolate chip/chunk	Pepperidge Farm Goldfish	0.5	oz.	0	1	1
chocolate chip/chunk	Pepperidge Farm Nantucket	0.6	pc.	0	1	1
chocolate chip/chunk	Smart Snackers	0.5	oz.	0	1	1
chocolate chip/chunk	Snackwell's Reduced Fat	5.7	pcs.	0	1	1
chocolate chip/chunk	Tastykake	0.4	pc.	0	1	1
chocolate chip/chunk, all varieties	Health Valley Healthy Chips Fat Free	1.4	pcs.	0	1	0
chocolate chip/chunk, bar	Tastykake	0.3	pc.	0	1	1
chocolate chip/chunk, chocolate	Barbara's	0.9	pc.	0	1	1
chocolate chip/chunk, walnut, soft	Pepperidge Farm	0.6	pc.	0	1	1
chocolate chip/chunk, crisps	Barbara's Small Indulgences	3	pcs.	0	1	1
chocolate chip/chunk, drop	Archway	0.8	pc.	0	1	3
chocolate chip/chunk, fudge	Grandma's Big	0.3	pc.	0	1	1
chocolate chip/chunk, fudge bar	Grandma's	0.3	pc.	0	1	1
chocolate chip/chunk, macadamia	Pepperidge Farm Sausalito	0.6	pc.	0	1	1

CARBOHYDRATES

FOOD ITEM	SPECIFICATIONS	BRAND NAME	QUANTITY	SIZE	PROTEIN BLOCKS	CARBOHYDRATE BLOCKS	FAT BLOCKS
	chocolate chip/chunk, macadamia, soft	Pepperidge Farm	0.6	pc.	0	1	1
	chocolate chip/chunk, macadamia, white	Pepperidge Farm Tahoe	0.6	pc.	0	1	1
	chocolate chip/chunk, mini	Sunshine	2.3	pcs.	0	1	1
	chocolate chip/chunk, rainbow	Chips Deluxe	0.9	pc.	0	1	1
	chocolate chip/chunk, snaps	Nabisco	2.6	pcs.	0	1	1
	chocolate chip/chunk, soft	Chips Deluxe	0.9	pc.	0	1	1
	chocolate chip/chunk, soft	Pepperidge Farm Chunk	0.6	pc.	0	1	1
	chocolate chip/chunk, soft sprinkled	Chips Ahoy!	1.1	pcs.	0	1	1
	chocolate chip/chunk, striped	Chips Ahoy!	0.9	pc.	0	1	1
	chocolate chip/chunk and toffee	Archway	0.5	pc.	0	1	1
	chocolate chip/chunk, toffee	Pepperidge Farm Charleston	0.6	pc.	0	1	1
	chocolate chip/chunk, walnut	Pepperidge Farm Beacon Hill	0.6	pc.	0	1	0
	chocolate sandwich	Elfin Delights Light	1	pc.	0	1	1
	chocolate sandwich	Hydrox	1.4	pcs.	0	1	1
	chocolate sandwich	Hydrox Fat Free	1.2	pcs.	0	1	1
	chocolate sandwich	Oreo	1.3	pcs.	0	1	1
	chocolate sandwich	Oreo Reduced Fat	1.1	pcs.	0	1	1
	chocolate sandwich	Oreo Double Stuff	1	pc.	0	1	1
	chocolate sandwich	Pepperidge Farm Bordeaux	1.8	pcs.	0	1	1
	chocolate sandwich	Pepperidge Farm Brussels	1.4	pcs.	0	1	1
	chocolate sandwich	Pepperidge Farm Lido	0.8	pc.	0	1	1
	chocolate sandwich	Pepperidge Farm Milano	1.3	pcs.	0	1	1
	chocolate sandwich	Smart Snackers	0.4	oz.	0	1	1
	chocolate sandwich	Snackwell's Reduced Fat	1	pc.	0	1	0
	chocolate sandwich	Vienna Fingers Reduced Fat	0.8	pc.	0	1	0
	chocolate sandwich, chocolate fudge	Keebler Classic Collection	0.8	pc.	0	1	1
	chocolate sandwich, chocolate fudge, double	Barbara's Cookies & Creme	1.1	pcs.	0	1	1

		Amount				
chocolate sandwich, double	Pepperidge Farm Milano	1.1	pcs.	0	1	1
chocolate sandwich, fudge coated	Oreo	0.6	pc.	0	1	1
chocolate sandwich, hazelnut	Pepperidge Farm Milano	1.2	pcs.	0	1	0
chocolate sandwich, milk	Pepperidge Farm Bordeaux	1.4	pcs.	0	1	1
chocolate sandwich, milk	Pepperidge Farm Milano	1.3	pcs.	0	1	1
chocolate sandwich, mint	Pepperidge Farm Brussels	1.3	pcs.	0	1	1
chocolate sandwich, mint	Pepperidge Farm Milano	1.1	pcs.	0	1	2
chocolate sandwich, orange	Pepperidge Farm Milano	1.1	pcs.	0	1	2
chocolate sandwich, raspberry or vanilla	Barbara's Cookies & Creme	1	pc.	0	1	1
chocolate sandwich, white fudge coated	Oreo	0.6	pc.	0	1	1
cinnamon, apple	Archway	0.5	pc.	0	1	1
cinnamon, honey heart	Archway Fat Free	1.1	pcs.	0	1	0
cinnamon snaps	Archway	2.3	pcs.	0	1	1
cocoa, Dutch	Archway	0.5	pc.	0	1	1
cocoa, mocha	Barbara's Fat Free Mini	2.6	pcs.	0	1	1
coconut	Dare Breaktime	1.7	pcs.	0	1	0
coconut macaroon	Archway	0.8	pc.	0	1	1
coffee cake crunch	Barbara's Small Indulgences	3	pcs.	0	1	1
cranberry bar	Archway Fat Free	0.6	pc.	0	1	0
cranberry bar	Newton's Fat Free	0.8	pc.	0	1	0
cranberry bar	Sunshine Golden Fruit	0.6	pc.	0	1	0
Danish	Nabisco Import	2.2	pcs.	0	1	1
devil's food cake	Snackwell's Fat Free	0.7	pc.	0	1	0
egg biscuit	Stella D'Oro Jumbo	1	pc.	0	1	0
egg biscuit	Stella D'Oro Low Sodium	1.4	pcs.	0	1	0
egg biscuit, Roman	Stella D'Oro	0.4	pc.	0	1	0
fig	Archway Fat Free	0.6	pc.	0	1	0
fig	Fig Newtons	1	pc.	0	1	0
fig	Fig Newtons Fat Free	0.9	pc.	0	1	0
fig	Smart Snackers	1.1	pcs.	0	1	0
fig	Sunshine Bar	1	pc.	0	1	0
fig	Sunshine Golden Fruit Fat Free	0.7	pc.	0	1	0
fortune	La Choy	1.4	pcs.	0	1	0

FOOD ITEM	SPECIFICATIONS	BRAND NAME	QUANTITY	SIZE	PROTEIN BLOCKS	CARBOHYDRATE BLOCKS	FAT BLOCKS
	fruit bar	Archway Fat Free	0.2	pc.	0	1	0
	fruit, cake	Archway	1.5	pcs.	0	1	1
	fruit, Hawaiian	Health Valley Fat Free	1.3	pcs.	0	1	0
	fruit, honey bar	Archway	0.5	pc.	0	1	1
	fruit, slices	Stella D'Oro Fat Free	0.8	pc.	0	1	0
	fudge	Stella D'Oro Swiss	1.1	pcs.	0	1	1
	fudge bar	Tastykake	0.3	pc.	0	1	1
	fudge, double, cake	Snackwell's Fat Free	0.8	pc.	0	1	0
	fudge, fudge filled	Keebler Truffles	1.3	pcs.	0	1	1
	fudge, mint patties	Sunshine	1.1	pcs.	0	1	1
	fudge, nut bar	Archway	0.5	pc.	0	1	1
	fudge, nutty	Grandma's Big	0.4	pc.	0	1	1
	ginger	Dare Breaktime	1.7	pcs.	0	1	1
	ginger	Pepperidge Farm Gingerman	1.7	pcs.	0	1	1
	ginger snaps	Archway	2.5	pcs.	0	1	1
	ginger snaps	Nabisco Import	1.7	pcs.	0	1	0
	ginger snaps	Sunshine	2.9	pcs.	0	1	1
	gingerbread, iced	Archway	1.2	pcs.	0	1	1
	gingerbread, iced	Sunshine	2.4	pcs.	0	1	1
	golden bar	Stella D'Oro	0.5	pc.	0	1	1
	graham	Bugs Bunny	4.2	pcs.	0	1	1
	graham	Keebler	3.1	pcs.	0	1	1
	graham	Nabisco	3.5	pcs.	0	1	0
	graham	Pepperidge Farm Goldfish	0.6	oz.	0	1	1
	graham, amaranth or oat bran	Health Valley Fat Free	5	pcs.	0	1	0
	graham, chocolate	Bugs Bunny	5.7	pcs.	0	1	1
	graham, chocolate	Keebler	3.3	pcs.	0	1	1
	graham, chocolate	Nabisco Pure	1.4	pcs.	0	1	1
	graham, chocolate-coated	Dunkaroos	0.5	1-oz. tray	0	1	1
	graham, cinnamon	Bugs Bunny	5	pcs.	0	1	1
	graham, cinnamon	Honey Maid	3.6	pcs.	0	1	0
	graham, cinnamon	Keebler Light	3.1	pcs.	0	1	0
	graham, cinnamon	Pepperidge Farm Goldfish	0.6	oz.	0	1	1

Food	Brand					
graham, cinnamon	Snackwell's Fat Free Snacks	7.1	pcs.	0	1	0
graham, cinnamon	Sunshine	0.8	pcs.	0	1	1
graham, French vanilla	Keebler Light	3	pcs.	0	1	0
graham, fudge coated	Keebler Deluxe	1.4	pcs.	0	1	1
graham, fudge coated	Nabisco Family Favorites	1.5	pcs.	0	1	1
graham, fudge coated	Keebler S'mores	1.3	pcs.	0	1	1
graham, fudge dipped	Sunshine	1.8	pcs.	0	1	1
graham, honey	Honey Maid	3.5	pcs.	0	1	0
graham, honey	Keebler Light	3.3	pcs.	0	1	0
graham, honey	Sunshine	1	pcs.	0	1	1
granola	Archway Fat Free	0.8	pcs.	0	1	0
granola, soft	Grandma's Bar	0.3	pc.	0	1	1
hazelnut	Pepperidge Farm	1.3	pcs.	0	1	1
hermits	Archway Cookie Jar	0.5	pc.	0	1	0
	Heyday Bar	0.7	pc.	0	1	1
	Sunshine Coolers	2.2	pcs.	0	1	1
lemon, almond	Barbara's Small Indulgences	3	pcs.	0	1	1
lemon bits	Grandma's	3.9	pcs.	0	1	1
lemon creme	Dare Breaktime	0.7	pcs.	0	1	1
lemon drop	Archway	0.5	pc.	0	1	1
lemon frosty	Archway	0.5	pc.	0	1	1
lemon nuggets	Archway Fat Free	2.1	pc.	0	1	1
lemon nut crunch	Pepperidge Farm	1.7	pcs.	0	1	0
lemon, sandwich	Barbara's Cookies & Creme	1	pcs.	0	1	2
lemon snaps	Archway	2.3	pcs.	0	1	1
marshmallow, chocolate	Mallomars	1.1	pcs.	0	1	1
marshmallow, chocolate	Pinwheels	0.4	pc.	0	1	1
marshmallow, fudge puffs	Nabisco	0.6	pc.	0	1	1
marshmallow, fudge twirls	Nabisco	0.5	pc.	0	1	1
mint sandwich	Mystic Mint	0.8	pc.	0	1	1
molasses	Archway	0.5	pc.	0	1	1
molasses	Archway Low Fat	0.4	pc.	0	1	1
molasses	Archway Old Fashion	0.5	pc.	0	1	1
molasses	Archway Super Pak	0.5	pc.	0	1	0
molasses	Grandma's Old Time Big	0.3	pc.	0	1	0
molasses, crisps	Pepperidge Farm	2.3	pcs.	0	1	1

FOOD ITEM	SPECIFICATIONS	BRAND NAME	QUANTITY	SIZE	PROTEIN BLOCKS	CARBOHYDRATE BLOCKS	FAT BLOCKS
	molasses, dark	Archway	0.5	pc.	0	1	1
	molasses, drop, soft	Archway	0.5	pc.	0	1	1
	molasses, iced	Archway Iowa	0.5	pc.	0	1	1
	molasses, iced	Archway Ohio	0.5	pc.	0	1	1
	molasses, iced	Archway Super Pak	0.5	pc.	0	1	1
	mud pie	Archway	0.6	pc.	0	1	1
	New Orleans cake	Archway	0.5	pc.	0	1	1
	nut	Archway Nutty Nougat	1.5	pcs.	0	1	2
	nut	Little Debbie Nutty Bars	1.1	pcs.	0	1	2
	oatmeal	Archway	0.5	pc.	0	1	0
	oatmeal	Dare Breaktime	2	pcs.	0	1	1
	oatmeal	Nabisco Family Favorites	0.8	pc.	0	1	1
	oatmeal	Ruth's	0.5	pc.	0	1	1
	oatmeal	Ruth's Golden	0.5	pc.	0	1	1
	oatmeal	Sunshine Country	1.2	pcs.	0	1	1
	oatmeal, apple filled	Archway	0.5	pc.	0	1	1
	oatmeal, apple spice	Grandma's Big	0.4	pc.	0	1	1
	oatmeal, apple spice bar	Grandma's	0.3	pc.	0	1	1
	oatmeal, butterscotch	Pepperidge Farm	1.3	pcs.	0	1	1
	oatmeal, chewy	Master Choice Southern Classics	1	pc.	0	1	0
	oatmeal, chocolate chip	Entenmann's Fat Free	1	pc.	0	1	1
	oatmeal, chocolate chip	Sunshine	1.3	pcs.	0	1	1
	oatmeal, date filled	Archway	0.5	pc.	0	1	1
	oatmeal, iced	Archway	0.5	pc.	0	1	1
	oatmeal, iced	Sunshine	1	pc.	0	1	1
	oatmeal, Irish	Pepperidge Farm	1.6	pcs.	0	1	1
	oatmeal, pecan	Archway	0.5	pc.	0	1	1
	oatmeal, raspberry	Archway Fat Free	0.4	pc.	0	1	0
	oatmeal raisin	Archway	0.5	pc.	0	1	1
	oatmeal raisin	Archway Bag	1.5	pcs.	0	1	1
	oatmeal raisin	Archway Fat Free	0.4	pc.	0	1	0
	oatmeal raisin	Barbara's	0.8	pc.	0	1	0
	oatmeal raisin	Barbara's Fat Free Mini	2.5	pcs.	0	1	0

Food	Brand	Amount	Unit			
oatmeal raisin	Entenmann's Fat Free	1	pc.	0	1	0
oatmeal raisin	Health Valley Fat Free	1.3	pcs.	0	1	0
oatmeal raisin	Little Debbie	0.7	pc.	1	1	0
oatmeal raisin	Pepperidge Farm Old Fashioned	1.3	pcs.	1	1	0
oatmeal raisin	Pepperidge Farm Soft	0.6	pc.	1	1	0
oatmeal raisin	Pepperidge Farm Santa Fe	0.5	pc.	1	1	0
oatmeal raisin	Smart Snackers	0.5	oz.	0	1	0
oatmeal raisin	Snackwell's Reduced Fat	1	pc.	0	1	0
oatmeal raisin, bran	Tastykake Bar	0.3	pc.	1	1	0
oatmeal raisin, iced	Archway	0.5	pc.	1	1	0
peach tart	Tastykake	0.3	pc.	1	1	0
peach-apricot	Pepperidge Farm	0.8	pc.	0	1	0
peanut	Stella D'Oro Sodium Free	0.7	pc.	1	1	0
peanut, crunch	Archway Jumble	0.6	pc.	1	1	0
peanut butter	Archway	3	pcs.	1	1	0
peanut butter	Archway	0.6	pc.	1	1	0
peanut butter	Archway Ol' Fashion	0.5	pc.	1	1	0
peanut butter	Grandma's Big	0.4	pc.	1	1	0
peanut butter bits	Little Debbie Bar	0.3	pc.	1	1	0
peanut butter chip	Grandma's	4.1	pcs.	1	1	0
peanut butter, chocolate chip	Archway	0.6	pc.	1	1	0
peanut butter, chocolate chip	Grandma's Bar	0.4	pc.	1	1	0
peanut butter, chunky	Grandma's Big	0.4	pc.	1	1	0
peanut butter, fudge	Tastykake Bar	0.5	pc.	2	1	0
peanut butter, patties	P.B. Fudgebuters	1.3	pcs.	1	1	0
peanut butter, sandwich	Nutter Butter	2.8	pcs.	1	1	0
peanut butter, sandwich	Grandma's	1.6	pcs.	2	1	0
peanut butter, sandwich	Nutter Butter	1	pc.	1	1	0
pecan	Nutter Butter Bites	4.8	pcs.	1	1	0
pecan, malted nougat	Archway Ice Box	0.5	pc.	1	1	0
pound cake	Archway	1.8	pcs.	1	1	0
prune pastry	Aunt Bea's	0.5	pc.	2	1	0
raisin	Stella D'Oro	0.7	pc.	1	1	0
raisin	Dare Sun Maid	1.3	pcs.	1	1	0
raisin	Health Valley Fat Free Jumbo	0.6	pc.	0	1	0
raspberry	Health Valley Fat Free Jumbo	0.6	pc.	0	1	0

FOOD ITEM	SPECIFICATIONS	BRAND NAME	QUANTITY	SIZE	PROTEIN BLOCKS	CARBOHYDRATE BLOCKS	FAT BLOCKS
	raspberry	Fruitastic Bar	0.8	pc.	0	1	0
	raspberry	Newtons Fat Free	0.8	pc.	0	1	0
	raspberry	Sunshine Oh! Berry	1.5	pcs.	0	1	1
	raspberry centers	Health Valley Fat Free	0.6	pc.	0	1	0
	raspberry filled	Archway	0.5	pc.	0	1	1
	raspberry filled	Pepperidge Farm Linzer	0.6	pc.	0	1	1
	raspberry filled	Smart Snackers	0.6	pc.	0	1	0
	raspberry hazelnut	Pepperidge Farm Chantilly	0.8	pc.	0	1	1
	rocky road	Archway Iowa	0.5	pc.	0	1	1
	rocky road	Archway Ohio	0.5	pc.	0	1	1
	sesame	Stella D'Oro Regina	1.4	pcs.	0	1	1
	shortbread	Lorna Doone	1.9	pcs.	0	1	1
	shortbread	Pepperidge Farm	1.1	pcs.	0	1	1
	shortbread	Simply Sandies	1	pc.	0	1	2
	shortbread, butter	Dare	1.3	pcs.	0	1	2
	shortbread, fudge coated	Nabisco Family Favorites	1.3	pcs.	0	1	1
	shortbread, fudge striped	Keebler	1.3	pcs.	0	1	1
	shortbread, fudge striped	Sunshine	1.4	pcs.	0	1	1
	shortbread, pecan	Pecan Passion	1	pc.	0	1	2
	shortbread, pecan	Pecan Sandies	1	pc.	0	1	2
	shortbread, pecan	Pepperidge Farm	1.4	pcs.	0	1	2
	shortbread, pecan	Social Tea	2.7	pcs.	0	1	1
	spice, pfeffernusse	Archway	0.6	pc.	0	1	0
	spice, pfeffernusse drops	Stella D'Oro	1.3	pcs.	0	1	0
	sprinkles	Dare Breaktime	1.7	pcs.	0	1	1
		Stella D'Oro Angelica Goodies	0.6	pc.	0	1	1
		Stella D'Oro Angel Wings	1.4	pcs.	0	1	2
		Stella D'Oro Anginetti	1.5	pcs.	0	1	1
		Stella D'Oro Como Delights	0.6	oz.	0	1	1
	strawberry	Newtons Fat Free	0.8	pc.	0	1	0
	strawberry	Pepperidge Farm	1.3	pcs.	0	1	1
	strawberry	Sunshine Oh! Berry Fat Free	0.5	oz.	0	1	0
	strawberry filled	Archway	0.6	pc.	0	1	1

Food	Brand	Amount	Unit			
strawberry filled	Archway Ohio	0.5	pc.	0	—	1
sugar	Archway	0.5	pc.	0	—	1
sugar	Archway Fat Free	0.5	pc.	0	—	0
sugar	Dare	1.4	pcs.	0	—	1
sugar	Keebler Classic Collection	1	pc.	0	—	1
sugar	Pepperidge Farm	1.4	pcs.	0	—	1
sugar, soft	Archway	0.5	pc.	0	—	1
sugar, wafer	Biscos	3.5	pcs.	0	—	1
sugar, wafer, chocolate	Sunshine	0.9	pc.	0	—	1
sugar, wafer, peanut butter	Sunshine	2	pcs.	0	—	2
sugar, wafer, vanilla	Sunshine	1.5	pcs.	0	—	1
sugar, waffle	Biscos	1	pc.	0	—	1
vanilla	Sunshine Jingles	2.5	pcs.	0	—	1
vanilla	Pepperidge Farm Goldfish	0.5	oz.	0	—	1
vanilla bits	Stella D'Oro Margherite	0.8	pc.	0	—	1
vanilla, raspberry tart	Grandma's	3.9	pcs.	0	—	1
vanilla wafer	Pepperidge Farm Wholesome Choice	0.8	pc.	0	—	0
vanilla wafer	Archway	2.1	pcs.	0	—	1
vanilla wafer	Keebler	3.6	pcs.	0	—	1
vanilla wafer	Keebler Light	2.9	pcs.	0	—	0
vanilla wafer	Nilla	3	pcs.	0	—	1
vanilla wafer	Sunshine	3.2	pcs.	0	—	1
vanilla sandwich	Cameo	0.9	pc.	0	—	1
vanilla sandwich	Cookie Break	1.2	pcs.	0	—	1
vanilla sandwich	Grandma's	1.6	pcs.	0	—	1
vanilla sandwich	Nabisco Family Favorites	1.1	pcs.	0	—	0
vanilla sandwich	Smart Snackers	0.4	oz.	0	—	0
vanilla sandwich	Snackwell's Reduced Fat	0.9	pc.	0	—	0
vanilla sandwich, French	Vienna Fingers	0.8	pc.	0	—	1
vanilla sandwich, raspberry or vanilla	Keebler Classic Collection	0.8	pc.	0	—	1
vanilla sandwich, raspberry or vanilla	Barbara's Cookies & Creme	1	pc.	0	—	1
wafer, fudge	Keebler Fudge Sticks	1.4	pcs.	0	—	1
Cookie refrigerated						
walnut, black	Archway Ice Box	0.6	pc.	0	—	1
candy	Pillsbury	0.5	oz.	0	—	1
chocolate chip	Pillsbury	0.5	oz.	0	—	1

FOOD ITEM	SPECIFICATIONS	BRAND NAME	QUANTITY	SIZE	PROTEIN BLOCKS	CARBOHYDRATE BLOCKS	FAT BLOCKS
Cookie mix	chocolate chip, chocolate	Pillsbury	0.5	oz.	0	1	1
	chocolate chip, oatmeal	Pillsbury	0.6	oz.	0	1	1
	peanut butter	Pillsbury	0.6	oz.	0	1	1
	sugar	Pillsbury	1	pc.	0	1	1
	chocolate chip	Arrowhead Mills	0.6	pc., prepared	0	1	0
	chocolate chip	Arrowhead Mills Wheat Free	0.6	pc., prepared	0	1	0
	espresso chip	Arrowhead Mills	0.6	pc., prepared	0	1	0
	oatmeal	Arrowhead Mills	0.6	pc., prepared	0	1	0
Corn	fresh, kernels, boiled, drained		0.3	cup	0	1	0
Corn, canned	baby	Roland	2.5	cup	1	1	0
	kernel	Del Monte	0.3	cup	0	1	0
	kernel	Del Monte Supersweet No Salt	0.6	cup	0	1	0
	kernel	Del Monte Supersweet No Sugar	0.6	cup	0	1	0
	kernel	Del Monte Supersweet Vac Pack	0.5	cup	0	1	0
	kernel	Del Monte Supersweet Vac Pack No Salt	0.5	cup	0	1	0
	kernel	Del Monte Fiesta	0.5	cup	0	1	0
	kernel	Goya	0.2	cup	0	1	0
	kernel	Green Giant	0.3	cup	0	1	0
	kernel	Green Giant less Salt	0.3	cup	0	1	0
	kernel	Green Giant Niblets	0.2	cup	0	1	0
	kernel	Green Giant Niblets Extra Sweet	0.4	cup	0	1	0
	kernel	Green Giant Niblets Less Sodium	0.2	cup	0	1	0
	kernel	Green Giant Niblets No Salt/No Sugar	0.3	cup	0	1	0
	kernel	S&W	0.4	cup	0	1	0
	kernel	S&W Sweet 'n Crisp	0.3	cup	0	1	0
	kernel	Stokely	0.4	cup	0	1	0
	kernel	Stokely No Salt	0.4	cup	0	1	0
	kernel	Stokely Vac Pac	0.3	cup	0	1	0
	kernel	Stokely Vac Pac No Salt	0.3	cup	0	1	0
	kernel, gold/white	Del Monte Supersweet	0.3	cup	0	1	0
	kernel, white	Del Monte	0.3	cup	0	1	0
	kernel, white	Green Giant	0.2	cup	0	1	0

Food	Description	Brand	Amount	Unit	P	C	F
	kernel, white	Stokely	0.4	cup	0	1	0
	kernel, white	Stokely No Salt	0.4	cup	0	1	0
	kernel, w/peppers	Green Giant Mexicorn	0.4	cup	0	1	0
	kernel, w/peppers	Stokely	0.2	cup	0	1	0
	cream style	Del Monte	0.3	cup	0	1	0
	cream style	Del Monte No Salt	0.3	cup	0	1	0
	cream style	Del Monte Supersweet	0.4	cup	0	1	0
	cream style	Del Monte Supersweet No Salt	0.4	cup	0	1	0
	cream style	Green Giant	0.2	cup	0	1	0
	cream style	S&W	0.2	cup	0	1	0
	cream style	Stokely	0.2	cup	0	1	0
	cream style, white	Del Monte	0.2	cup	0	1	0
Corn, freeze-dried		AlpineAire	0.3	cup	0	1	0
		Mountain House	0.3	cup	0	1	0
Corn, frozen	on the cob	John Cope's	0.5	ear	0	1	0
	on the cob	Green Giant Extra Sweet	2.5	ear	1	1	2
	on the cob	Green Giant Nibblers	2.5	ear	1	1	1
	on the cob	Green Giant Niblets	1.1	ear	0	1	1
	on the cob	Ore-Ida Mini-Gold	0.5	ear	0	1	0
	on the cob, white	John Cope's	0.3	ear	0	1	0
	kernel	Green Giant Harvest Fresh Niblets	0.4	cup	0	1	0
	kernel	Green Giant Niblets	0.4	cup	0	1	0
	kernel	Green Giant Niblets Extra Sweet	0.6	cup	0	1	0
	kernel	Stilwell	0.3	cup	0	1	0
	kernel, white	Green Giant	0.4	cup	0	1	0
	kernel, white	Green Giant Extra Sweet	0.8	cup	0	1	0
	kernel, white	Green Giant Harvest Fresh	0.5	cup	0	1	0
	kernel, white	John Cope's	0.2	cup	0	1	0
	cream style	Green Giant	0.2	cup	0	1	0
	cream style, white	John Cope's Sweet 'N Creamy	0.2	cup	0	1	0
	in butter sauce	Green Giant Niblets	0.3	cup	0	1	0
	in butter sauce, white	Green Giant	0.4	cup	0	1	0
		John Cope's	0.2	cup	0	1	0
Corn, dried	crude		0.4	oz	0	1	0
Corn, whole grain	crude		0.1	cup	0	1	0
Corn bran	crude		33.3	oz	8	1	3
	crude		10	cup	6	1	2

FOOD ITEM	SPECIFICATIONS	BRAND NAME	QUANTITY	SIZE	PROTEIN BLOCKS	CARBOHYDRATE BLOCKS	FAT BLOCKS
Corn chips and puffs		Barbara's Pinta Chips	0.5	oz.	0	1	1
		Barrel O'Fun Chip	0.6	oz.	0	1	2
		Bugels	0.7	cup	0	1	2
		Bugels Light	0.6	cup	0	1	0
		Dipsey Doodles	0.6	oz.	0	1	2
		Fritos King Size	0.6	oz.	0	1	2
		Fritos Original/Wild 'N Mild	0.6	oz.	0	1	2
		Fritos Scoops	0.6	oz.	0	1	2
		Old Dutch Chips	0.7	oz.	0	1	2
		Old Dutch Chips	0.8	oz.	0	1	3
		Old Dutch Puffcorn Curls	0.7	oz.	0	1	3
		Planters Chips	0.6	oz.	0	1	2
		Sunchips Original	0.6	oz.	0	1	2
	barbeque	Fritos	0.6	oz.	0	1	2
	barbeque	Old Dutch	0.7	oz.	0	1	2
	barbeque	Old Dutch	0.7	oz.	0	1	2
	barbeque	Smart Snackers Curls	0.5	oz.	0	1	0
	blue corn	Barbara's	0.6	oz.	0	1	1
	blue corn	Barbara's Pinta Blues	0.6	oz.	0	1	1
	blue corn, light salt	Barbara's Amazing Bakes	0.4	oz.	0	1	0
	blue corn, picante	Barbara's Pinta	0.6	oz.	0	1	1
	blue corn, salsa	Barbara's Pinta	0.5	oz.	0	1	1
	caramel coated	Old Dutch Puffcorn	0.4	oz.	0	1	0
	cheese	Cheese Doodles	0.5	oz.	0	1	1
	cheese	Chee*tos Cheesy Checkers	0.6	oz.	0	1	2
	cheese	Chee*tos Crunchy	0.6	oz.	0	1	2
	cheese, cheddar	Sunchips Harvest	0.6	oz.	0	1	1
	cheese, chili, w/corn shell	Combos	0.6	oz.	0	1	1
	cheese, fried	Cheese Doodles	0.6	oz.	0	1	2
	cheese, hot	Chee*tos Flamin'	0.6	oz.	0	1	2
	cheese, nacho	Barbara's Pinta	0.6	oz.	0	1	1
	cheese, nacho	Doodle Twisters	0.6	oz.	0	1	2
	cheese, nacho	Combos	0.6	oz.	0	1	1

Food	Brand	Amount	Unit	Protein	Carbohydrate	Fat
cheese, nacho, w/tortilla shell	Combos	0.5	oz.	0	1	1
cheese and pepperoni	Combos	0.5	oz.	0	1	1
cheese balls	Barrel O'Fun	0.6	oz.	0	2	1
cheese balls	Planters Cheez	0.6	oz.	0	2	1
cheese balls	Planters Cheez	0.6	oz.	0	2	1
cheese balls, puffed	Chee*tos	0.7	oz.	0	2	1
cheese curls	Barrel O'Fun Baked	0.6	oz.	0	2	1
cheese curls	Barrel O'Fun Crunchy	0.6	oz.	0	2	1
cheese curls	Chee*tos	0.6	oz.	0	1	1
cheese curls	Old Dutch Crunchy	0.5	oz.	0	2	1
cheese curls	Planters Cheez	0.6	oz.	0	2	1
cheese curls	Planters Cheez	0.6	oz.	0	1	1
cheese curls	Smart Snackers	0.5	oz.	0	2	1
cheese puffs	Barbara's Original	0.6	oz.	0	3	1
cheese puffs	Barbara's Bakes	0.8	oz.	0	0	1
cheese puffs	Barrel O'Fun Light	0.4	oz.	0	2	1
cheese puffs	Chee*tos	0.6	oz.	0	0	1
cheese puffs, cheddar	No Fries	0.4	oz.	0	1	1
cheese puffs, cheddar	Barbara's Less Fat	0.5	oz.	0	1	1
cheese puffs, jalapeno New York	Barbara's	0.6	oz.	0	2	1
cheese puffs, Monterey Jack and green chili	Barbara's Less Fat	0.5	oz.	0	1	1
chili cheese	Fritos	0.6	oz.	0	2	1
onion, French	Sunchips	0.6	oz.	0	1	1
onion flavor rings	Borden	0.5	oz.	0	1	1
pizza curls	Smart Snackers	0.5	oz.	0	1	1
ranch	Combos	0.6	oz.	0	1	1
ranch	Smart Snackers	0.5	oz.	0	1	1
ranch, puffs	No Fries	0.4	oz.	0	0	1
sour cream and onion	Bugles	0.7	cup	0	2	1
taco	Taco Bell Supreme	0.5	oz.	0	1	1
tortilla	Doritos Dunkers	0.5	oz.	0	1	1
tortilla	Doritos Toasted	0.5	oz.	0	1	1
tortilla	Mesa	0.6	oz.	0	0	1
tortilla	Nachips	0.6	oz.	0	2	1

CARBOHYDRATES

FOOD ITEM	SPECIFICATIONS	BRAND NAME	QUANTITY	SIZE	PROTEIN BLOCKS	CARBOHYDRATE BLOCKS	FAT BLOCKS
	tortilla	No Fries Natural	0.4	oz.	0	1	0
	tortilla	Old Dutch Restaurant	0.5	oz.	0	1	1
	tortilla	Sanitas Chips	0.5	oz.	0	1	1
	tortilla	Sanitas Strips	0.5	oz.	0	1	1
	tortilla	Tostitos Baked	0.4	oz.	0	1	0
	tortilla	Tostitos Bite Size	0.6	oz.	0	1	2
	tortilla	Tostitos Crispy Round	0.6	oz.	0	1	2
	tortilla	Tostitos Restaurant/Santa Fe Gold	0.5	oz.	0	1	1
	tortilla	Tyson	0.5	oz.	0	1	1
	tortilla	Tyson Yellow Corn	0.5	oz.	0	1	1
	tortilla, crisps	Mr. Phipps	0.5	oz.	0	1	1
	tortilla, crisps	Pepperidge Farm	0.6	oz.	0	1	1
	tortilla, 5 grain	Kettle Tias	0.6	oz.	0	1	1
	tortilla, hot	Doritos Flamin'	0.6	oz.	0	1	2
	tortilla, lime and chili	Kettle Tias	0.6	oz.	0	1	1
	tortilla, lime and chili	Tostitos	0.5	oz.	0	1	1
	tortilla, pizza	Doritos Cravers	0.5	oz.	0	1	1
	tortilla, ranch	Doritos Cooler	0.5	oz.	0	1	1
	tortilla, ranch	Doritos Cooler Reduced Fat	0.5	oz.	0	1	1
	tortilla, ranch	No Fries	0.4	oz.	0	1	0
	tortilla, ranch	Tostitos Baked	0.5	oz.	0	1	0
	tortilla, salsa crisps	Pepperidge Farm	0.6	oz.	0	1	1
	tortilla, salsa and sour	No Fries	0.4	oz.	0	1	0
	tortilla, tomato basil	Kettle Tias	0.6	oz.	0	1	1
	tortilla, tostados	Old Dutch	0.6	oz.	0	1	1
	tortilla, blue corn	Barbara's Less Fat	0.5	oz.	0	1	1
	tortilla, blue corn	Kettle Tias	0.6	oz.	0	1	1
	tortilla, blue corn, hot salsa	Barbara's Less Fat	0.5	oz.	0	1	1
	tortilla, blue corn, cheddar jalapeno	No Fries	0.4	oz.	0	1	0
	tortilla, cheese	Doritos Chester's	0.5	oz.	0	1	1
	tortilla, cheese, cheddar, white	Barbara's Less Fat	0.5	oz.	0	1	1
	tortilla, cheese, chili crisps	Pepperidge Farm	0.6	oz.	0	1	1

Food	Brand	Amount	Unit	Protein	Carbohydrate	Fat
tortilla, cheese, nacho	Barrel O'Fun	0.5	oz.	0	1	1
tortilla, cheese, nacho	Borden	0.6	oz.	0	1	2
tortilla, cheese, nacho	Doritos Cheesier	0.5	oz.	0	1	1
tortilla, cheese, nacho	Doritos Cheesier Reduced Fat	0.5	oz.	0	1	1
tortilla, cheese, nacho	Old Dutch	0.6	oz.	0	1	1
tortilla, cheese, nacho	Old Dutch	0.6	oz.	0	1	1
tortilla, cheese, nacho	Tyson	0.5	oz.	0	1	1
tortilla, cheese, nacho	Mr. Phipps	0.5	oz.	0	1	1
tortilla, flour, cheese and salsa	Barrel O'Fun	0.5	oz.	0	1	1
tortilla, flour, nacho	Barrel O'Fun	0.5	oz.	0	1	1
tortilla, flour, white	Barrel O'Fun	0.5	oz.	0	1	1
tortilla, flour, white, mini-rounds	Barrel O'Fun	0.5	oz.	0	1	1
tortilla, flour, yellow	Barrel O'Fun Tostada	0.5	oz.	0	1	1
tortilla, flour, yellow, mini	Barrel O'Fun Tostada	0.5	oz.	0	1	1
tortilla, white corn	Barbara's Less Fat	0.5	oz.	0	1	1
tortilla, white corn	Kettle Tias	0.6	oz.	0	1	1
tortilla, white corn	Old Dutch	0.6	oz.	0	1	1
tortilla, white corn	Old El Paso	0.6	oz.	0	1	2
tortilla, white corn	Santitas 100%	0.5	oz.	0	1	1
tortilla, white corn, ranch	Barbara's Less Fat	0.5	oz.	0	1	1
Corn flake crumbs	Kellogg's	2	Tbsp.	0	1	0
Corn flour	whole grain	0.5	oz.	0	1	0
Corn flour	whole grain	0.1	cup	0	1	0
masa		0.5	oz.	0	1	0
masa		0.1	cup	0	1	0
Corn grits						
dry	Albers Quick Hominy	0.1	cup	0	1	0
dry	Goya	0.1	cup	0	1	0
instant	Quaker Original	0.4	pkg.	0	1	0
instant bacon bits	Quaker	0.4	pkg.	0	1	0
instant, butter flavor	Quaker	0.5	pkg.	0	1	0
instant, cheddar	Quaker	0.5	pkg.	0	1	0
instant, cheddar, zesty	Quaker	0.5	pkg.	0	1	0
instant, ham bits	Quaker	0.5	pkg.	0	1	0
instant, sausage bits	Quaker	0.5	pkg.	0	1	0
white	Arrowhead Mills	0.1	cup	0	1	0

FOOD ITEM	SPECIFICATIONS	BRAND NAME	QUANTITY	SIZE	PROTEIN BLOCKS	CARBOHYDRATE BLOCKS	FAT BLOCKS
	white	Quaker Hominy	0.1	cup	0	1	0
	white	Quaker Quick Hominy	0.1	cup	0	1	0
	yellow	Arrowhead Mills	0.1	cup	0	1	0
	yellow	Quaker Quick Hominy	0.1	cup	0	1	0
Corn pudding mix		Goya	0.2	cup, prepared	0	1	0
Corn relish		Green Giant	1.7	Tbsp.	0	1	0
		Nance's	2.9	Tbsp.	0	1	0
		Pickle Eater's	1.7	Tbsp.	0	1	0
Corn souffle	frozen	Stouffer's	2.2	oz.	0	1	1
Corn syrup	dark	Karo	0.6	Tbsp.	0	1	0
	light	Karo	0.6	Tbsp.	0	1	0
Cornmeal	blue or hi-lysine	Arrowhead Mills	0.1	cup	0	1	0
	blue and red	Frieda's	0.1	cup	0	1	0
	coarse	Goya	1.1	Tbsp.	0	1	0
	fine	Goya	1.3	Tbsp.	0	1	0
	self-rising, white	Aunt Jemima	1.4	Tbsp.	0	1	0
	self-rising, white	Aunt Jemima, Mix	1.5	Tbsp.	0	1	0
	self-rising, white, buttermilk	Aunt Jemima, Mix	1.6	Tbsp.	0	1	0
	self-rising, yellow	Aunt Jemima, Mix	1.5	Tbsp.	0	1	0
	white	Arrowhead Mills	0.1	cup	0	1	0
	white	Goya	1	Tbsp.	0	1	0
	white	Albers	0.8	Tbsp.	0	1	0
	yellow	Arrowhead Mills	0.1	cup	0	1	0
	yellow	Goya	0.9	Tbsp.	0	1	0
Cornstarch		Argo/Kingsford	1.3	Tbsp.	0	1	0
Cottonseed kernels	roasted		5	Tbsp.	2	1	6
Cottonseed meal	partially defatted	Durkee	0.8	oz.	1	1	0
Country gravy mix		French's	2.5	Tbsp.	0	1	1
		Loma Linda Gravy Quick	0.4	cup, prepared	0	1	1
		Arrowhead Mills	2.5	Tbsp.	0	1	1
Couscous	dry	Fantastic Foods	0.1	cup	0	1	0
	dry, whole wheat	Fantastic Foods	0.1	cup	0	1	0
	cooked		0.2	cup	0	1	0

Food	Description	Brand	Amount	Unit	P	C	F
Couscous mix	almond chicken, vegetarian	Near East Moroccan	0.3	cup, prepared	0	1	0
	asparagus au gratin	Casbah	0.3	pkg.	0	1	0
	black bean salsa	Casbah	0.3	pkg.	0	1	0
	cheddar, broccoli, creamy	Fantastic Cup	0.2	pkg.	0	1	0
	cheddar, nacho	Casbah	0.4	pkg.	0	1	0
	corn, sweet	Fantastic Cup	0.3	pkg.	0	1	0
	w/lentils	Fantastic Cup	0.3	pkg.	0	1	0
	pilaf	Fantastic Only A Pinch Cup	0.4	pkg.	0	1	0
	savory pilaf	Casbah	0.5	oz.	0	1	0
	tomato Parmesan	Fantastic Foods	0.2	cup	0	1	0
	vegetable, creole	Casbah	0.3	oz.	0	1	0
Cowpeas	fresh, raw, trimmed	Fantastic Cup	0.3	oz.	1	1	0
	fresh, boiled, drained		0.5	cup	1	1	0
	mature, boiled		0.4	cup	1	1	0
	frozen, boiled, drained		0.4	cup	1	1	0
Crabapple, canned	sliced		0.3	cup	0	1	0
	sliced	S&W	1.3	pcs.	0	1	0
	sliced	Apple Time	1.1	oz.	0	1	0
Cracker	bacon flavor	Nabisco	0.5	oz.	0	1	1
	butter/butterflavor	Barbara's Rite Lite	3.8	pcs.	0	1	0
	butter/butterflavor	Goya Tropical	1.7	oz.	0	1	1
	butter/butterflavor	Hi-Ho	0.5	pcs.	0	1	1
	butter/butterflavor	Keebler Club Partners	4	pcs.	0	1	1
	butter/butterflavor	Ritz	4.5	pcs.	0	1	1
	butter/butterflavor	Ritz Low Sodium	4.5	oz.	0	1	1
	butter/butterflavor	Toasted Complements Buttercrisp	0.5	pcs.	0	1	1
	butter/butterflavor, mini	Town House	5	oz.	0	1	2
	butter/butterflavor, thins	Ritz Bits	0.6	pcs.	0	1	2
	cheese	Pepperidge Farm	3.6	pcs.	0	1	1
	cheese	Appeteasers Original	0.6	pcs.	0	1	1
	cheese	Barbara's Bites Original/Hot & Spicy	0.4	oz.	0	1	0
	cheese	Krispy Mild Cheddar	0.5	oz.	0	1	1
	cheese	Nips	0.6	oz.	0	1	1
	cheese	Snackwells	0.5	oz.	0	1	0
	cheese	Tid-Bit	0.6	oz.	0	1	1
	cheese, chili	Munch 'ems	0.5	oz.	0	1	1

FOOD ITEM	SPECIFICATIONS	BRAND NAME	QUANTITY	SIZE	PROTEIN BLOCKS	CARBOHYDRATE BLOCKS	FAT BLOCKS
	cheese, garlic herb	Appeteasers	0.6	oz.	0	1	1
	cheese, Parmesan	Goldfish	0.6	oz.	0	1	1
	cheese, Swiss	Nabisco Swiss	0.6	oz.	0	1	1
	cheese, zesty	Snackwell's	0.5	oz.	0	1	0
	cheese, cheddar	Better Cheddars	0.6	oz.	0	1	1
	cheese, cheddar	Better Cheddars Low Sodium	0.6	oz.	0	1	1
	cheese, cheddar	Better Cheddars Reduced Fat	0.5	oz.	0	1	1
	cheese, cheddar	Cheez-It	0.6	oz.	0	1	2
	cheese, cheddar	Cheez-It Low Sodium	0.6	oz.	0	1	2
	cheese, cheddar	Cheez-It Reduced Fat	0.5	oz.	0	1	1
	cheese, cheddar	Combos	0.6	oz.	0	1	2
	cheese, cheddar	Munch 'ems	0.5	oz.	0	1	1
	cheese, cheddar	Goldfish	0.5	oz.	0	1	1
	cheese, cheddar	Goldfish Less Sodium	0.6	oz.	0	1	1
	cheese, cheddar	Snorkels	0.6	oz.	0	1	1
	cheese, cheddar, double	Appeteasers	0.6	oz.	0	1	2
	cheese, cheddar, hot and spicy	Cheez-It	0.6	oz.	0	1	2
	cheese, cheddar, white	Cheez-It	0.6	oz.	0	1	1
	cheese, cheddar, white	Wheatables	0.5	oz.	0	1	2
	cheese sandwich	Little Debbie	0.6	oz.	0	1	2
	cheese sandwich	Handi-Snacks Cheez'n Crackers	0.9	pc.	0	1	2
	cheese sandwich	Ritz	0.6	oz.	0	1	2
	cheese sandwich	Ritz Bits	0.6	oz.	0	1	2
	cheese sandwich, bacon	Frito-Lay	0.4	pkg.	0	1	1
	cheese sandwich, cheddar, golden toast	Frito-Lay	0.4	pkg.	0	1	2
	cheese sandwich, cheddar, jalapeno	Frito-Lay	0.4	pkg.	0	1	1
	cheese sandwich, cream cheese and chive, golden toast	Frito-Lay	0.4	pkg.	0	1	2
	cheese sandwich, wheat	Frito-Lay	0.4	pkg.	0	1	1
		Chicken In A Biskit	0.6	oz.	0	1	2
croissant		Carr's	0.6	oz.	0	—	0

Food	Brand / Description	Amount	Unit	Protein	Carbohydrate	Fat
flatbread	J.J. Flats Flavorall	0.9	pc.	0	1	0
flatbread	Lavosh Hawaii Classic	0.5	oz.	0	1	0
flatbread	New York	1.4	pcs.	0	1	0
flatbread	New York Everything	1.3	pcs.	0	1	0
flatbread	New York Fat Free	1.1	pcs.	0	1	0
flatbread, Cajun	New York	1.3	pcs.	0	1	0
flatbread, caraway rye	Lavosh Hawaii	0.5	oz.	0	1	0
flatbread, cracked pepper	New York Fat Free	1.1	oz.	0	1	0
flatbread, garlic	California Crisps	2	pcs.	0	1	1
flatbread, garlic	J.J. Flats	0.9	pc.	0	1	0
flatbread, garlic, roasted, or honey cinnamon	New York Fat Free	1.1	pcs.	0	1	0
flatbread, herb, Italian	J.J. Flats	1	pc.	0	1	1
flatbread, oat bran	J.J. Flats	0.9	pc.	0	1	0
flatbread, onion or poppy	California Crisps	1.8	pcs.	0	1	1
flatbread, onion	J.J. Flats	0.8	pc.	0	1	0
flatbread, onion	New York	1.4	pcs.	0	1	0
flatbread, onion, slightly	Lavosh Hawaii	0.5	oz.	0	1	0
flatbread, peppercorn	Lavosh Hawaii	0.5	oz.	0	1	0
flatbread, poppy	J.J. Flats	0.9	pc.	0	1	0
flatbread, poppy	New York	1.3	pcs.	0	1	0
flatbread, pumpernickel	New York Fat Free	1.1	pcs.	0	1	0
flatbread, pumpernickel onion	New York	1.4	pcs.	0	1	0
flatbread, pumpernickel	New York	1.3	pcs.	0	1	1
flatbread, rosemary garlic	Lavosh Hawaii	0.5	oz.	0	1	0
flatbread, sesame	J.J. Flats	1	pc.	0	1	0
flatbread, sesame	New York	1.3	pcs.	0	1	1
flatbread, 10 grain	California Crisps	1.8	pcs.	0	1	0
flatbread, 10 grain	Lavosh Hawaii	0.5	oz.	0	1	0
flatbread, vegetable, garden	New York Fat Free	1.1	pcs.	0	1	0
golden	Snackwell's Classic	5	pcs.	0	1	0
	Goldfish Original	0.5	oz.	0	1	1
	Goya Snack	4.8	pcs.	0	1	1
	Goya Tropical	1.7	pcs.	0	1	1
matzo	Manichewitz Unsalted	0.4	oz.	0	1	0

FOOD ITEM	SPECIFICATIONS	BRAND NAME	QUANTITY	SIZE	PROTEIN BLOCKS	CARBOHYDRATE BLOCKS	FAT BLOCKS
	matzo	Manichewitz Everything	0.5	oz.	0	1	0
	matzo, garlic	Manichewitz Savory	0.5	oz.	0	1	0
	matzo, rye	Manichewitz	0.5	oz.	0	1	0
	melba rounds/snacks, plain	Devonsheer	4.2	pcs.	0	1	0
	melba rounds/snacks, bacon	Old London	5	pcs.	0	1	1
	melba rounds/snacks, cheese	Old London	4.5	pcs.	0	1	0
	melba rounds/snacks, garlic	Devonsheer	4.5	pcs.	0	1	0
	melba rounds/snacks, garlic	Old London	5	pcs.	0	1	1
	melba rounds/snacks, herb, savory	Devonsheer	4.5	pcs.	0	1	0
	melba rounds/snacks, honey bran	Devonsheer	4.2	pcs.	0	1	0
	melba rounds/snacks, onion	Devonsheer	4.5	pcs.	0	1	0
	melba rounds/snacks, onion	Old London	5	pcs.	0	1	1
	melba rounds/snacks, Mexican corn	Old London	5.6	pcs.	0	1	1
	melba rounds/snacks, rye	Old London	4.5	pcs.	0	1	0
	melba rounds/snacks, sesame	Devonsheer	5	pcs.	0	1	1
	melba rounds/snacks, sesame	Old London	5.6	pcs.	0	1	1
	melba rounds/snacks, 12 grain	Devonsheer	4.2	pcs.	0	1	0
	melba rounds/snacks, vegetable	Devonsheer	4.2	pcs.	0	1	0
	melba rounds/snacks, white	Old London	5	pcs.	0	1	1
	melba rounds/snacks, whole grain	Old London	5	pcs.	0	1	1
	melba toast, plain, rye or wheat	Devonsheer	4.5	pcs.	0	1	0
	melba toast, plain or wheat	Devonsheer No Salt	4.5	pcs.	0	1	0
	melba toast, onion	Old London	4.5	pcs.	0	1	0
	melba toast, rye	Devonsheer	4.5	pcs.	0	1	0
	melba toast, rye	Old London	4.5	pcs.	0	1	0
	melba toast, sesame	Devonsheer	1.1	oz.	0	1	0

Food	Brand	Amount	Unit	Protein	Carbohydrate	Fat
melba toast, sesame	Devonsheer/Old London No Salt	1.2	oz.	0	1	1
melba toast, sesame	Old London	1.2	oz.	0	1	1
melba toast, 12 grain or vegetable	Devonsheer	1	oz.	0	1	0
melba toast, wheat	Old London	1.1	oz.	0	1	0
melba toast, white	Old London	1	oz.	0	1	0
melba toast, whole grain	Old London	1.1	oz.	0	1	0
milk	Royal Lunch	1.1	pcs.	0	1	1
multigrain	Hi-Ho	0.6	oz.	0	1	2
multigrain	Wheat Thins	0.5	oz.	0	1	1
multigrain 5	Harvest Crisps	0.5	oz.	0	1	1
oat	Munch' ems	0.5	oz.	0	1	1
oat	Harvest Crisps	0.5	oz.	0	1	1
onion	Oat Thins	0.6	oz.	0	1	1
onion, French	Toasted Complements	0.5	oz.	0	1	0
onion, French	Snackwell's	0.5	oz.	0	1	1
peanut butter	Wheatables	0.5	oz.	0	1	2
peanut butter	Combos	0.7	oz.	0	1	3
peanut butter, graham	Handi-Snacks	0.9	oz.	0	1	2
peanut butter sandwich	Handi-Snacks Graham Stick	0.8	oz.	0	1	2
peanut butter sandwich, cheese	Ritz	0.6	oz.	0	1	2
peanut butter sandwich, cheese	Little Debbie	0.6	oz.	0	1	1
peanut butter sandwich, cheese	Frito-Lay	0.4	pkg.	0	1	1
peanut butter sandwich, cheese	Nabs	0.5	oz.	0	1	1
peanut butter sandwich, toast	Planters	0.6	oz.	0	1	1
peanut butter sandwich, toast	Frito-Lay	0.4	pkg.	0	1	1
peanut butter sandwich, toast	Little Debbie	0.6	oz.	0	1	1
peanut butter sandwich, toast	Nabs	0.5	oz.	0	1	1
peanut butter sandwich, toast	Planters	0.6	pkg.	0	1	1
peanut butter sandwich, toast	Sunshine	0.6	pkg.	0	1	2
pizza	Goldfish	0.6	oz.	0	1	1
pizza, all varieties	Health Valley	6	pcs.	0	1	0

FOOD ITEM	SPECIFICATIONS	BRAND NAME	QUANTITY	SIZE	PROTEIN BLOCKS	CARBOHYDRATE BLOCKS	FAT BLOCKS
	pizza bites	Barbara's	0.4	oz.	0	1	0
	potato au gratin	No Fries	0.4	oz.	0	1	0
	potato, barbeque	No Fries	0.4	oz.	0	1	0
	potato, sour cream and chives	No Fries	0.4	oz.	0	1	0
	ranch	Munch 'ems	0.5	oz.	0	1	1
	rice, bran	Health Valley	0.6	oz.	0	1	1
	rice, brown	Eden	0.5	oz.	0	1	0
	salsa	Munch 'ems	0.5	oz.	0	1	1
	saltines	Dux	2.2	pcs.	0	1	0
	saltines	Krispy	4.5	pcs.	0	1	0
	saltines	Krispy Fat Free	3.8	pcs.	0	1	0
	saltines	Krispy Unsalted Top	4.5	pcs.	0	1	0
	saltines	Premium	4.5	pcs.	0	1	0
	saltines	Premium Fat Free	4.2	pcs.	0	1	0
	saltines	Premium Low Sodium	4.5	pcs.	0	1	0
	saltines	Premium Unsalted Top	4.5	pcs.	0	1	1
	saltines	Zesta	4.5	pcs.	0	1	0
	saltines, cracked pepper	Krispy	4.5	pcs.	0	1	1
	saltines, mini	Premium Bits	0.5	oz.	0	1	1
	sesame	Brenton	0.6	oz.	0	1	1
	sesame	Pepperidge Farm	3.8	oz.	0	1	1
	sesame	Toasted Complements	0.5	oz.	0	1	1
	sesame cheese	Twigs	0.6	oz.	0	1	1
		Sociables	7	oz.	0	1	1
	soup and oyster	Krispy	0.4	oz.	0	1	0
	soup and oyster	Oysterettes	0.5	oz.	0	1	1
	soup and oyster	Premium	0.5	oz.	0	1	0
	sour cream and onion	Munch 'ems	0.5	oz.	0	1	1
		Uneeda	1.7	pcs.	0	1	0
	vegetable	Garden Crisps	0.5	oz.	0	1	1
	vegetable	Vegetable Thins	0.6	oz.	0	1	2
	water or soda	Brenton	0.5	oz.	0	1	1
	water or soda	Brenton Less Salt	0.5	oz.	0	1	1

Description	Brand	Amount	Unit			
water or soda	Brenton Light	0.4	oz.	1	1	0
water or soda	Cabaret	0.5	oz.	1	1	0
water or soda	Carr's Table Water	3.6	pcs.	0	1	0
water or soda	Crown Pilot	0.7	.6-oz. pc.	0	1	0
water or soda	Dux	2.2	pcs.	0	1	0
water or soda	Hi-Ho	0.6	oz.	2	1	0
water or soda	Pepperidge Farm Original	0.4	oz.	0	1	0
water or soda	Vivant	0.5	oz.	1	1	0
water or soda, cracked pepper	Carr's Table Water	3.6	pcs.	0	1	0
water or soda, cracked pepper	Hi-Ho	0.6	oz.	2	1	0
water or soda, cracked pepper	Pepperidge Farm	0.4	oz.	0	1	0
water or soda, cracked pepper	Snackwell's	0.4	oz.	0	1	0
water or soda, poppy sesame	Carr's	0.5	oz.	1	1	0
water or soda, sesame	Brenton	0.6	oz.	1	1	0
water or soda, sesame	Carr's Table Water	3.6	pcs.	0	1	0
wheat	Snackwell's Fat Free	0.4	oz.	0	1	0
wheat	Stoned Wheat Thins	1.8	pcs.	0	1	0
wheat	Stoned Wheat Thins Lower Sodium	1.8	pcs.	0	1	0
wheat	Toasted Complements	0.5	oz.	0	1	0
wheat	Triscuit	0.6	oz.	1	1	0
wheat	Triscuit Low Sodium	0.6	oz.	1	1	0
wheat	Triscuit Reduced Fat	0.5	oz.	1	1	0
wheat	Waverly	0.5	oz.	0	1	0
wheat	Wheat Thins	0.6	oz.	1	1	0
wheat	Wheat Thins Low Salt	0.6	oz.	1	1	0
wheat	Wheat Thins Reduced Fat	0.5	oz.	1	1	0
wheat	Wheatables	0.6	oz.	1	1	0
wheat	Wheatsworth	0.6	oz.	1	1	0
wheat, all varieties	Barbara's Wheatines	0.8	1/2-oz. sq.	0	1	0
wheat, cracked	Pepperidge Farm	2	pcs.	1	1	0
wheat, hearty	Pepperidge Farm	3	pcs.	1	1	0
wheat, herb, garden	Triscuit	0.6	oz.	1	1	0
wheat, and rye	Triscuit Deli	0.6	oz.	1	1	0
wheat, whole	Carr's	1.8	pcs.	1	1	0
wheat, whole	Health Valley No Salt	5	pcs.	0	1	0
wheat, whole	Hi-Ho	0.6	oz.	2	1	0

FOOD ITEM	SPECIFICATIONS	BRAND NAME	QUANTITY	SIZE	PROTEIN BLOCKS	CARBOHYDRATE BLOCKS	FAT BLOCKS
	wheat, whole	Krispy	4.5	pcs.	0	1	0
	wheat, whole, all varieties	Health Valley	5	pcs.	0	1	0
	wheat, whole, and bran	Triscuit	0.6	oz.	0	1	1
		Zwieback	5	oz.	0	1	1
Cracker crumbs and meal	crumbs	Ritz	0.2	cup	0	1	1
	crumbs, saltine	Premium Fat Free	0.1	cup	0	1	0
	matzo meal	Manischewitz	0.1	cup	0	1	0
	matzo meal	Streit's	0.1	cup	0	1	0
Cranberry, fresh, raw	whole		1.3	cup	0	1	0
	chopped		1	cup	0	1	0
Cranberry, dried		Sonoma	0.1	cup	0	1	0
Cranberry bean	boiled		0.2	cup	0	1	0
	canned		0.2	cup	0	1	0
Cranberry drink		Farmer's Market	2.4	fl. oz.	0	1	0
		Tropicana Punch	2.1	fl. oz.	0	1	0
		Tropicana Punch	2.1	fl. oz.	0	1	0
		Tropicana Ruby Red	2.4	fl. oz.	0	1	0
	spiced	J.M.S. Cooler	2.4	fl. oz.	0	1	0
Cranberry drink blends	hibiscus	Heinke's	2.4	fl. oz.	0	1	0
	hibiscus	R.W. Knudsen	2.4	fl. oz.	0	1	0
	lemon	Santa Cruz	2.5	fl. oz.	0	1	0
	raspberry	After the Fall	3.1	fl. oz.	0	1	0
	raspberry	R.W. Knudsen	2	fl. oz.	0	1	0
	raspberry-strawberry	Tropicana Twister	2.4	fl. oz.	0	1	0
	raspberry-strawberry	Tropicana Twister Light	6.7	fl. oz.	0	1	0
Cranberry juice		After the Fall Cape Cod	3	fl. oz.	0	1	0
		After the Fall Nantucket	4.7	fl. oz.	0	1	0
		Apple Eve Naturally Cranberry	2.4	fl. oz.	0	1	0
		Heinke's 100%	5	fl. oz.	0	1	0
		Ocean Spray Cocktail	2.1	fl. oz.	0	1	0
		R.W. Knudsen Concentrate	5.7	fl. oz.	0	1	0
		R.W. Knudsen Just Cranberry	5	fl. oz.	0	1	0
		R.W. Knudsen Yankee	2.4	fl. oz.	0	1	0

Category	Food	Brand / Note	Amount	Unit			
Cranberry juice blends	apple	Season's Best Medley	2.5	fl. oz.	0	1	0
	apricot	Snapple	2.4	fl. oz.	0	1	0
	blueberry	Cranapple	1.8	fl. oz.	0	1	0
		Cranicot	1.8	fl. oz.	0	1	0
		Cran*Blueberry	1.7	fl. oz.	0	1	0
	grape	Apple & Eve	2.1	fl. oz.	0	1	0
	grape	Cran*Grape	1.7	fl. oz.	0	1	0
	grapefruit	After the Fall	2.5	fl. oz.	0	1	0
	kiwi	After the Fall	2.8	fl. oz.	0	1	0
	mango	After the Fall	2.8	fl. oz.	0	1	0
	orange	After the Fall	2.6	fl. oz.	0	1	0
	punch	Crantastic	2	fl. oz.	0	1	0
	raspberry	After the Fall	3.1	fl. oz.	0	1	0
	strawberry	After the Fall	2.8	fl. oz.	0	1	0
	strawberry	Ocean Spray	2.1	fl. oz.	0	1	0
Cranberry nectar		Heinke's	2.4	fl. oz.	0	1	0
		R.W. Knudsen	1.9	fl. oz.	0	1	0
		Santa Cruz	2.7	fl. oz.	0	1	0
	guava	Santa Cruz	3	fl. oz.	0	1	0
Cranberry sauce		Ocean Spray	0.8	oz.	0	1	0
		R.W. Knudsen	1.4	Tbsp.	0	1	0
		S&W	0.1	cup	0	1	0
Cranberry sauce blends	w/orange or raspberry	Cran*Fruit	0.8	oz.	0	1	0
	w/strawberry	Cran*Fruit	0.8	oz.	0	1	0
Cranberry-orange relish	in jars	New England	0.1	cup	0	1	0
Cream of tartar		Tone's	10	Tbsp.	0	1	0
Cress, garden	raw		5	cup	0	1	0
	boiled, drained		2.5	cup	0	1	1
Croissant	butter	Awrey's	1.1	oz.	1	1	1
	butter	Awrey's	1.1	oz.	1	1	2
	butter	Awrey's Tip-to-Tip	0.3	pc.	0	1	2
	butter	Pepperidge Farm Petite	0.7	pc.	0	1	2
	margarine	Awrey's Tip-to-Tip	0.6	pc.	0	1	2
	margarine, sandwich	Awrey's	0.9	oz.	0	1	2
	margarine, sandwich	Awrey's	1	oz.	0	1	2
	margarine, sandwich, wheat	Awrey's	0.4	pc.	0	1	2
	frozen	Sara Lee	0.5	pc.	0	1	1

CARBOHYDRATES

FOOD ITEM	SPECIFICATIONS	BRAND NAME	QUANTITY	SIZE	PROTEIN BLOCKS	CARBOHYDRATE BLOCKS	FAT BLOCKS
Crookneck squash	fresh, sliced, raw, ends trimmed		2.5	cup	1	1	1
	fresh, sliced, boiled, drained		1.7	cup	0	1	0
	canned, cut, drained, no salt		2.5	cup	1	1	0
	frozen, boiled, sliced		1	cup	0	1	0
Croutons	Caesar	Brownberry	0.6	oz.	0	1	1
	Caesar	Pepperidge Farm	0.6	oz.	0	1	1
	cheddar	Brownberry	0.6	oz.	0	1	1
	cheddar and Romano	Pepperidge Farm	0.6	oz.	0	1	1
	cheese and garlic	Arnold Crispy	0.4	oz.	0	1	1
	cheese and garlic	Brownberry	0.4	oz.	0	1	1
	cheese and garlic	Pepperidge Farm	0.6	oz.	0	1	1
	cracked pepper and Parmesan	Pepperidge Farm	0.6	oz.	0	1	1
	garlic	Old London Restaurant Style	0.6	oz.	0	1	1
	herb, fine	Arnold Crispy	0.4	oz.	0	1	1
	Italian	Arnold Crispy	0.6	oz.	0	1	1
	Italian	Old London Restaurant Style	0.6	oz.	0	1	1
	Italian, zesty	Pepperidge Farm	0.6	oz.	0	1	1
	olive oil and garlic	Pepperidge Farm	0.4	oz.	0	1	1
	onion and garlic	Arnold Crispy	0.4	oz.	0	1	1
	onion and garlic	Brownberry	0.6	oz.	0	1	1
	onion and garlic	Pepperidge Farm	0.4	oz.	0	1	1
	ranch	Arnold Crispy	0.4	oz.	0	1	1
	ranch	Brownberry	0.6	oz.	0	1	1
	ranch	Pepperidge Farm	0.6	oz.	0	1	1
	seasoned	Arnold Crispy	0.4	oz.	0	1	1
	seasoned	Brownberry	0.6	oz.	0	1	1
	seasoned	Pepperidge Farm	0.6	oz.	0	1	1
	sourdough	Old London Restaurant Style	0.6	oz.	0	1	1
	sourdough, cheese	Pepperidge Farm	0.6	oz.	0	1	1
	toasted	Brownberry	0.4	oz.	0	1	1
Cucumber, w/peel	sliced		1.4	medium	0	1	0
	sliced		5	cup	0	1	0
Cucumber dip	creamy	Kraft Premium	10	Tbsp.	0	1	7

CARBOHYDRATES

Food	Description	Brand	Amount	Unit	Protein	Carbohydrate	Fat
Cucumber salad		Rosoff/Schorr's	3.3	oz.	0	1	0
Cumin seed			10	tsp.	0	1	2
Currant	fresh, black, Europe		0.8	cup	0	1	0
Currant	fresh, red or white		0.8	cup	0	1	0
Currant	dried, zante		0.1	cup	0	1	0
Currant	dried, zante	S&W	0.1	cup	0	1	0
Curry powder			3.3	Tbsp.	0	1	1
Curry sauce, cooking		Kylin Thai	0.4	cup	0	1	0
	hot, madras	Patak's	0.3	cup	0	1	5
	hot, tikka masala	Patak's	0.4	cup	0	1	5
	hot, vindaloo	Patak's	0.4	cup	0	1	8
	jalfrezzi	Patak's	0.4	cup	0	1	3
	Masala	Shahi Cream	0.6	cup	0	1	3
	Masala	Shahi Curry	0.8	cup	0	1	4
	rogan josh	Patak's	0.6	cup	0	1	6
Curry sauce mix		Knorr	0.5	pkg.	0	1	1
Custard apple	trimmed		1.4	oz.	0	1	0
Daiquiri mixer	bottled	Holland House/Mr. & Mrs. "T"	1.1	fl. oz.	0	1	0
	bottled, strawberry	Holland House	0.9	fl. oz.	0	1	0
	frozen, prepared, strawberry	Barcardi	2.1	fl. oz.	0	1	0
	mix	Bar-Tenders	0.6	pkts.	0	1	0
Dandelion greens	raw, chopped		2.5	cup	1	1	1
	boiled, drained, chopped		2.5	cup	1	1	1
Danish, cake, ring, or twist	all varieties	Awrey's Petite	0.6	pc.	0	1	2
	apple	Awrey's Grande	0.2	pc.	0	1	2
	apple	Hostess	0.2	pc.	0	1	1
	apple	Hostess Fruit Roll	0.3	pc.	0	1	0
	apple	Hostess Twist	0.2	pc.	0	1	0
	apple, cheese, cinnamon swirl, or strawberry	Awrey's	0.3	pc.	0	1	2
	caramel pecan swirl	Hostess	0.4	pc.	0	1	2
	cheese	Awrey's Grande	0.2	pc.	0	1	0
	cheese	Tastykake Pocket	0.3	pc.	0	1	2
	cheese, cherry or lemon	Awrey's Marquise	0.2	pc.	0	1	2
	cheese, cinnamon	Awrey's Marquise	0.1	pc.	0	1	1
	cheese, raspberry swirl	Awrey's Grande	0.2	pc.	0	1	1

FOOD ITEM	SPECIFICATIONS	BRAND NAME	QUANTITY	SIZE	PROTEIN BLOCKS	CARBOHYDRATE BLOCKS	FAT BLOCKS
	cinnamon swirl	Awrey's Grande	0.2	pc.	0	1	1
	pecan	Hostess Spinners	0.6	pc.	0	1	1
	raspberry	Hostess	0.4	pc.	0	1	0
	strawberry	Awrey's Grande	0.2	pc.	0	1	2
Danish, frozen	apple or raspberry	Pepperidge Farm	0.3	pc.	0	1	1
or refrigerated	cheese	Pepperidge Farm	0.4	pc.	0	1	1
Date, dehydrated	course ground	Dole	0.4	oz.	0	1	0
Date, dried, pitted		Del Monte	0.5	oz.	0	1	0
		Dole	0.1	cup	0	1	0
	chopped	Sonoma	0.5	oz.	0	1	0
		Del Monte	0.4	oz.	0	1	0
		Dole	0.1	cup	0	1	0
	natural, dry		1.6	dates	0	1	0
Date nut pastry		Awrey's	0.5	pc.	0	1	1
Demi-glace sauce mix		Knorr	2.5	Tbsp.	0	1	1
Dessert mix, no bake	banana cream	Betty Crocker	0.03	pkg.	0	1	0
	chocolate French silk	Betty Crocker	0.03	pkg.	0	1	0
	coconut cream	Betty Crocker	0.03	pkg.	0	1	1
	cookies 'n creme	Betty Crocker	0.03	pkg.	0	1	0
	lemon supreme	Betty Crocker	0.02	pkg.	0	1	0
Diable sauce		Escoffier	2.5	Tbsp.	0	1	0
Dill seed	dried		10	tsp.	0	1	1
Dill weed			10	tsp.	0	1	0
Dock	boiled, drained		10	oz.	1	1	1
Donut	plain	Awrey's	0.7	oz.	0	1	2
	plain	Awrey's	0.9	oz.	0	1	2
	plain	Hostess	0.7	oz.	0	1	1
	plain	Hostess Jumbo	0.7	oz.	0	1	1
	plain	Hostess Old Fashion	0.4	pc.	0	1	1
	plain	Tastykake Assorted	0.5	pc.	0	1	2
	assorted	Hostess	0.4	pc.	0	1	1
	cinnamon	Hostess	0.6	pc.	0	1	1
	cinnamon	Hostess Gems	1.2	pcs.	0	1	1

Food	Brand	Amount	Unit	Protein	Fat	Carbohydrate
cinnamon	Tastykake Assorted	0.4	pc.	0	1	2
cinnamon, sugar	Entenmann's Variety Pack	0.3	pc.	0	1	2
coconut top	Awrey's	0.4	pc.	0	1	1
crumb	Entenmann's	0.3	pc.	0	1	1
crumb	Entenmann's Variety Pack	0.2	pc.	0	1	1
crumb	Hostess	0.6	pc.	0	1	2
crunch	Awrey's	0.3	pc.	0	1	1
crunch top	Awrey's	0.5	pc.	0	1	1
devil's food crumb	Entenmann's	0.3	pc.	0	1	1
frosted/iced, chocolate	Awrey's	0.7	oz.	0	1	2
frosted/iced, chocolate	Awrey's	0.7	oz.	0	1	2
frosted/iced, chocolate	Hostess	0.7	oz.	0	1	2
frosted/iced, chocolate	Hostess Gems	1.4	pcs.	0	1	2
frosted/iced, chocolate	Hostess Jumbo	0.7	oz.	0	1	2
frosted/iced, chocolate, chocolate	Awrey's	0.6	oz.	0	1	1
frosted/iced, chocolate, chocolate	Awrey's	0.7	oz.	0	1	1
frosted/iced, chocolate, chocolate, mini	Hostess	1.4	pcs.	0	1	1
frosted/iced, chocolate, custard Bismark	Awrey	0.3	pc.	0	1	2
frosted/iced, chocolate, mini	Sonoma	0.8	pcs.	0	1	3
frosted/iced, chocolate, rich	Entenmann's	0.3	pc.	0	1	2
frosted/iced, chocolate, rich	Entenmann's Variety Pack	0.3	pc.	0	1	2
frosted/iced, chocolate, rich	Tastykake	0.3	pc.	0	1	2
frosted/iced, chocolate, rich, mini	Tastykake	1.3	pcs.	0	1	2
frosted/iced, chocolate, rich, w/raspberry	Entenmann's	0.3	pc.	0	1	2
frosted/iced, chocolate, ring	Awrey's	0.3	pc.	0	1	2
frosted/iced, chocolate, sour cream	Awrey's	0.2	pc.	0	1	1
glazed	Entenmann's Popems	1.6	pcs.	0	1	1
glazed	Hostess Old Fashion	0.3	pc.	0	1	1
glazed	Hostess Party	0.2	pc.	0	1	1

FOOD ITEM	SPECIFICATIONS	BRAND NAME	QUANTITY	SIZE	PROTEIN BLOCKS	CARBOHYDRATE BLOCKS	FAT BLOCKS
	glazed	Hostess Whirl	0.3	pc.	0	1	1
	glazed, buttermilk	Entenmann's	0.3	pc.	0	1	1
	glazed, chocolate	Entenmann's Popems	1.3	pcs.	0	1	1
	glazed, honey, devil's food	Awrey's	0.2	pc.	0	1	2
	glazed, honey, ring	Awrey's	0.3	pc.	0	1	1
	glazed, honey wheat	Hostess Old Fashion	0.3	pc.	0	1	1
	glazed, orange	Tastykake	0.3	pc.	0	1	1
	glazed, sour cream	Awrey's	0.2	pc.	0	1	1
	honey wheat	Tastykake	0.3	pc.	0	1	1
	honey wheat, mini	Tastykake	1.4	pcs.	0	1	1
	powdered sugar	Awrey's	0.7	oz.	0	1	2
	powdered sugar	Awrey's	0.5	oz.	0	1	2
	powdered sugar	Hostess	0.6	oz.	0	1	1
	powdered sugar	Hostess Jumbo	0.6	oz.	0	1	1
	powdered sugar	Hostess Gems	1.2	pcs.	0	1	1
	powdered sugar	Tastykake Assorted	0.4	pc.	0	1	1
	powdered sugar, jelly Bismark	Awrey's	0.3	pc.	0	1	2
	powdered sugar, mini	Tastykake	1.4	pcs.	0	1	1
	powdered sugar, raspberry fill	Hostess O's	0.3	pc.	0	1	1
	sour creme, plain	Awrey's	0.2	pc.	0	1	2
	sprinkle topped	Awrey's	0.5	pc.	0	1	1
	strawberry filled, frosted	Hostess Gems	1	pcs.	0	1	1
	strawberry filled, powdered	Hostess Gems	0.9	pcs.	0	1	1
	vanilla iced	Awrey's Long John	0.3	pc.	0	1	2
	vanilla iced, jelly Bismark	Awrey's	0.3	pc.	0	1	2
	white iced	Awrey's	0.4	pc.	0	1	1
Donut, frozen	glazed	Rich's	0.6	pc.	0	1	1
Eclair	chocolate, frozen	Rich's	0.4	1 pc.	0	1	1
	shrimp	Chung King	0.4	3-oz. roll	0	1	1
	shrimp	La Choy	0.4	3-oz. roll	0	1	1
	shrimp, mini	Chung King	2.1	rolls	0	1	1
	shrimp, mini	La Choy	2.1	rolls	0	1	0
	vegetables, w/lobster, mini	La Choy	2.3	rolls	0	1	1

Food	Description	Brand	Amount	Unit			
Egg roll, frozen	chicken	Empire Kosher	0.3	3-oz. roll	0	1	1
	chicken	Empire Kosher Mini	1.5	rolls	0	1	1
	chicken	Chun King	0.5	3-oz. roll	1	1	1
	chicken, sweet and sour	La Choy	0.5	3-oz. roll	1	1	1
	chicken, mini	La Choy	0.3	3-oz. roll	0	1	0
	chicken, mini	Chung King	2	rolls	0	1	1
	pork	La Choy	2	rolls	0	1	1
	pork	Chung King	0.5	3-oz. roll	1	1	1
	pork, moo shu	La Choy	0.5	3-oz. roll	1	1	1
	pork and shrimp, mini	La Choy	0.3	3-oz. roll	0	1	1
	pork and shrimp, mini	Chung King	2	rolls	0	1	1
	pork and shrimp, mini, bite size	La Choy	2.3	rolls	0	1	1
		La Choy	5	rolls	0	1	1
Egg roll, vegetarian	frozen	Worthington	0.5	rolls	0	1	1
Egg roll wrapper		Frieda's	0.7	pcs.	0	1	0
Eggnog, dairy		Nasoya	0.6	oz.	0	1	0
		Borden	0.3	cup	0	1	2
		Borden Light	0.2	cup	0	1	1
		Crowley	0.2	cup	0	1	1
		Crowley Light	0.2	cup	0	1	0
		Crowley Nonfat	0.2	cup	0	1	0
Eggplant		Frieda's	2.5	cup	0	1	0
	fresh, raw		2.5	cup	0	1	0
	boiled, drained		5.8	oz.	0	1	0
	Japanese, raw, w/peel		1.7	Tbsp.	0	1	0
	roasted		0.9	Tbsp.	0	1	0
Eggplant appetizer		Frieda's	0.6	cup	0	1	0
Eggplant pickle relish		Peloponnese	0.3	pcs.	0	1	1
Elderberry		Patak's Brinjal	1.2	pcs.	0	1	0
Empanadilla, frozen	plain		0.3	pcs.	0	1	1
	plain, cocktail size		0.8	cup	0	1	1
	pizza flavor		0.8	cup	0	1	2
Enchilada sauce		Chi-Chi's	2.5	cup	0	1	1
		La Victoria	0.8	cup	0	1	2
	green chili	Las Palmas	0.8	cup	0	1	2
		Rosarita					1
		Las Palmas					2

FOOD ITEM	SPECIFICATIONS	BRAND NAME	QUANTITY	SIZE	PROTEIN BLOCKS	CARBOHYDRATE BLOCKS	FAT BLOCKS
	green chili	Old El Paso	0.8	cup	0	1	2
	hot	Las Palmas	1.3	cup	0	1	1
	hot	Old El Paso	0.6	cup	0	1	1
	mild	Old El Paso	0.6	cup	0	1	1
Enchilada seasoning mix		Durkee	7.5	tsp.	0	1	0
		Lawry's	5	tsp.	0	1	0
		Old El Paso	10	tsp.	0	1	0
Endive	chopped		12.5	cup	1	1	1
Eppaw			0.3	cup	0	1	0
Etouffee dinner mix		Luzianne	0.1	pkg.	0	1	0
	and marinade	World Harbors Guadalupe	1.8	Tbsp.	0	1	0
	skillet	Lawry's	10	Tbsp.	0	1	0
Fajita seasoning mix		Lawry's	6.7	tsp.	0	1	0
	beef	Durkee Easy	0.4	pkg.	0	1	0
Falafel mix		Casbah	0.1	pkg.	0	1	1
		Fantastic Falafil	0.1	cup	0	1	0
		Near East	1.8	fried patties	1	1	4
Farina, whole grain	dry		0.4	oz.	0	1	0
	cooked		0.4	cup	0	1	0
Fennel seed			10	tsp.	0	1	1
Fenugreek seed			5	tsp.	1	1	1
Fettuccine entree mix	refrigerated	Contadina	0.3	cup	0	1	0
	w/creamy basil sauce	Noodle Roni	0.2	cup, prepared	0	1	2
		Knorr Cup	0.2	pkg.	0	1	0
Fig	fresh		0.9	large	0	1	0
	fresh		1.1	medium	0	1	0
	fresh, Calimyrna	Frieda's	1.7	oz.	0	1	0
	canned, in syrup		0.2	cup	0	1	0
	canned, in syrup, Kadota	S&W Southwestern	1.6	figs	0	1	0
	dried		0.9	figs	0	1	0
	dried, California		1.2	figs	0	1	0
	dried, Clamata string	Agora	0.1	cup	0	1	0
	dried, Calimyrna or Mission	Blue Ribbon/Sun-Maid	1.5	figs	0	1	0

Food	Variety	Brand	Amount	Unit			
Filo pastry	frozen	Apollo	0.03	pkg.	0	1	0
Fish sauce mix	lemon butter	Weight Watcher's	2.5	cup, prepared	0	1	0
Fish seasoning	batter seasoning, Cajun	Tone's	3.3	tsp.	0	1	0
	seafood	Tone's	10	tsp.	1	1	2
Fish seasoning and coating mix		Shake'n Bake	0.2	pkt.	0	1	0
	lemon butter	Durkee/French's Roasting Bag	0.4	pkt.	0	1	0
	lemon pepper-dill	Durkee Easy	0.4	pkt.	0	1	1
	tomato basil	Durkee Easy	0.4	pkt.	0	1	0
Frosting, ready to spread	caramel pecan	Pillsbury Supreme/Creamy Supreme	1	Tbsp.	0	1	1
	chocolate	Betty Crocker Creamy Deluxe	0.7	Tbsp.	0	1	1
	chocolate	Pillsbury Creamy Supreme	0.9	Tbsp.	0	1	1
	chocolate	Pillsbury Supreme	0.9	Tbsp.	0	1	1
	chocolate	Pillsbury Supreme/Creamy Supreme Confetti	0.8	Tbsp.	0	1	1
	chocolate, dark	Pillsbury Supreme/Creamy Supreme	0.9	Tbsp.	0	1	1
	chocolate, fudge	Pillsbury Creamy Supreme	0.9	Tbsp.	0	1	1
	chocolate, fudge	Pillsbury Supreme	0.9	Tbsp.	0	1	1
	chocolate, fudge	Pillsbury Supreme/Creamy Supreme Reduced Fat	0.7	Tbsp.	0	1	0
	chocolate, milk	Betty Crocker Creamy Deluxe	0.7	Tbsp.	0	1	1
	chocolate, milk	Pillsbury Supreme/Creamy Supreme	0.9	Tbsp.	0	1	1
	chocolate, milk	Pillsbury Supreme/Creamy Supreme Lovin' Lites	0.7	Tbsp.	0	1	0
	chocolate, milk, swirl w/ fudge glaze	Pillsbury Supreme/Creamy Supreme	0.8	Tbsp.	0	1	1
	chocolate, Swiss almond	Betty Crocker Creamy Deluxe	0.7	Tbsp.	0	1	1
	coconut, almond	Pillsbury Supreme	1	Tbsp.	0	1	2
	coconut, pecan	Pillsbury Supreme/Creamy Supreme	1.1	Tbsp.	0	1	2
	cookie	Pillsbury Supreme/Creamy Supreme Oreo	0.8	Tbsp.	0	1	1
	cream cheese	Betty Crocker Creamy Deluxe	0.7	Tbsp.	0	1	1
	cream cheese	Pillsbury Supreme/Creamy Supreme	0.7	Tbsp.	0	1	1
	creamy candy	Pillsbury Supreme/Creamy Supreme	0.8	Tbsp.	0	1	1
	lemon creme	Pillsbury Supreme/Creamy Supreme	0.7	Tbsp.	0	1	1
	rainbow chip	Betty Crocker Creamy Deluxe	0.7	Tbsp.	0	1	1
	strawberry creme	Pillsbury Supreme/Creamy Supreme	0.7	Tbsp.	0	1	1

FOOD ITEM	SPECIFICATIONS	BRAND NAME	QUANTITY	SIZE	PROTEIN BLOCKS	CARBOHYDRATE BLOCKS	FAT BLOCKS
	vanilla	Betty Crocker Creamy Deluxe	0.7	Tbsp.	0	1	1
	vanilla	Pillsbury Supreme/Creamy Supreme	0.8	Tbsp.	0	1	1
	vanilla	Pillsbury Creamy Supreme Funfetti	0.7	Tbsp.	0	1	1
	vanilla	Pillsbury Supreme Funfetti	0.7	Tbsp.	0	1	1
	vanilla	Pillsbury Supreme/Creamy Supreme Lovin' Lites	0.6	Tbsp.	0	1	0
	vanilla, French	Betty Crocker Creamy Deluxe	0.7	Tbsp.	0	1	1
	vanilla, French	Pillsbury Creamy Supreme	0.9	Tbsp.	0	1	1
	vanilla, French	Pillsbury Supreme	0.7	Tbsp.	0	1	1
	vanilla, pink	Pillsbury Supreme/Creamy Supreme Funfetti	0.7	Tbsp.	0	1	1
	vanilla, swirl, w/fudge glaze	Pillsbury Supreme/Creamy Supreme	0.7	Tbsp.	0	1	1
Fructose		Estee	2.5	tsp.	0	1	0
Fruit, mixed, candied		S&W Glace	0.8	Tbsp.	0	1	0
		White Swan	0.5	Tbsp.	0	1	0
		White Swan Deluxe	0.7	Tbsp.	0	1	0
	fruit and peel mis	Paradise Old English	0.5	Tbsp.	0	1	0
	cake mix	Queen Anne/Paradise Extra Fancy	0.7	Tbsp.	0	1	0
Fruit, mixed, canned	in juice, chunky	Del Monte Naturals	0.3	cup	0	1	0
	in juice, chunky	Libby's Lite	1.7	cup	0	1	0
	in juice, chunky	S&W Natural	0.3	cup	0	1	0
	in juice or extra light syrup	Del Monte Lite/Snack Cups	0.3	cup	0	1	0
	in light syrup	Del Monte Snack Cup	1.8	oz.	0	1	0
	in heavy syrup	Del Monte Snack Cup	1.9	oz.	0	1	0
	in heavy syrup, chunky	Del Monte	0.2	cup	0	1	0
	tropical salad, in light syrup	Del Monte	0.2	cup	0	1	0
	tropical salad, in light syrup	Dole	0.2	cup	0	1	0
	tropical salad, in heavy syrup	Dole	0.2	cup	0	1	0
Fruit, mixed, dried		Del Monte	0.1	cup	0	1	0
		Dole Sun Giant	0.7	cup	0	1	0
		Sonoma	0.5	oz.	0	1	0
	diced	Sonoma	0.1	oz.	0	1	0
Fruit, mixed, frozen		Big Valley	0.5	cup	0	1	0
		Stilwell	0.5	cup	0	1	0

Category	Flavor	Brand	Amount	Unit	Protein	Carbohydrate	Fat
Fruit bar, frozen	all flavors	Dole	1.5	oz.	0	1	0
	all flavors	Dole 'n Sugar	2.5	oz.	0	1	0
	all flavors, except coconut	Edy's	0.4	pc.	0	1	0
	all flavors	Starburst	0.8	pc.	0	1	0
	banana cream	Frozfruit	0.5	pc.	0	1	1
	cantaloupe	Frozfruit	0.6	pc.	0	1	0
	cherry	Frozfruit	0.5	pc.	0	1	0
	coconut	Dole Fruit 'n Juice	0.3	pc.	0	1	1
	coconut	Edy's Calypso	0.3	pc.	0	1	1
	coconut cream	Frozfruit	0.6	pc.	0	1	2
	cranberry-apple	Frozfruit	0.5	pc.	0	1	0
	guava-pineapple	Frozfruit	0.5	pc.	0	1	0
	kiwi-strawberry	Frozfruit	0.4	pc.	0	1	0
	lemon	Frozfruit	0.4	pc.	0	1	0
	lemon, iced tea	Frozfruit	0.5	pc.	0	1	0
	lemonade	Dole Fruit 'n Juice	0.3	pc.	0	1	0
	lime	Frozfruit	0.4	pc.	0	1	0
	orange	Frozfruit	0.4	pc.	0	1	0
	peach passion	Dole Fruit 'n Juice	0.5	pc.	0	1	0
	pina colada, cream	Frozfruit	0.4	pc.	0	1	0
	pine-coconut	Dole Fruit 'n Juice	0.3	pc.	0	1	1
	pine-orange-banana	Dole Fruit 'n Juice	1.4	oz.	0	1	0
	pine-orange-banana	Dole Fruit 'n Juice	1.3	oz.	0	1	0
	pineapple	Frozfruit	0.5	pc.	0	1	0
	raspberry	Dole Fruit 'n Juice	0.6	pc.	0	1	0
	raspberry	Frozfruit	0.5	pc.	0	1	0
	strawberry	Dole Fruit 'n Juice	1.3	oz.	0	1	0
	strawberry	Dole Fruit 'n Juice	1.4	oz.	0	1	0
	strawberry	Frozfruit	0.5	pc.	0	1	0
	strawberry cream	Frozfruit	0.5	pc.	0	1	1
	strawberry-banana cream	Frozfruit	0.5	pc.	0	1	0
	tropical	Frozfruit	0.4	pc.	0	1	1
	watermelon	Frozfruit	0.8	pc.	0	1	0
Fruit cocktail, canned		Del Monte Very Cherry	0.2	cup	0	1	0
		Hunt's	0.2	cup	0	1	0
	in extra light syrup	Del Monte Lite	0.3	cup	0	1	0

FOOD ITEM	SPECIFICATIONS	BRAND NAME	QUANTITY	SIZE	PROTEIN BLOCKS	CARBOHYDRATE BLOCKS	FAT BLOCKS
	in juice	Del Monte Natural	0.3	cup	0	1	0
	in juice	Libby's Lite	0.3	cup	0	1	0
	in juice	S&W Natural	0.3	cup	0	1	0
	in heavy syrup	Del Monte	0.2	cup	0	1	0
	in heavy syrup	S&W Natural	0.2	cup	0	1	0
	honey flavor	Del Monte Natural	0.2	cup	0	1	0
	in light syrup		0.3	cup	0	1	0
Fruit dip	caramel	Smucker's Fat Free	0.6	Tbsp.	0	1	0
	chocolate	Smucker's Fat Free	0.1	cup	0	1	0
Fruit drink blends		Capri Sun Mountain Cooler	2.3	fl. oz.	0	1	0
		Capri Sun Pacific Cooler	2.1	fl. oz.	0	1	0
		Capri Sun Surfer Cooler	2.3	fl. oz.	0	1	0
		Dole Fruit Fiesta	3.6	fl. oz.	0	1	0
		Dole Lanai/Tropical Breeze	2.4	fl. oz.	0	1	0
		Hi-C Ecto Cooler	2.2	fl. oz.	0	1	0
		Lincoln Party	2.1	fl. oz.	0	1	0
		Snapple Bali Blast	2.4	fl. oz.	0	1	0
		Snapple Samoan Splash	2.5	fl. oz.	0	1	0
		Tropicana	2.2	fl. oz.	0	1	0
		Veryfine Avalanche	2.8	fl. oz.	0	1	0
		Veryfine Tropical Breeze	2.4	fl. oz.	0	1	0
	nectar	Kern's Tropical	2.2	fl. oz.	0	1	0
	punch	Capri Sun	2.3	fl. oz.	0	1	0
	punch	Capri Sun Maui	2.2	fl. oz.	0	1	0
	punch	Capri Sun Safari	2.4	fl. oz.	0	1	0
	punch	Dole Paradise	2.4	fl. oz.	0	1	0
	punch	Dole Tropical	2.7	fl. oz.	0	1	0
	punch	Farmer's Market Tropical	2.5	fl. oz.	0	1	0
	punch	Heinke's California/Paradise	2.6	fl. oz.	0	1	0
	punch	Heinke's Macchu Pichu	2.4	fl. oz.	0	1	0
	punch	Hi-C	2.2	fl. oz.	0	1	0
	punch	Hi-C Hula	2.4	fl. oz.	0	1	0
	punch	Minute Maid	2.4	fl. oz.	0	1	0

Category	Type	Brand/Product	Amount	Unit	P	C	F
		punch	Minute Maid Box	2.2	fl. oz.	0	1	0
		punch	R.W. Knudsen Rain Forest/Tropical	2.5	fl. oz.	0	1	0
		punch	Snapple Tree Top	2.6	fl. oz.	0	1	0
		frozen, prepared	Dole Fruit Fiesta	2.2	fl. oz.	0	1	0
		frozen, prepared	Dole Lanai/Tropical Breeze	2.1	fl. oz.	0	1	0
		frozen, prepared	R.W. Knudsen Tropical	2.4	fl. oz.	0	1	0
		frozen, prepared, punch	Minute Maid	2.5	fl. oz.	0	1	0
Fruit juice blends			R.W. Knudsen Morning Blend	2.4	fl. oz.	0	1	0
			R.W. Knudsen Natural Breakfast	2.4	fl. oz.	0	1	0
			R.W. Knudsen Vita	2.7	fl. oz.	0	1	0
			Season's Best Medley	2.5	fl. oz.	0	1	0
			Snapple Vitamin Supreme	2.2	fl. oz.	0	1	0
		punch	After the Fall Maui	2.4	fl. oz.	0	1	0
		punch	After the Fall Sangria de la Noche	3.1	fl. oz.	0	1	0
		punch	Apple & Eve Nothin' But Juice	2.4	fl. oz.	0	1	0
		punch	Juicy Juice	2.5	fl. oz.	0	1	0
		punch	Tree Top	2.2	fl. oz.	0	1	0
		punch	Veryfine Juice-Ups	2.4	fl. oz.	0	1	0
		tropical fruit	Dole	2	fl. oz.	0	1	0
		tropical fruit	Dole	2.1	fl. oz.	0	1	0
		tropical fruit	Juicy Juice	2	fl. oz.	0	1	0
		tropical fruit frozen, prepared	Dole	2.5	fl. oz.	0	1	0
Fruit pectin		all varieties	Sure*Jell	2.5	tsp.	0	1	0
Fruit protector		all varieties	EverFresh	2.5	tsp.	0	1	0
Fruit snack		all varieties	Fruit Roll Ups	0.4	oz.	0	1	0
		all varieties	Roller Blade	0.4	oz.	0	1	0
		all varieties	Smart Snackers	0.8	oz.	0	1	0
		all varieties	String Thing	0.3	oz.	0	1	0
		apple	Stretch Island	0.3	oz.	0	1	0
		apple, organic	Stretch Island	3.3	fl. oz.	0	1	0
		apricot	Stretch Island	3.5	fl. oz.	0	1	0
		blackberry, cherry, grape, or raspberry	Stretch Island	3.3	fl. oz.	0	1	0
		grape, organic	Stretch Island	3.3	fl. oz.	0	1	0
		raspberry, organic	Stretch Island	3.1	fl. oz.	0	1	0

FOOD ITEM	SPECIFICATIONS	BRAND NAME	QUANTITY	SIZE	PROTEIN BLOCKS	CARBOHYDRATE BLOCKS	FAT BLOCKS
Fruit spreads	tropical	Stretch Island	3.5	fl. oz.	0	1	0
	all varieties	Kraft Reduced Calorie	1.7	Tbsp.	0	1	0
	all varieties	Polaner	0.9	Tbsp.	0	1	0
	all varieties	R.W. Knudsen	0.7	Tbsp.	0	1	0
	all varieties	Simply Fruit	0.9	Tbsp.	0	1	0
	all varieties	Slenderella Reduced Calorie	1.7	Tbsp.	0	1	0
	all varieties	Smucker's Bagel Toppers	0.9	Tbsp.	0	1	0
	and peanuts	Smucker's Super Spreaders	0.9	Tbsp.	0	1	0
Fruit syrup		Smucker's	0	cup	0	1	0
	light	Smucker's	0.1	cup	0	1	0
	and maple	R.W. Knudsen	0.1	cup	0	1	0
Fusilli pasta mix	w/creamy pesto	Knorr	0.1	cup	0	1	0
Garbanzo flour		Arrowhead Mills	0.2	cup	0	1	0
Garden salad	dill	S&W	0.4	cup	0	1	0
	marinated	S&W	0.5	cup	0	1	0
Garlic	trimmed		1	oz.	0	1	0
			10	clove	0	1	0
	crushed	Christopher Ranch	10	tsp.	0	1	0
	crushed	Frieda's	1	oz.	0	1	0
	granulated/minced		3.3	tsp.	0	1	0
	granulated/minced	Tone's	2.5	tsp.	0	1	0
	roasted and onion	Marie's Fat Free	2.9	Tbsp.	0	1	0
Garlic pepper			5	tsp.	0	1	0
Garlic pickle relish		Patak's	2.5	Tbsp.	0	1	3
Garlic powder			3.3	tsp.	0	1	0
Garlic salt			10	tsp.	0	1	0
Gelatin dessert	all flavors	Del Monte Snack	0.2	cup	0	1	0
	all flavors	Hunt's Snack Pack	0.2	cup	0	1	0
	all flavors	Jell-O Snacks	0.3	cup	0	1	0
	all flavors, except strawberry	Kraft Handi-Snacks	0.2	cup	0	1	0
	strawberry	Kraft Handi-Snacks	0.2	cup	0	1	0
	black raspberry	Jell-O	0.2	cup	0	1	0
Gelatin dessert mix, prepared	strawberry	Jell-O 1-2-3	0.2	cup	0	1	0

Food	Brand / Description	Amount	Unit	Protein	Carbohydrate	Fat
Ginger	trimmed root	2.5	oz.	0	1	0
Ginger	trimmed root, sliced	0.8	cup	0	1	0
Ginger, candied or crystallized	Frieda's	0.4	oz.	0	1	0
Ginger, ground	Paradise/White Swan	1.1	pcs.	0	1	0
Ginger drink		10	tsp.	0	1	0
Ginger drink	Santa Cruz Hawaiian	2.7	fl. oz.	0	1	0
Ginkgo nut, shelled	raw	0.8	oz.	1	1	0
Glaze, fruit	canned, drained	2.5	oz.	0	1	0
Glaze, fruit	Marie's, for banana, creamy	2.2	Tbsp.	0	1	0
Glaze, fruit	Marie's, for blueberries	1.8	Tbsp.	0	1	0
Glaze, fruit	Marie's, for peaches	1.8	Tbsp.	0	1	0
Glaze, fruit	Marie's, for strawberries	2	Tbsp.	0	1	0
Glaze, fruit	Smucker's, pie, strawberries	0.9	oz.	0	1	0
Gooseberry	fresh	1	cup	0	1	0
Gooseberry	canned, light syrup	0.2	cup	0	1	0
Goulash seasoning mix	Knorr Recipe	1.9	Tbsp.	0	1	0
Gourd, boiled	dishcloth, 1" sliced	0.4	cup	0	1	0
Gourd, boiled	white-flower, 1" cubes	1.7	cup	0	1	0
Granola cereal bar	Rice Krispies Treats, all varieties	0.5	bar	0	1	0
Granola cereal bar	Health Valley Fat Free Granola, all varieties	0.3	bar	0	1	0
Granola cereal bar	Health Valley Healthy Breakfast Bakes Fat Free	0.4	bar	0	1	0
Granola cereal bar	Health Valley Healthy Cereal Bars No Fat, all varieties	0.4	bar	0	1	0
Granola cereal bar	Health Valley Healthy Energy Bars, all varieties	0.3	bar	0	1	0
Granola cereal bar	Kellogg's Low Fat, all varieties	0.6	bar	0	1	0
Granola cereal bar	Nature's Choice Fat Free Granola, all varieties	0.4	bar	0	1	0
Granola cereal bar	Nature's Choice Real Fruit, all varieties	0.7	bar	0	1	0
Granola cereal bar	Nutri-Grain, all varieties except apple berry and oatmeal cookie	0.3	bar	0	1	0
Granola cereal bar	Quaker Chewy Lowfat, all varieties, scones	0.4	bar	0	1	0
Granola cereal bar	Health Valley, w/almonds, chewy	0.2	bar	0	1	0
Granola cereal bar	Little Debbie	0.4	bar	0	1	0
Granola cereal bar	Nature's Choice Fat Free Cereal, apple, blueberry, or peach filled	0.4	bar	0	1	0
Granola cereal bar	Quaker Chewy Lowfat, apple berry	0.4	bar	0	1	0

FOOD ITEM	SPECIFICATIONS	BRAND NAME	QUANTITY	SIZE	PROTEIN BLOCKS	CARBOHYDRATE BLOCKS	FAT BLOCKS
	blueberry	Kudo's Low Fat	0.6	bar	0	1	0
	carob chip	Nature's Choice Granola	0.6	bar	0	1	0
	chocolate chip	Kudos	0.8	bar	0	1	1
	chocolate chip	Kudos Enrobed	0.5	bar	0	1	1
	chocolate chip	Carnation Chewy	0.4	bar	0	1	1
	chocolate chip	Little Debbie	0.3	bar	0	1	1
	chocolate chip	Nature's Choice Grrr-Nola Treats	0.6	bar	0	1	0
	chocolate chip	Quaker Chewy	0.5	bar	0	1	1
	chocolate chip	Rice Krispies	0.5	bar	0	1	1
	chocolate chip, chunk	Carnation Granola	0.4	bar	0	1	0
	cinnamon and oats	Barbara's Granola	0.3	bar	0	1	2
	cinnamon raisin	Nature's Choice Granola	0.7	bar	0	1	1
	coconut almond	Barbara's Granola	0.5	bar	0	1	3
	cranberry, raspberry or strawberry filled	Nature's Choice Fat Free Cereal	0.4	bar	0	1	0
	fudge, nutty	Kudos	0.5	bar	0	1	1
	fudge dipped, macaroon	Little Debbie	0.3	bar	0	1	2
	fudge dipped, w/peanuts	Little Debbie	0.3	bar	0	1	1
	milk and cookies	Kudo's	0.5	bar	0	1	1
	oats and honey	Carnation Granola	0.4	bar	0	1	1
	oats and honey	Little Debbie	0.3	bar	0	1	1
	oats and honey	Nature's Choice Granola	0.7	bar	0	1	1
	oatmeal cookie	Quaker Chewy Lowfat	0.4	bar	0	1	0
	oatmeal raisin	Little Debbie	0.3	bar	0	1	0
	oatmeal raisin	Sweet Success	0.5	bar	0	1	1
	peanut butter	Barbara's Granola	0.4	bar	0	1	2
	peanut butter	Kudo's	0.5	bar	0	1	1
	peanut butter	Nature's Choice Granola	0.8	bar	0	1	1
	peanut butter, chocolate chip	Carnation Chewy	0.5	bar	0	1	0
	peanut butter, chocolate chip	Quaker Chewy	0.5	bar	0	1	1
	peanut butter, and jelly	Nature's Choice Grrr-Nola	0.8	bar	0	1	1
	strawberry	Kudo's Low Fat	0.6	bar	0	1	0

Food	Description	Brand	Amount	Unit			
Grape	fresh, American type (slipskin)		25	medium	0	1	0
	fresh, American type (slipskin), peeled and seeded		0.6	cup	0	1	0
	fresh, European type (adherent skin), seeded		0.1	lb.	0	1	0
	fresh, European type (adherent skin), seedless		10	medium	0	1	0
	fresh, European type (adherent skin), seedless or seeded		0.3	cup	0	1	0
	canned, seedless, heavy syrup	S&W	0.2	cup	0	1	0
	canned, seedless, heavy syrup	S&W Fancy Jubilee	0.2	cup	0	1	0
	canned, seedless, heavy syrup		0.1	cup	0	1	0
Grape drink		Capri Sun	2.2	oz.	0	1	0
		Dole	2.4	fl. oz.	0	1	0
		Hi-C	2.2	fl. oz.	0	1	0
		Lincoln	2.2	fl. oz.	0	1	0
		Veryfine Glacial	2.6	fl. oz.	0	1	0
		Snapple	2.6	fl. oz.	0	1	0
		Minute Maid	2.2	fl. oz.	0	1	0
Grape drink blends	grapeade	Tree Top	2.1	fl. oz.	0	1	0
	apple	Minute Maid	2.2	fl. oz.	0	1	0
	punch	Minute Maid	2.2	fl. oz.	0	1	0
Grape drink mix	frozen, prepared	Kool-Aid	2.9	fl. oz., prepared	0	1	0
	punch, frozen, prepared	Kool-Aid w/Sugar	4.4	fl. oz., prepared	0	1	0
Grape juice		After the Fall Concord	2.4	fl. oz.	0	1	0
		Goya	2.1	fl. oz.	0	1	0
		Juicy Juice	2.2	fl. oz.	0	1	0
		Lucky Leaf	2.1	fl. oz.	0	1	0
		R.W. Knudsen	2	fl. oz.	0	1	0
		R.W. Knudsen Concord	1.8	fl. oz.	0	1	0
		Season's Best	1.9	fl. oz.	0	1	0
		Veryfine	2	fl. oz.	0	1	0
		Veryfine Juice-Ups	2.2	fl. oz.	0	1	0
Grape leaves, stuffed	in jars	Perfecta Dolmadakia	2.6	oz.	0	1	3
Grapefruit, fresh	pink or red, California or Arizona		0.4	medium	0	1	0

FOOD ITEM	SPECIFICATIONS	BRAND NAME	QUANTITY	SIZE	PROTEIN BLOCKS	CARBOHYDRATE BLOCKS	FAT BLOCKS
	pink or red, California or Arizona, sections w/juice		0.5	cup	0	1	0
	pink or red, Florida		0.6	medium	0	1	0
	pink or red, Florida, sections w/juice		0.6	cup	0	1	0
	white, California		0.5	medium	0	1	0
	white, California, sections w/juice		0.5	cup	0	1	0
	white, Florida		0.5	medium	0	1	0
	white, Florida, sections, w/juice		0.5	cup	0	1	0
Grapefruit, canned	in juice	S&W Natural Style	0.4	cup	0	1	0
Grapefruit drink	pink	Ocean Spray	0.4	cup	0	1	0
	pink	Tree Top Desert Ice	2.6	fl. oz.	0	1	0
	pink	Tropicana Twister	2.5	fl. oz.	0	1	0
	pink	Tropicana Twister	2.5	fl. oz.	0	1	0
	pink	Tropicana Twister Light	2.6	fl. oz.	0	1	0
	pink	Tropicana Twister Light	7.3	fl. oz.	0	1	0
	ruby red	Ocean Spray	2.2	fl. oz.	0	1	0
	ruby red and tangerine	Ocean Spray	2.2	fl. oz.	0	1	0
Grapefruit juice	fresh		3.2	fl. oz.	0	1	0
		Dole	3.1	fl. oz.	0	1	0
		Goya	2.1	fl. oz.	0	1	0
		Ocean Spray	3	fl. oz.	0	1	0
		S&W	4	fl. oz.	0	1	0
		S&W	2.9	fl. oz.	0	1	0
		Tree Top	2.9	fl. oz.	0	1	0
		Veryfine	3.6	fl. oz.	0	1	0
	blend	Dole Sunripe	2.4	fl. oz.	0	1	0
	blend, cranberry	Apple & Eve Ruby Red	2.4	fl. oz.	0	1	0
	golden	Tropicana	3.1	fl. oz.	0	1	0
	pink or white	R.W. Knudsen	3.1	fl. oz.	0	1	0
	red	R.W. Knudsen Rio	2.1	fl. oz.	0	1	0

Food	Variety / Preparation	Brand	Amount	Unit			
	ruby red	Tropicana Carton	3.1	fl. oz.	0	1	0
	ruby red	Tropicana Plastic	2.9	fl. oz.	0	1	0
	frozen, prepared	Minute Maid	3	fl. oz.	1	1	1
Great northern beans	dried, boiled	Goya	0.4	cup	1	1	1
	canned, w/liquid		0.3	cup	0	1	0
	canned	Allens	0.4	cup	0	1	0
	canned	Eden Organic	0.3	cup	0	1	0
	canned	Goya	0.4	cup	0	1	0
	canned	Green Giant/Joan of Arc	0.4	cup	0	1	0
	canned	Stokely	0.3	cup	0	1	0
	canned	Sun-Vista	0.4	cup	1	1	1
	canned, w/sausage	Trappey's	0.4	cup	1	1	1
Green beans, fresh	raw		2.5	cup	0	1	0
	boiled drained		1.7	cup	0	1	0
Green beans, canned	all varieties	Allens Shells Out	1.3	cup	0	1	0
	whole, cut, jar French	Goya	2.5	cup	0	1	0
		Green Giant Kitchen Sliced	1.7	cup	0	1	0
		Green Giant Kitchen Sliced Less Sodium	2.5	cup	0	1	0
	cut	Stokely	1.7	cup	0	1	0
		Del Monte	2.5	cup	0	1	0
		S&W	2.5	cup	0	1	0
		Allens No Salt	5	cup	0	1	0
		Allens/Sunshine/Alma/Crest Top	1.7	cup	0	1	0
		Green Giant	2.5	cup	0	1	0
	w/wax beans	S&W	5	cup	0	1	0
	French style	Allens	2.5	cup	0	1	0
	French style	Green Giant	2.5	cup	0	1	0
	Italian cut	Allens/Sunshine	1.3	cup	0	1	0
	Italian cut	Del Monte	1.7	cup	0	1	0
	w/potatoes	Allens/Sunshine	0.8	cup	0	1	0
		S&W	2.5	oz.	0	1	0
		Mountain House	2.2	cup	0	1	0
Green beans, dilled		Seabrook	5	cup	0	1	0
Green beans, freeze dried	cut	Green Giant	2.2	cup	0	1	0
Green beans, frozen	cut	Green Giant Harvest Fresh	2.2	cup	0	1	0
	sliced	Stilwell	3.3	cup	0	1	0

FOOD ITEM	SPECIFICATIONS	BRAND NAME	QUANTITY	SIZE	PROTEIN BLOCKS	CARBOHYDRATE BLOCKS	FAT BLOCKS
Green bean combinations, frozen	and almonds	Green Giant Harvest Fresh	2.2	cup	1	1	3
Greens	mushroom casserole	Stouffer's	3.2	oz.	0	1	2
	mixed, canned	Allens/Sunshine	1.3	cup	0	1	1
Grenadine syrup		Mr. & Mrs. "T"	1	Tbsp.	0	1	0
		Rose's	0.8	Tbsp.	0	1	0
Grilling sauce	Chardonnay	Knorr	10	Tbsp.	0	1	4
	herb, Tuscan	Knorr	10	Tbsp.	0	1	4
	mandarin ginger	Knorr, Microwave	6.7	Tbsp.	0	1	4
	Parmesano	Knorr, Microwave	10	Tbsp.	0	1	4
	plum, spicy	Knorr	2	Tbsp.	0	1	1
	tequila lime	Knorr	3.3	Tbsp.	0	1	1
Ground cherry			0.8	cup	0	1	0
Guacamole seasoning		Lawry's	5	tsp.	0	1	0
Guanabana	frozen chunks	Goya	0.3	pkg.	0	1	0
Guanabana nectar	canned	Goya	1.9	fl. oz.	0	1	0
Guava			1.7	medium	0	1	0
			0.8	cup	0	1	0
	strawberry		0.3	cup	0	1	0
Guava drink		Mauna La'i	2.2	fl. oz.	0	1	0
		Snapple Guava Mania	2.5	fl. oz.	0	1	0
		After the Fall Maya	2.8	fl. oz.	0	1	0
Guava juice		Goya	1.9	fl. oz.	0	1	0
Guava nectar		Kern's	1.9	fl. oz.	0	1	0
		Libby's/Kern's	1.9	fl. oz.	0	1	0
Guava paste		Goya	0.4	3/4-in. slice	0	1	0
Guava sauce		Goya	0.6	cup	0	1	0
Gumbo dinner mix		Luzianne	0.1	pkg.	0	1	0
Gyro mix		Casbah	0.1	pkg.	0	1	0
Hamburger entree mix, dry	beef pasta	Hamburger Helper	0.2	cup	0	1	0
	beef taco	Hamburger Helper	0.2	cup	0	1	0
	w/cheese	Hamburger Mate	0.1	pkg.	0	1	0
	cheeseburger macaroni	Hamburger Helper	0.1	cup	0	1	1

Food	Description	Brand	Amount	Unit	P	C	F
chili		Hamburger Mate	0.1	pkg.	0	1	0
fettuccini alfredo		Hamburger Helper	0.2	cup	0	1	0
Italian, zesty		Hamburger Helper	0.1	cup	0	1	0
lasagna		Hamburger Helper	0.2	cup	0	1	0
w/noodles		Hamburger Mate	0.1	pkg.	0	1	0
w/pasta and tomato sauce		Hamburger Mate	0.1	pkg.	0	1	0
pizza pasta		Hamburger Helper	0.2	cup	0	1	0
stroganoff		Hamburger Helper	0.2	cup	0	1	0
Ham glaze		Crosse & Blackwell	1.1	Tbsp.	0	1	0
Hoisin sauce		Marzetti	2	Tbsp.	0	1	0
		House of Tsang	3.3	tsp.	0	1	0
		Lee Kum Kee	0.7	Tbsp.	0	1	0
Hollandaise sauce mix		Durkee	0.5	pkg.	0	1	0
		French's	10	Tbsp.	0	1	0
Homestyle gravy mix		Knorr	0.5	pkg.	0	1	0
		Durkee	0.8	cup, prepared	0	1	0
		French's	0.8	cup, prepared	0	1	0
		Pillsbury	0.8	cup, prepared	0	1	0
Hominy, canned	golden	Allens/Uncle William	0.2	cup	0	1	0
	golden	Goya	0.2	cup	0	1	0
	golden	Sun-Vista	0.3	cup	0	1	0
	golden	Van Camp's	0.3	cup	0	1	0
	Mexican	Allens/Uncle William	0.2	cup	0	1	0
	white	Allens/Uncle William	0.3	cup	0	1	0
	white	Goya	0.3	cup	0	1	0
	white	Sun-Vista	0.3	cup	0	1	0
	white	Van Camp's	0.3	cup	0	1	0
Honey		Aunt Sue's/Grandma's/Sue Bee	0.5	Tbsp.	0	1	0
Honey butter		Downey's	0.6	oz.	0	1	0
Honey mustard sauce		Rice Road	2.5	Tbsp.	0	1	0
Honeycomb		Frieda's	0.4	oz.	0	1	0
Honeydew			0.1	melon 7"x2"	0	1	0
Honeydew	pulp, cubed		0.6	cup	0	1	0
Hors d'oeuvre kit, frozen			1.8	sheets	0	1	2
beef Stroganoff		Pepperidge Farm	0.4	filled sheet	1	1	4
chicken a la king		Pepperidge Farm	0.4	filled sheet	1	1	3

FOOD ITEM	SPECIFICATIONS	BRAND NAME	QUANTITY	SIZE	PROTEIN BLOCKS	CARBOHYDRATE BLOCKS	FAT BLOCKS
Horseradish, fresh	shrimp Newburg	Pepperidge Farm	0.3	filled sheet	0		2
	leafy tips, raw, chopped		5	cup	1	1	0
	leafy tips, boiled, drained, chopped		2.5	cup	1	1	1
	pods, raw, sliced		1.7	cup	0	1	0
	pods, boiled, drained, sliced		1.7	cup	0	1	0
		Reese's	5	Tbsp.	0	1	8
Hubbard squash	raw		2.5	cup	0	1	0
	baked, cubed		0.6	cup	0	1	0
	boiled, drained, mashed		1	cup	0	1	0
Hummus		Casbah	1.4	oz.	1	1	2
Hushpuppies	frozen	Stilwell	1.6	pcs.	0	1	1
Ice, Italian	cherry	Luigi's	1.9	fl. oz.	0	1	0
	chocolate fudge	Luigi's	1.4	fl. oz.	0	1	0
	grape	Luigi's	2.1	fl. oz.	0	1	0
	lemon	Luigi's	2.1	fl. oz.	0	1	0
	strawberry	Luigi's	2.1	fl. oz.	0	1	0
Ice cream cone or cup	cone	Oreo	0.9	pc.	0	1	0
	cone, cinnamon	Teddy Grahams	0.7	pc.	0	1	0
	cone, sugar	Comet	0.8	pc.	0	1	0
	cone, waffle	Comet	0.7	pc.	0	1	0
	cup	Comet	0.2	pc.	0	1	0
Italian beans	in sauce	Joan of Arc	0.2	cup	0	1	0
Jackfruit	trimmed		1.4	oz.	0	1	0
Jam and preserves	all varieties	Knott's Berry Farm	2.5	tsp.	0	1	0
	all varieties	Smucker's	0.7	Tbsp.	0	1	0
	all varieties	Smucker's Reduced Sugar	1.4	Tbsp.	0	1	0
	all varieties	Smucker's Light	1.7	Tbsp.	0	1	0
	apricot, raspberry, or strawberry	Kraft	0.7	Tbsp.	0	1	0
	blackberry	Kraft	0.7	Tbsp.	0	1	0
	grape	Kraft	0.6	Tbsp.	0	1	0
	mango	Goya	0.8	Tbsp.	0	1	0

			Amount	Unit	Brand	Food
0	1	0	0.6	Tbsp.	Crosse & Blackwell	orange marmalade
0	1	0	0.6	Tbsp.	Kraft	orange marmalade
0	1	0	0.7	Tbsp.	Smucker's	orange marmalade
0	1	0	0.8	Tbsp.	Goya	papaya
0	1	0	0.8	Tbsp.	Goya	passion fruit
0	1	0	0.6	Tbsp.	Kraft	peach or pineapple
0	1	0	0.8	Tbsp.	Goya	pineapple
0	1	0	0.7	Tbsp.	Kraft	plum, red
0	1	0	0.8	Tbsp.	Goya	strawberry
0	1	0	0.7	Tbsp.	Kraft	strawberry
0	1	0	15	medium		Java plum
0	1	0	0.4	cup	Knott's Berry Farm	Jelly seeded
0	1	0	2.5	Tbsp.	Smucker's	all fruit flavors
0	1	0	0.7	Tbsp.	Kraft	all fruit flavors
0	1	0	0.7	Tbsp.		all fruit flavors except apple, grape, and strawberry
0	1	0	0.6	Tbsp.	Kraft	apple or strawberry
0	1	0	0.7	Tbsp.	Crosse & Blackwell	apple mint
0	1	0	0.6	Tbsp.	Crosse & Blackwell	currant, red
0	1	0	0.8	Tbsp.	Goya	grape
0	1	0	0.6	Tbsp.	Kraft	grape
0	1	0	0.8	Tbsp.	Goya	guava
0	1	0	0.6	Tbsp.	Tabasco	pepper, mild
0	1	0	0.8	Tbsp.	Tabasco	pepper, spicy
0	1	0	1.8	Tbsp.	World Harbors Blue Morning	Jerk sauce
0	1	0	0.4	cup		Jerusalem artichoke sliced
0	1	0	1.7	cup		Kale fresh, raw, chopped
0	1	0	1.7	cup		fresh, boiled, drained, chopped
0	1	2	5	cup	Allens/Sunshine	canned
0	1	2	30	oz.	Seabrook	frozen
0	1	0	1.7	cup		Kale, Scotch raw, chopped
0	1	0	1.7	cup		boiled, drained, chopped
2	1	0	0.1	cup	Arrowhead Mills	Kamut flour
0	1	0	2.5	Tbsp.	Del Monte	
0	1	0	5	Tbsp.	Healthy Choice	Ketchup

FOOD ITEM	SPECIFICATIONS	BRAND NAME	QUANTITY	SIZE	PROTEIN BLOCKS	CARBOHYDRATE BLOCKS	FAT BLOCKS
		Heinz	2.5	Tbsp.	0	1	0
		Hunt's	3.3	Tbsp.	0	1	0
		Hunt's No Salt	3.3	Tbsp.	0	1	0
		Smucker's	1.3	Tbsp.	0	1	0
Kidney beans	dry, boiled		0.3	cup	1	1	0
	dry, uncooked		0.1	cup	1	1	0
	canned, red, w/liquid		0.4	cup	0	1	0
	canned, red	Arrowhead Mills	0.6	cup	1	1	0
	canned, red	Eden Organic	0.3	cup	0	1	0
	canned, red	Hunt's	0.4	cup	0	1	0
	canned, red	Progresso	0.2	cup	1	1	0
	canned, red, baked	B&M	0.2	cup	1	1	0
	canned, red, baked	Friends	0.3	cup	1	1	0
	canned, red, dark	Allens/East Texas Fair/Trappey's	0.4	cup	0	1	0
	canned, red, dark	Goya	0.3	cup	1	1	0
	canned, red, dark	Van Camp's	0.3	cup	0	1	0
	canned, red, dark or light	Green Giant/Joan of Arc	0.3	cup	0	1	0
	canned, red, dark or light	Stokely	0.3	cup	0	1	0
	canned, red, dark or light	Stokely No Sugar	0.3	cup	0	1	0
	canned, red, light	Allens/Trappey's	0.3	cup	0	1	0
	canned, red, light	Van Camp's	0.3	cup	0	1	0
	canned, red, w/bacon, light	Trappey's New Orleans	0.3	cup	0	1	1
	canned, red, w/chili gravy	Trappey's	0.4	cup	0	1	0
	canned, red, w/jalapenos, light	Trappey's	0.4	cup	0	1	0
	canned, red, in tomato sauce	Goya Guisadas	0.4	cup	0	1	0
	canned, white	Progresso Cannellini	0.4	cup	1	1	0
Kidney beans, sprouted	raw		1.3	cup	1	1	0
Kishka		Hebrew National	2.2	oz.	1	1	4
Kiwi			0.8	large	0	1	0
			1	medium	0	1	0
Kiwi, dried		Sonoma	0.5	oz.	0	1	0
Kiwi punch		After the Fall	3	fl. oz.	0	1	0
Kiwi-strawberry drink		Snapple	2.5	fl. oz.	0	1	0
		Snapple Diet	13.3	fl. oz.	0	1	0

Food	Description	Brand	Amount	Unit	P	C	F
Kohlrabi	raw, sliced		2.5	cup	1	1	0
	boiled, drained, sliced		1	cup	0	1	0
Kumquat	seeded		5	medium	0	1	0
Lasagna entree mix	dry	Master-A-Meal	3.3	oz.	0	1	0
			0.1	pkg.	0	1	0
Leek	fresh, raw		0.6	9.9-oz. leek	0	1	0
	fresh, raw, chopped		0.7	cup	0	1	0
	fresh, boiled, drained, chopped		1.3	cup	0	1	0
Lemon	peeled		0.8	2 1/8" lemon, 3.9 oz.	0	1	0
			3.3	wedge, 1/4 medium 2 1/8" lemon	0	1	0
Lemon herb sauce mix		Knorr	2.5	Tbsp.	1	1	1
Lemon juice	fresh		2.5	Tbsp.	0	1	0
	fresh		10	Tbsp.	0	1	0
Lemon peel	candied		25	Tbsp.	0	1	0
	candied, diced	S&W	0.5	oz.	0	1	0
Lemon pepper			1	Tbsp.	0	1	0
Lemon sauce		Paradise/White Swan	10	tsp.	0	1	0
		House of Tsang	1.1	Tbsp.	0	1	0
Lemonade		After the Fall	3.1	fl. oz.	0	1	0
		Heinke's Old Fashion	2.5	fl. oz.	0	1	0
		Minute Maid	2.4	fl. oz.	0	1	0
		R.W. Knudsen	2.5	fl. oz.	0	1	0
		Santa Cruz Hawaiian	2.5	fl. oz.	0	1	0
		Snapple	2.5	fl. oz.	0	1	0
		Tropicana	2.5	fl. oz.	0	1	0
		Tropicana	2.7	fl. oz.	0	1	0
		Veryfine Chillers	2.3	fl. oz.	0	1	0
	pink	Minute Maid	2.4	fl. oz.	0	1	0
	pink	Snapple	2.5	fl. oz.	0	1	0
	pink	Snapple Diet	20	fl. oz.	0	1	0
	pink	Veryfine Chillers	2.3	fl. oz.	0	1	0
	frozen, prepared	Minute Maid	2.4	fl. oz.	0	1	0
Lemonade fruit blends	all fruit flavors	R.W. Knudsen	2.5	fl. oz.	0	1	0
	all fruit flavors	Santa Cruz	2.5	fl. oz.	0	1	0

FOOD ITEM	SPECIFICATIONS	BRAND NAME	QUANTITY	SIZE	PROTEIN BLOCKS	CARBOHYDRATE BLOCKS	FAT BLOCKS
	cherry	Snapple	2.4	fl. oz.	0	1	0
	cherry	Veryfine Chillers	2.5	fl. oz.	0	1	0
	cranberry	Heinke's	2.5	fl. oz.	0	1	0
	cranberry	Minute Maid	2.2	fl. oz.	0	1	0
	cranberry, frozen, prepared	Minute Maid	2.4	fl. oz.	0	1	0
	ginger	R.W. Knudsen Echinecea	2.9	fl. oz.	0	1	0
	lime	Veryfine Chillers	2.5	fl. oz.	0	1	0
	peach	Snapple	2.4	fl. oz.	0	1	0
	peach	Veryfine Chillers	2.4	fl. oz.	0	1	0
	raspberry	Minute Maid	2.2	fl. oz.	0	1	0
	raspberry, frozen, prepared	Minute Maid	2.4	fl. oz.	0	1	0
	strawberry	Snapple	2.5	fl. oz.	0	1	0
	strawberry	Veryfine Chillers	2.4	fl. oz.	0	1	0
	tangerine	Veryfine Chillers	2.4	fl. oz.	0	1	0
	tropical	Minute Maid	2.2	fl. oz.	0	1	0
Lemonade mix, prepared		Country Time	4.2	fl. oz.	0	1	0
		Country Time Punch	4.4	fl. oz.	0	1	0
		Hi-C Pink	2.8	fl. oz.	0	1	0
		Kool-Aid Presweetened	4.2	fl. oz.	0	1	0
	w/sugar	Kool-Aid	2.9	fl. oz.	0	1	0
Lentil	dry, green or red	Arrowhead Mills	0.1	cup	1	1	0
	dry, red	Goya	0.1	cup	1	1	0
	cooked		0.4	cup	1	1	0
	raw		0.6	cup	0	1	0
Lentil, sprouted		Patak's Moong Dhal	0.3	cup	0	1	1
Lentil dishes, canned		Spice Islands Quick Meal	0.3	pkg.	0	1	0
Lentil dishes mix	hearty, and wild rice	Eastern Traditions	0.5	oz.	0	1	0
	and herb	Casbah	0.5	oz.	0	1	0
	pilaf	Near East	0.3	cup, prepared	0	1	0
	pilaf, almond	Spice Islands Quick Meal	0.3	pkg.	0	1	0
Lentil rice loaf	frozen, prepared	Natural Touch	0.9	1" slice	1	1	3
Lettuce	bibb or Boston		5	head, 5" diam.	1	1	1
	butter	Dole	5	head	1	1	0

Food	Brand	Amount	Unit	P	C	F
cos or romaine		100	inner leaf	2	1	0
cos or romaine, shredded	Dole	15	cups	1	1	3
iceberg		2.5	head, 6" diam.	1	1	1
iceberg		100	leaf, .7 oz.	2	1	0
iceberg, precut	Dole	13.6	oz.	0	1	0
looseleaf, shredded		5	cup	0	1	0
fresh, raw, trimmed		0.4	cup	0	1	0
fresh, boiled, drained, chopped		0.3	cup	0	1	0
Lima beans mature, baby, boiled		0.3	cup	0	1	0
mature, large, boiled		0.4	cup	1	1	0
canned	Goya	0.4	cup	0	1	0
canned	Green Giant/Joan of Arc Butterbeans	0.4	cup	1	1	0
canned	S&W Butterbeans	0.4	cup	0	1	0
canned	Stokely	0.4	cup	0	1	0
canned	Stokely No Salt	0.4	cup	0	1	0
canned	Van Camp's Butterbeans	0.3	cup	0	1	0
canned, baby	Allens Butterbeans	0.3	cup	0	1	0
canned, green	Allens/East Texas Fair/Sunshine Limas/Butterbeans	0.3	cup	0	1	0
canned, green	Del Monte	0.4	cup	0	1	0
canned, green	Goya	0.4	cup	0	1	0
canned, green and white	Allens	0.4	cup	1	1	0
canned, large	Allens Butterbeans	0.4	cup	1	1	0
canned, mature, baby, green or butterbeans	Stokely	0.3	cup	0	1	0
canned, w/bacon, baby green	Trappey's Limas	0.3	cup	0	1	0
canned, w/bacon, baby white	Trappey's Limas	0.3	cup	0	1	0
canned, w/ham and sauce	Nalley	0.5	cup	1	1	1
canned, w/sausage, large white	Trappey's Butterbeans	0.3	cup	0	1	0
frozen, baby	Green Giant Harvest Fresh	0.4	cup	0	1	0
frozen, baby	Seabrook	0.3	cup	0	1	0
frozen, baby	Stilwell	0.3	cup	0	1	0
frozen, baby butter sauce	Green Giant	0.5	cup	0	1	1
frozen, Fordhook	Stilwell	0.4	cup	0	1	0
frozen, plain or speckled	Stilwell Butterbeans	0.3	cup	0	1	0

FOOD ITEM	SPECIFICATIONS	BRAND NAME	QUANTITY	SIZE	PROTEIN BLOCKS	CARBOHYDRATE BLOCKS	FAT BLOCKS
Lime	peeled, seeded		1.7	2"-diam. lime	0	1	0
Lime juice	fresh		5	oz.	0	1	0
Lime drink		After the Fall Key West	10	Tbsp.	0	1	0
		R.W. Knudsen Cactus Cooler	2.9	fl. oz.	0	1	0
		Minute Maid Limeade	2.5	fl. oz.	0	1	0
	frozen, prepared		2.8	fl. oz.	0	1	0
	refrigerated	Contadina	0.3	cup	0	1	0
Lingine entree, mix	refrigerated, tomato herb	Contadina	0.3	cup	0	1	0
	w/chicken, broccoli	Noodle Roni	0.2	cup, prepared	0	1	1
Loganberry	fresh		0.4	cup	0	1	0
	frozen		0.7	cup	0	1	0
Longan, shelled	fresh, seeded		2.5	oz.	0	1	0
	dried		0.4	oz.	0	1	0
Loquat			10	medium	0	1	0
	peeled, seeded		3.3	oz.	0	1	0
Lotus root	raw trimmed	Frieda's	2.5	oz.	0	1	0
	boiled, drained		2.5	oz.	0	1	0
Lychee, shelled	raw, seeded		2	oz.	0	1	0
	raw, peeled	Frieda's	2	oz.	0	1	0
	dried		0.5	oz.	0	1	0
Macaroni, see also Pasta	uncooked		0.4	oz.	0	1	0
	uncooked	Creamette	0.5	oz.	0	1	0
	uncooked, elbow		0.1	cup	0	1	0
	uncooked, elbow, regular or whole wheat	Eden	0.5	oz.	0	1	0
	uncooked, elbow		0.2	oz.	0	1	0
	cooked		1.2	oz.	0	1	0
	cooked, elbow		0.2	cup	0	1	0
	cooked, small shells		0.3	cup	0	1	0
	cooked, spirals		0.3	cup	0	1	0
	cooked, vegetable (tricolor)		1.4	oz.	0	1	0
	whole-wheat		1.4	oz.	0	1	0

Food	Brand / Variety	Amount	Unit	P	C	F
Macaroni entrée, mix, dry and cheese	Creamette	0.1	pkg.	0	1	0
and cheese	Kraft Original Dinner	0.5	oz.	0	1	0
and cheese	Kraft Original Deluxe Dinner	0.7	oz.	0	1	1
and cheese	Kraft Thick'n Creamy	0.5	oz.	0	1	0
and cheese, alfredo	Annie's	0.1	cup	0	1	0
and cheese, all varieties except original and white cheddar	Kraft Dinner	0.5	2 1/2 oz.	0	1	0
and cheese, cheddar	Golden Grain	0.2	cup, prepared	0	1	1
and cheese, cheddar, white, mild	Kraft Dinner	0.5	oz.	0	1	0
and cheese, cheddar or Parmesan	Fantastic	0.1	cup	0	1	0
and cheese, rotini, w/broccoli	Velveeta	0.9	oz.	0	1	1
and cheese, shells	Velveeta Original	0.8	oz.	0	1	1
and cheese, shells, w/bacon	Velveeta	0.9	oz.	0	1	1
and cheese, shells, w/salsa	Velveeta Original	0.8	oz.	0	1	1
and cheese, three cheese	Knorr Cup	0.2	pkg.	0	1	0
Mace, ground		10	tsp.	0	1	2
Mai tai drink mixer, bottled	Mr. & Mrs. "T"	1.2	fl. oz.	0	1	0
Malt beverage	Goya	2.8	fl. oz.	0	1	0
Malt cooler, berry	Bartles & Jaymes	3.2	oz.	0	1	0
black cherry	Bartles & Jaymes	3.3	oz.	0	1	0
Fuzzy Navel	Bartles & Jaymes	2.8	oz.	0	1	0
iced tea, Long Island	Bartles & Jaymes	2.5	oz.	0	1	0
Mai Tai	Bartles & Jaymes	2.7	oz.	0	1	0
margarita	Bartles & Jaymes	2.4	oz.	0	1	0
original	Bartles & Jaymes	3.8	oz.	0	1	0
peach	Bartles & Jaymes	3.2	oz.	0	1	0
pina colada	Bartles & Jaymes	2.3	oz.	0	1	0
sangria, red	Bartles & Jaymes	3.5	oz.	0	1	0
strawberry	Bartles & Jaymes	3.2	oz.	0	1	0
strawberry daiquiri	Bartles & Jaymes	3	oz.	0	1	0
tropical	Bartles & Jaymes	2.9	oz.	0	1	0
Malted milk powder, natural	Kraft	1.6	Tbsp.	0	1	0
natural	Nestlé Original	1.8	Tbsp.	0	1	0
chocolate	Kraft	1.8	Tbsp.	0	1	0

FOOD ITEM	SPECIFICATIONS	BRAND NAME	QUANTITY	SIZE	PROTEIN BLOCKS	CARBOHYDRATE BLOCKS	FAT BLOCKS
	chocolate	Nestle	1.5	Tbsp.	0	1	0
Mammy apple	fresh, peeled, seeded		3.3	oz.	0	1	0
Mango	frozen, chunks	Goya	0.1	pkg.	0	1	0
	fresh		0.3	10.6 oz. fruit	0	1	0
	fresh, peeled		2	oz.	0	1	0
	fresh, peeled, sliced		0.4	cup	0	1	0
	dried	Sonoma	0.4	oz.	0	1	0
	frozen, chunks	Goya	0.1	pkg.	0	1	0
Mango drink		Snapple Madness	2.5	fl. oz.	0	1	0
		Snapple Madness Diet	13.3	fl. oz.	0	1	0
		Tree Top More Mango	2.5	fl. oz.	0	1	0
Mango juice	tangerine	Veryfine	2.7	fl. oz.	0	1	0
		After the Fall Montage	2.7	fl. oz.	0	1	0
	peach	R.W. Knudsen	2.4	fl. oz.	0	1	0
Mango nectar		Goya	2	fl. oz.	0	1	0
	orange	Libby's/Kern's	2.1	fl. oz.	0	1	0
		Kern's	2.1	fl. oz.	0	1	0
Manhattan mixer	bottled	Holland House/Mr. & Mrs. "T"	1.2	fl. oz.	0	1	0
Manicotti	frozen	Celentano	1.9	oz.	1	1	2
	frozen, mini	Celentano	1.3	oz.	0	1	1
Maple syrup		Cary's/Maple Orchard's/ MacDonald's Pure	0	cup	0	1	0
Margarita mixer	bottled	Holland House/Mr. & Mrs. "T"	1.3	fl. oz.	0	1	0
	bottled, strawberry	Holland House/Mr. & Mrs. "T"	0.9	fl. oz.	0	1	0
	frozen, prepared	Bacardi	2.9	fl. oz.	0	1	0
	mix	Bar-Tenders	0.9	pkts.	0	1	0
Marinade		House of Tsang Classic	1.3	Tbsp.	0	1	0
		House of Tsang Mandarin	1.4	Tbsp.	0	1	0
	Hawaiian	Lawry's	2.5	Tbsp.	0	1	0
	lemon butter dill, seafood	Ken's Steak House	3.3	Tbsp.	0	1	5
	lemon pepper	Lawry's	10	Tbsp.	0	1	2
	red wine	Lawry's	10	Tbsp.	0	1	0
	and stir-fry sauce	Mary Rose Sari	10	Tbsp.	0	1	0
Marinade seasoning mix	meat	Lawry's Carne Asada	10	tsp.	0	1	0

Food	Description	Brand	Amount	Unit	P	C	F
Marjoram	dried		25	tsp.	0	1	0
Marrow squash	raw, trimmed		10	oz.	0	1	0
Marshmallow topping	creme	Smucker's	0.6	Tbsp.	0	1	0
Marshmallow topping	all varieties	Kraft	1.8	Tbsp.	0	1	0
Marshmallow topping		Marshmallow Fluff	3.3	Tbsp.	0	1	0
Meat loaf seasoning mix		Durkee Pouch	0.4	pkt.	0	1	0
Meat loaf seasoning mix		Durkee/French's Roasting Bag	0.6	pkg.	0	1	0
Meat loaf seasoning mix		Lawry's	1.3	Tbsp.	0	1	0
Meat tenderizer	unseasoned	Tone's	10	tsp.	0	1	0
Meatball seasoning mix	Italian	Durkee Pouch	0.7	pkt.	0	1	0
Melon balls, frozen	cantaloupe, honeydew	Stilwell	0.7	cup	0	1	0
Melon drink blend		Tree Top Wonder Melon	0.7	cup	0	1	0
Melonberry juice cocktail		Snapple	2.4	fl. oz.	0	1	0
Menudo	canned	Goya	2.5	fl. oz.	0	1	0
Mesquite sauce		S&W	0.9	cup	0	1	0
Mexican beans, canned		Allen's/Brown Beauty	3.3	Tbsp.	0	1	0
Mexican beans, canned		Chi-Chi's Ranchero	0.4	cup	0	1	0
Mexican beans, canned		Green Giant/Joan of Arc	0.3	cup	0	1	0
Mexican beans, canned		Old El Paso Mexe Beans	0.3	cup	0	1	0
Mexican beans, canned		Stokely Red	0.4	cup	0	1	0
Mexican beans, canned	w/jalapenos	Brown Beauty	0.3	cup	0	1	0
Mexican beans, canned	w/jalapenos	Trappey's MexiBeans	0.3	cup	0	1	0
Mexican seasoning mix		Chi-Chi's Mix	0.3	cup	0	1	0
Millet	raw	Arrowhead Mills	0.3	tsp.	0	1	0
Millet	cooked		10	oz.	0	1	0
Millet flour	hulled	Arrowhead Mills	0.5	oz.	0	1	0
Mint sauce		Crosse & Blackwell	1.4	cup	0	1	0
Mocha drink	chilled	Nestle Mocha Cooler	0.1	cup	0	1	0
Mocha drink	canned, café	Carnation Instant Breakfast	0.1	tsp.	0	1	0
Molasses		Grandma's 4-Star	10	oz.	0	1	0
Molasses	bead	La Choy	0.4	fl. oz.	0	1	0
Molasses	blackstrap	New Morning	2.6	Tbsp.	0	1	0
Molasses	dark or light	Br'er Rabbit	0.6	Tbsp.	0	1	0
Molasses	gold	Grandma's	0.8	Tbsp.	0	1	0
Molasses	green	Grandma's	0.7	Tbsp.	0	1	0
Molasses			0.6	Tbsp.	0	1	0
Molasses			0.6	Tbsp.	0	1	0
Molasses			0.8	Tbsp.	0	1	0

FOOD ITEM	SPECIFICATIONS	BRAND NAME	QUANTITY	SIZE	PROTEIN BLOCKS	CARBOHYDRATE BLOCKS	FAT BLOCKS
Mothbean	boiled		1.5	oz.	0	1	0
Muffin		Arnold Bran'nola	0.3	pc.	0	1	0
		Arnold Extra Crisp	0.4	pc.	0	1	1
	almond poppyseed	Aunt Fanny's	0.4	pcs.	0	1	1
	apple	Awrey's	0.8	oz.	0	1	1
	apple	Awrey's	0.5	oz.	0	1	2
	apple, bran	Aunt Fanny's	0.4	2 pcs.	0	1	1
	apple oatmeal	Pepperidge Farm Wholesome Choice	0.4	pc.	0	1	0
	banana nut	Aunt Fanny's	0.4	pcs.	0	1	1
	banana nut	Awrey's Grande	0.2	pc.	0	1	1
	banana nut	Tastykake	0.7	oz.	0	1	2
	banana nut	Tastykake Family	0.3	pc.	0	1	1
	banana nut	Weight Watchers	0.3	pc.	0	1	0
	banana nut, mini	Hostess	1.6	pcs.	0	1	2
	blueberry	Aunt Fanny's	0.4	pcs.	0	1	1
	blueberry	Awrey's	0.7	oz.	0	1	1
	blueberry	Awrey's	0.8	oz.	0	1	1
	blueberry	Awrey's Grande	0.2	pc.	0	1	1
	blueberry	Entenmann's	0.4	pc.	0	1	1
	blueberry	Entenmann's Fat Free	0.3	pc.	0	1	0
	blueberry	Pepperidge Farm Wholesome Choice	0.4	pc.	0	1	0
	blueberry	Tastykake	0.6	oz.	0	1	1
	blueberry	Tastykake Family	0.3	pc.	0	1	1
	blueberry	Tastykake Low Fat	0.6	oz.	0	1	0
	blueberry	Weight Watchers	0.3	pc.	0	1	0
	blueberry, loaf	Hostess	0.6	oz.	0	1	1
	blueberry, mini	Hostess	1.5	pcs.	0	1	1
	blueberry, top	Awrey's	0.8	oz.	0	1	1
	bran, harvest honey	Weight Watchers	0.2	pc.	0	1	0
	bran, w/raisins	Pepperidge Farm Wholesome Choice	0.3	pc.	0	1	0
	carrot raisin	Awrey's Grande	0.2	pc.	0	1	1
	cheese streusel	Awrey's Grande	0.2	pc.	0	1	1

Food	Brand	Amount	Unit	Protein	Carbohydrate	Fat
chocolate chip, chocolate	Awrey's Grande	0.2	pc.	0	1	2
chocolate chip, mini	Hostess	1.6	pcs.	0	1	2
chocolate, chocolate chip	Weight Watchers	0.2	pc.	0	1	0
cinnamon apple, mini	Hostess	1.6	pcs.	0	1	2
corn	Awrey's	0.7	oz.	0	1	1
corn	Awrey's	0.7	oz.	0	1	1
corn	Pepperidge Farm Wholesome Choice	0.3	pc.	0	1	0
corn	Tastykake	0.6	oz.	0	1	1
cranberry orange	Tastykake Golden Family	0.3	pc.	0	1	1
cranberry nut	Tastykake Low Fat	0.6	oz.	0	1	0
English	Awrey's	0.5	pc.	0	1	1
English	Awrey's	0.3	pc.	0	1	0
English	Pepperidge Farm	0.4	pc.	0	1	0
English	Roman Meal	0.4	pc.	0	1	0
English	Tastykake	0.4	pc.	0	1	0
English, blueberry	Thomas'	0.4	pc.	0	1	0
English, cinnamon raisin	Thomas'	0.3	pc.	0	1	0
English, cinnamon raisin	Pepperidge Farm	0.3	pc.	0	1	0
English, cranberry	Tastykake	0.5	pc.	0	1	0
English, honey wheat	Thomas'	0.3	pc.	0	1	0
English, oat bran	Thomas'	0.4	pc.	0	1	0
English, raisin	Thomas'	0.4	pc.	0	1	0
English, sandwich size	Thomas'	0.3	pc.	0	1	0
English, sandwich size	Thomas' 4 Pack	0.3	pc.	0	1	0
English, seven grain	Thomas' Twin	0.2	pc.	0	1	0
English, sourdough	Pepperidge Farm	0.4	pc.	0	1	0
English, sourdough	Pepperidge Farm	0.4	pc.	0	1	0
English, sourdough	Tastykake	0.4	pc.	0	1	0
English, sourdough, sandwich size	Thomas'	0.2	pc.	0	1	0
English, wheat, sandwich size	Thomas' Em's	0.3	pc.	0	1	0
lemon poppyseed	Awrey's	0.1	pc.	0	1	0
lemon poppyseed	Awrey's Grande	0.2	pc.	0	1	2
oat bran	Hostess	0.4	pc.	0	1	1

FOOD ITEM	SPECIFICATIONS	BRAND NAME	QUANTITY	SIZE	PROTEIN BLOCKS	CARBOHYDRATE BLOCKS	FAT BLOCKS
	oat bran, banana nut	Hostess	0.4	pc.	0	1	1
	onion, sandwich size	Thomas 'Em's	0.2	pc.	0	1	0
	raisin	Arnold	0.3	pc.	0	1	1
	raisin bran	Awrey's	0.8	oz.	0	1	1
	raisin bran	Awrey's	0.8	oz.	0	1	1
	raisin bran	Awrey's Grande	0.2	pc.	0	1	1
	raisin bran	Tastykake Low Fat	0.5	oz.	0	1	0
	raisin bran, top	Awrey's	0.3	pc.	0	1	1
	sourdough	Arnold	0.4	pc.	0	1	0
Muffin Mix, dry	blueberry, wild	Betty Crocker Fat Free	1	Tbsp.	0	1	0
	blueberry, wild	Betty Crocker	0.1	cup	0	1	0
	bran, multi	Buckeye	0	pkg.	0	1	0
	bran, wheat	Arrowhead Mills	0.2	cup, dry	0	1	1
	bran, oat	Arrowhead Mills	0.2	cup, dry	0	1	0
	corn	Flako	0.1	cup	0	1	0
	lemon poppy seed	Betty Crocker	0.1	cup	0	1	0
Mulberry			100	berries	0	1	0
Mung beans	dry		0.1	cup	1	1	0
	boiled		0.4	cup	1	1	0
Mung beans, sprouted	raw	Arrowhead Mills	10	oz.	1	1	1
	raw	Jonathan's	2.5	cup	1	1	1
	boiled, drained		2.5	cup	1	1	0
Mungo beans	boiled		0.4	cup	1	1	0
Mushroom	fresh, raw, pieces		5	cup	1	1	0
	fresh, boiled, drained, pieces		1.7	cup	1	1	0
	canned, all varieties except w/garlic	BinB	21.3	oz.	2	1	0
	canned, all varieties	Green Giant	2.5	cup	2	1	0
	canned, w/garlic, sliced	BinB	14.2	oz.	1	1	1
	freeze-dried	Tone's	3.3	cup	1	1	0
Mushroom breaded, frozen		Empire Kosher	4.1	pcs.	0	1	0
Mushroom, enoki	trimmed		5	oz.	0	1	0
			25	large, 4 1/8" long	0	1	0

Food	Description	Brand	Amount	Unit			
Mushroom, Japanese honey	trimmed	Frieda's	10	oz.	1	1	0
Mushroom, oyster	fresh or dried	Frieda's	10	oz.	1	1	0
Mushroom, portobello	fresh	Frieda's	10	oz.	1	1	0
	dried	Frieda's	1.3	oz.	1	1	0
Mushroom, shiitake	fresh, raw	Frieda's	3.3	oz.	1	1	0
	fresh, cooked		4	medium or 1/2 cup pcs.	0	1	0
Mushroom gravy	dried		3.6	medium, 1/2 oz.	0	1	0
		Franco-American	0.8	cup	1	1	1
	country or w/wine	Pepperidge Farm	0.6	cup	0	1	1
	creamy	Franco-American	0.6	cup	1	1	1
Mushroom gravy mix		Durkee	0.8	cup, prepared	0	1	0
		French's	0.8	cup, prepared	0	1	0
		Loma Linda Gravy Quick	3.3	Tbsp.	0	1	0
	brown	Durkee	0.8	cup, prepared	0	1	0
	hunter	Knorr	2.5	Tbsp.	0	1	1
Mushroom sauce		House of Tsang	5	Tbsp.	0	1	1
Mushroom sauce mix		Knorr	1	pkg.	0	1	2
Mustard greens	fresh, chopped, raw		10	oz.	1	1	0
	canned	Allens/Sunshine	2.5	cup	1	1	1
Mustard sauce mix	herb	Knorr	1.7	Tbsp.	1	1	1
Mustard seeds			10	tsp.	1	1	3
Nacho dip		McCormick	25	tsp.	2	1	7
	mild	Guiltless Gourmet	3.3	Tbsp.	0	1	0
Nacho dip mix		Knorr	5	tsp.	0	1	0
Natto			0.6	cup	2	1	4
Navy beans	boiled		0.2	cup	0	1	0
	canned, w/liquid		0.2	cup	0	1	0
	canned	Allens	0.4	cup	0	1	0
	canned	Eden Organic	0.4	cup	1	1	0
	canned	Stokely	0.3	cup	0	1	0
	canned, bacon or bacon/jalapeno	Trappey's	0.5	cup	1	1	0
Navy beans sprouted	raw		0.6	cup	0	1	0

FOOD ITEM	SPECIFICATIONS	BRAND NAME	QUANTITY	SIZE	PROTEIN BLOCKS	CARBOHYDRATE BLOCKS	FAT BLOCKS
Nectarine	sliced		0.7	medium, 2 1/2" diam.	0	1	0
Newburg sauce mix		Knorr	0.6	cup	0	1	0
Noodle, Chinese		Nasoya	0.8	pkg.	0	1	1
	cellophane or long rice, dry		0.6	oz.	0	1	0
	chow mein	Mee Tu	0.4	oz.	0	1	2
	chow mein	La Choy	0.4	cup	0	1	1
	chow mein	La Choy	0.3	cup	0	1	1
	crispy, wide	House of Tsang	0.3	cup	0	1	2
	egg, dried	La Choy	0.4	oz.	0	1	0
	rice		0.2	cup	0	1	0
Noodle, egg	uncooked	Creamette/Penn Dutch	0.5	oz.	0	1	0
	uncooked	Kluski	0.5	oz.	0	1	0
	uncooked, all varieties	Manischewitz	0.4	oz.	0	1	0
	uncooked, all varieties	Creamette/Goodman's	0.5	oz.	0	1	0
	uncooked, bow ties	Eden Organic	0.5	oz.	0	1	0
	uncooked, and spinach	Mueller's	0.5	oz.	0	1	0
	uncooked, yolk free	Prince Paglia E Fieno	0.5	oz.	0	1	0
	cooked	Borden	0.5	oz.	0	1	0
	cooked, spinach		0.2	cup	0	1	0
Noodle, egg-free	frozen	Morninstar Farms Homestyle	0.3	cup	0	1	0
Noodle, Japanese, dry		Nasoya	0.1	cup	0	1	0
	soba, buckwheat	Eden 100%	0.2	cup	0	1	0
	soba, buckwheat	Eden 40%	0.5	oz.	0	1	0
	soba, lotus root	Eden	0.5	oz.	0	1	0
	soba, mugwort	Eden	0.5	oz.	0	1	0
	soba, wild yam	Eden	0.5	oz.	0	1	0
	soba, cooked	Eden	0.5	oz.	0	1	0
	somen		0.4	cup	0	1	0
	somen, cooked		0.5	oz.	0	1	0
	spinach	Nasoya	0.2	cup	0	1	0

Category	Food	Brand	Amount	Unit			
Noodle dishes, mix	udon	Eden	0.5	oz.	0	1	0
	udon, cooked	Eden	1.5	oz.	0	1	0
	udon, brown rice	Eden	0.5	oz.	1	1	0
	Alfredo	Lipton Noodles & Sauce	0.1	pkg.	1	1	0
	Alfredo, carbonara	Lipton Noodles & Sauce	0.1	pkg.	1	1	0
	Alfredo, broccoli	Lipton Noodles & Sauce	0.1	pkg.	1	1	0
	beef	Lipton Noodles & Sauce	0.1	pkg.	0	1	0
	broccoli, au gratin	Noodle Roni	0.2	cup, prepared	1	1	0
	broccoli, and mushroom	Noodle Roni	0.2	cup, prepared	2	1	0
	butter	Lipton Noodles & Sauce	0.1	pkg.	1	1	0
	butter and herb	Lipton Noodles & Sauce	0.1	pkg.	1	1	0
	cheddar	Kraft Dinner	0.5	oz.	0	1	0
	cheddar	Master-A-Meal	0.1	pkg.	0	1	0
	cheddar, bacon	Nissin Noodles and Sauce	0.5	oz.	1	1	0
	cheddar, mild	Lipton Noodles & Sauce	0.1	pkg.	0	1	0
	cheese	Noodle Roni	0.2	cup, prepared	1	1	0
	chicken/chicken flavor	Lipton Noodles & Sauce	0.1	pkg.	0	1	0
	chicken/chicken flavor	Kraft Dinner	0.5	oz.	1	1	0
	chicken/chicken flavor	Lipton Noodles & Sauce	0.1	pkg.	0	1	0
	chicken/chicken flavor	Nissin Noodles and Sauce	0.6	oz.	0	1	0
	chicken/chicken flavor, broccoli	Noodles Roni	0.2	cup, prepared	0	1	0
	chicken/chicken flavor, creamy	Lipton Noodles & Sauce	0.1	pkg.	1	1	0
	chicken/chicken flavor, tetrazzini	Lipton Noodles & Sauce	0.1	pkg.	1	1	0
	garlic, creamy	Noodle Roni	0.2	cup, prepared	0	1	0
	herb and butter	Noodle Roni	0.2	cup, prepared	0	1	0
	Oriental	Knorr Cup	0.2	pkg.	0	1	0
	Oriental	Noodle Roni	0.3	cup, prepared	2	1	0
	Parmesan	Lipton Noodles & Sauce	0.1	pkg.	2	1	0
	Parmesan	Noodle Roni	0.2	cup, prepared	0	1	0
	Romanoff	Lipton Noodles & Sauce	0.1	pkg.	1	1	0
	Romanoff	Noodle Roni	0.2	cup, prepared	1	1	0
	sour cream and chive	Lipton Noodles & Sauce	0.1	pkg.	1	1	0

FOOD ITEM	SPECIFICATIONS	BRAND NAME	QUANTITY	SIZE	PROTEIN BLOCKS	CARBOHYDRATE BLOCKS	FAT BLOCKS
	Stroganoff	Lipton Noodles & Sauce	0.1	pkg.	0	1	0
	Stroganoff	Noodle Roni	0.2	cup, prepared	0	1	1
	tomato, Italian	Nissin Noodles and Sauce	0.6	oz.	0	1	1
Nutmeg	ground		10	tsp.	0	1	3
Oat, see also "Cereal"	whole grain		0.5	oz.	0	1	0
	flakes, rolled	Arrowhead Mills	0.2	cup, prepared	0	1	0
	rolled or oatmeal, dry		0.6	oz.	0	1	0
	rolled or oatmeal, cooked		0.4	cup	0	1	0
Oat bran	steel cut	Arrowhead Mills	0.1	cup	0	1	0
	dry		0.6	oz.	0	1	0
Oat flour	dry	Arrowhead Mills	0.2	cup	0	1	0
Oat groats		Arrowhead Mills	0.2	cup	0	1	0
Oheloberry		Arrowhead Mills	0.1	cup	0	1	0
Oil substitute		Baking Healthy	1	cup	0	1	0
Okra	fresh, raw, sliced		1.3	Tbsp.	0	1	0
	fresh, boiled, drained		1.7	cup	1	1	0
	fresh, boiled, drained, sliced		20	8 pods, 3" x 5/8"	1	1	0
	canned, cut		1.3	cup	0	1	0
	canned, w/tomatoes		1.7	cup	1	1	0
	canned, w/tomatoes and corn		2.5	cup	0	1	0
	canned, creole gumbo		2.5	cup	1	1	0
	frozen, boiled, drained, sliced		1.7	cup	1	1	0
	frozen, whole	Seabrook	1	1/2 cup	0	1	0
	frozen, whole	Stilwell	45	pods	1	1	0
	frozen, cut	Stilwell	45	pods	1	1	0
	frozen, and tomatoes	Stilwell	7.5	cup	2	1	1
	bottled	Holland House	3.3	cup	1	1	0
Old-fashioned drink mixer			0.9	fl. oz.	0	1	0
Onion, mature	fresh or stored, raw		5	oz.	0	1	0
	fresh or stored, raw, chopped		0.8	cup	0	1	0
	fresh or stored, raw, chopped		10	Tbsp.	0	1	0
	fresh or stored, boiled, drained, chopped		0.5	cup	0	1	0

Food	Description	Brand	Amount	Unit	Protein	Carbohydrate	Fat
Onion	canned, or in jars, whole	Green Giant	2.5	cup	0	1	0
	canned, or in jars, whole	S&W	0.6	cup	0	1	0
	canned, or in jars, cocktail	Crosse & Blackwell	10	Tbsp.	0	1	0
	canned, or in jars, cocktail	S&W 4 oz.	120	pcs.	0	1	0
	canned, or in jars, cocktail	S&W 16 oz.	80	pcs.	0	1	0
	canned, or in jars, sweet, in sauce	Boar's Head Vidalia	5	Tbsp.	0	1	0
	canned, or in jars, wild, marinated	Krinos Volvi	10	oz.	0	1	2
	frozen, chopped	Ore-Ida	1.3	cup	0	1	0
	frozen, chopped, boiled drained	Ore-Ida	10	Tbsp.	0	1	0
Onion, dried	flakes		2.5	Tbsp.	0	1	0
	minced		5	tsp.	0	1	0
Onion, green (scallion)	raw, trimmed, w/top, chopped		1.7	cup	0	1	0
	raw, trimmed, w/top, chopped		50	Tbsp.	0	1	0
Onion, Welch	and chive		5	oz.	0	1	0
Onion dip mix	roasted, and garlic	Knorr	5	tsp.	0	1	0
Onion gravy	zesty	Pepperidge Farm	0.6	cup	0	1	1
		Heinz Home Style	2.5	cup	0	1	1
	mix, prepared	Durkee	0.8	cup	1	1	0
	mix, prepared	French's	0.6	cup	0	1	1
	mix, prepared	Loma Linda Gravy Quick	0.8	cup	1	1	0
	brown	Durkee	0.6	cup	0	1	1
	brown, Lyonnaise	Knorr	0.6	cup	0	1	0
Onion powder			5	tsp.	0	1	0
Onion rings, frozen		Mrs. Paul's Old Fashioned	2.3	rings	0	1	1
		Ore-Ida Classic	1.5	rings	0	1	1
		Ore-Ida Gourmet	2.5	rings	0	1	1
		Ore-Ida Onion Ringers	2.2	rings	0	1	2
Onion sprouts		Jonathan's	3.3	cup	0	1	0
Orange	California navel		0.7	2 7/8" orange	0	1	0
	California navel, sections w/out membrane		0.6	cup	0	1	0
	California Valencia		0.8	2 5/8" orange	0	1	0

FOOD ITEM	SPECIFICATIONS	BRAND NAME	QUANTITY	SIZE	PROTEIN BLOCKS	CARBOHYDRATE BLOCKS	FAT BLOCKS
Orange drink	California Valencia, sections w/out membranes		0.6	cup	0	1	0
	Florida		0.7	2 11/16" orange	0	1	0
	Florida, sections w/out membrane		0.6	cup	0	1	0
		Bright & Early	2.4	fl. oz.	0	1	0
		Capri Sun	2.3	fl. oz.	0	1	0
		Hi-C	2.2	fl. oz.	0	1	0
		Lincoln	2.2	fl. oz.	0	1	0
	orangeade	Snapple	2.5	fl. oz.	0	1	0
	punch	Kool-Aid Bursts	2.5	fl. oz.	0	1	0
	tropical	Farmer's Market	2.5	fl. oz.	0	1	0
Orange drink blends	cranberry	Tropicana Twister	2.2	fl. oz.	0	1	0
	cranberry	Tropicana Twister Light	10	fl. oz.	0	1	0
	guava nectar	Kern's	2	fl. oz.	0	1	0
	peach	Tropicana Twister	2.4	fl. oz.	0	1	0
	pineapple	Lincoln	2.2	fl. oz.	0	1	0
	punch	Minute Maid	2.2	fl. oz.	0	1	0
	raspberry	Tropicana Twister	2.4	fl. oz.	0	1	0
	raspberry	Tropicana Twister Light	8	fl. oz.	0	1	0
	strawberry-banana	Tropicana Twister	2.5	fl. oz.	0	1	0
	strawberry-banana	Tropicana Twister Light	8	fl. oz.	0	1	0
	strawberry-guava	Tropicana Twister	2.5	fl. oz.	0	1	0
		Kool-Aid w/ sugar	4.4	fl. oz.	0	1	0
Orange drink mix, prepared		Tang	3	fl. oz.	0	1	0
		Tang Sugar Free	80	fl. oz.	0	1	0
Orange juice	fresh		2.9	fl. oz.	0	1	0
		Apple & Eve	2.8	fl. oz.	0	1	0
		Dole	2.7	fl. oz.	0	1	0
		Minute Maid Box	2.6	fl. oz.	0	1	0
		R.W. Knudsen	3.1	fl. oz.	0	1	0
		S&W	2.5	fl. oz.	0	1	0

Food	Description	Brand	Amount	Unit	P	C	F
Orange juice blends	chilled, all varieties except calcium rich and not concentrate	Tree Top	2.6	fl. oz.	0	1	0
		Tree Top	2.5	fl. oz.	0	1	0
		Tropicana Pure Premium	2.7	fl. oz.	0	1	0
		Tropicana Pure Premium + Fiber	2.6	fl. oz.	0	1	0
		Tropicana Ruby Red Pure Premium	2.6	fl. oz.	0	1	0
	chilled, calcium rich	Veryfine	3	fl. oz.	0	1	0
		Veryfine	3	fl. oz.	0	1	0
	chilled, not concentrate	Minute Maid Premium	2.7	fl. oz.	0	1	0
	frozen, prepared, all varieties, except calcium rich	Minute Maid Premium	2.7	fl. oz.	0	1	0
		Minute Maid Premium	2.7	fl. oz.	0	1	0
		Minute Maid Premium	2.7	fl. oz.	0	1	0
	calcium rich	Minute Maid Premium	2.7	fl. oz.	0	1	0
	Kiwi-passion fruit	Tropicana Tropics	2.8	fl. oz.	0	1	0
	mango	R.W. Knudsen	2.4	fl. oz.	0	1	0
	peach-mango	Tropicana Tropics	2.6	fl. oz.	0	1	0
	pineapple	Tropicana Tropics	2.7	fl. oz.	0	1	0
	punch	Juicy Juice	2.4	fl. oz.	0	1	0
	punch	Veryfine Juice-Ups	2.1	fl. oz.	0	1	0
		R.W. Knudsen	2.2	fl. oz.	0	1	0
Orange juice float			5	Tbsp.	0	1	0
Orange Peel	peel		0.4	oz.	0	1	0
	candied	S&W	22.3	pcs.	0	1	0
	candied, diced	Paradise/White Swan	0.9	Tbsp.	0	1	0
Orange sauce	mandarin	Ka-Me	25	tsp.	0	1	0
Oregano			1.7	Tbsp.	0	1	0
Oriental sauce		House of Tsang Imperial	5	tsp.	0	1	0
		House of Tsang Namasu	3.3	tsp.	0	1	0
	dried	House of Tsang	40	fl. oz.	0	1	0
Oriental 5-spice	brown, spicy	Tone's	5	tsp.	0	1	0
Oyster and shrimp sauce		Tryme Caribean Clipper	45	oz.	0	1	0
Palm	hearts of, canned	Haddon House	2.5	cup	0	1	2
		Goya	1.1	pcs.	0	1	1
Pancake, frozen		Aunt Jemima Lowfat	0.7	pcs.	0	1	0
		Aunt Jemima Original		pcs.	0	1	0

FOOD ITEM	SPECIFICATIONS	BRAND NAME	QUANTITY	SIZE	PROTEIN BLOCKS	CARBOHYDRATE BLOCKS	FAT BLOCKS
	blueberry	Downyflake	0.6	pcs.	0	1	0
	blueberry	Hungry Jack Microwave Original	0.6	pcs.	0	1	0
	blueberry	Aunt Jemima	0.7	pcs.	0	1	0
	buttermilk	Hungry Jack Microwave	0.6	pcs.	0	1	0
	buttermilk	Aunt Jemima	0.8	pcs.	0	1	0
	buttermilk, mini	Hungry Jack Microwave	0.6	pcs.	0	1	0
Pancake mix, dry		Hungry Jack Microwave	2.3	pcs.	0	1	0
		Aunt Jemima Original	0.1	cup	0	1	0
		Aunt Jemima Complete	0.1	cup	0	1	0
		Hungry Jack Original	0.1	cup	0	1	0
		Hungry Jack Premeasured	0.1	pkt.	0	1	0
		Hungry Jack Extra Lights	0.1	cup	0	1	0
		Hungry Jack Hungry Lights Complete	0.1	cup	0	1	0
	buckwheat	Arrowhead Mills	0.2	cup	0	1	0
	buckwheat	Aunt Jemima	0.1	cup	0	1	0
	buttermilk	Arrowhead Mills	0.1	cup	0	1	0
	buttermilk	Aunt Jemima	0.1	cup	0	1	0
	buttermilk	Aunt Jemima Complete Reduced Calorie	0.1	cup	0	1	0
	buttermilk	Hungry Jack	0.1	cup	0	1	0
	buttermilk	Hungry Jack Complete	0.1	cup	0	1	0
	corn, blue	Arrowhead Mills	0.1	cup	0	1	0
	gluten-free	Arrowhead Mills	0.1	cup	0	1	0
	kamut	Arrowhead Mills	0.1	cup	0	1	0
	multigrain	Arrowhead Mills	0.1	cup	0	1	0
	oat bran	Arrowhead Mills	0.2	cup	0	1	0
	wild rice	Arrowhead Mills	0.1	cup	0	1	0
	whole grain	Arrowhead Mills	0.1	cup	0	1	0
	whole wheat	Aunt Jemima	0.1	cup	0	1	0
Pancake syrup	table blends		0.6	Tbsp.	0	1	0
	table blends, w/butter		0.6	Tbsp.	0	1	0
	table blends, w/2% maple		0.7	Tbsp.	0	1	0
		Aunt Jemima	0.04	cup	0	1	0
		Aunt Jemima Lite	0.1	cup	0	1	0

Food	Description	Brand	Amount	Unit	Protein Blocks	Carbohydrate Blocks	Fat Blocks
		Country Kitchen	0.04	cup	0	1	0
		Country Kitchen Lite	0.1	cup	0	1	0
		Golden Griddle	0.04	cup	0	1	0
		Hungry Jack	0.1	cup	0	1	0
		Hungry Jack Lite	0.3	cup	0	1	0
		Karo	0.04	cup	0	1	0
		Log Cabin	0.04	cup	0	1	0
		Log Cabin Lite	0.1	cup	0	1	0
		Mrs. Richardson's	0.04	cup	0	1	0
		Mrs. Richardson's Lite	0.1	cup	0	1	0
		Smucker's Diet Breakfast Syrup	2.5	oz.	0	1	0
	butter flavor	Aunt Jemima Rich	0.04	cup	0	1	0
	butter flavor	Aunt Jemima Butterlite	0.1	cup	0	1	0
	butter flavor	Country Kitchen	0.04	cup	0	1	0
	butter flavor, maple	Hungry Jack	0.1	cup	0	1	0
	butter flavor, maple	Hungry Jack Lite	0.3	cup	0	1	0
	butter flavor, or maple	S&W Reduced Calorie	0.1	cup	0	1	0
Papaya	fresh		0.4	lb. fruit	0	1	0
	fresh, peeled, cubed		0.8	cup	0	1	0
	peeled	Frieda's	3.3	oz.	0	1	0
	dried		0.5	pcs.	0	1	0
	frozen, slices		0.3	pkg.	0	1	0
Papaya, creamed	colada	Goya	1.8	fl. oz.	0	1	0
Papaya drink	juice	R.W. Knudsen	2.2	fl. oz.	0	1	0
	nectar	Farmer's Market	2.5	fl. oz.	0	1	0
	nectar	Snapple	2.9	fl. oz.	0	1	0
	nectar	After the Fall Pele's	1.9	fl. oz.	0	1	0
	nectar	Goya	2	fl. oz.	0	1	0
	nectar	Libby's/Kern's	2.1	fl. oz.	0	1	0
	nectar	R.W. Knudsen	2.6	fl. oz.	0	1	0
	punch	Santa Cruz	2.2	fl. oz.	0	1	0
Pappadum		Patak's	3	pcs.	1	1	0
		Tamarind Tree	17.6	pcs.	0	1	0
Paprika			10	tsp.	0	1	1
Parsley	fresh, chopped		5	cup	1	1	1
Parsnip	raw, sliced		0.5	cup	0	1	0

FOOD ITEM	SPECIFICATIONS	BRAND NAME	QUANTITY	SIZE	PROTEIN BLOCKS	CARBOHYDRATE BLOCKS	FAT BLOCKS
	boiled, drained		0.4	medium	0	1	0
	boiled, drained, sliced		0.4	cup	0	1	0
Passion fruit	fresh, purple		3.3	medium	0	1	0
	fresh, purple, trimmed	Frieda's	2.5	oz.	0	1	0
	fresh, purple		1.5	oz.	0	1	0
	frozen, chunks	Goya	0.2	pkg.	0	1	0
Passion fruit juice	fresh, purple		2.1	fl. oz.	0	1	0
	fresh, yellow		2.1	fl. oz.	0	1	0
		Snapple	2.3	fl. oz.	0	1	0
		Heinke's	2.2	fl. oz.	0	1	0
Passion fruit-mango drink							
Pasta, dry, uncooked	plain		0.4	oz.	0	1	0
	all varieties	Creamette/Prince	0.5	oz.	0	1	0
	all varieties	Delverde	0.5	oz.	0	1	0
	all varieties	Goya Estrellas	0.4	oz.	0	1	0
	all varieties	Mueller's	0.4	oz.	0	1	0
	all varieties, w/egg	Herb's	0.5	oz.	0	1	0
	all varieties, kamut	Eden	0.6	oz.	0	1	0
	fettuccine	Prince	0.5	oz.	0	1	0
	kadzu and sweet potato	Eden	0.4	oz.	0	1	0
	linguine, tomato-basil	Prince	0.5	oz.	0	1	0
	mung bean	Eden	0.4	oz.	0	1	0
	noodl-style, yolk free	Mueller's	0.4	oz.	0	1	0
	penne, tomato-pepper-basil	Prince	0.5	oz.	0	1	0
	ribbons, durum wheat, all varieties	Eden	0.4	oz.	0	1	0
	ribbons, regular or spinach, whole wheat	Eden	0.5	oz.	0	1	0
	ribbons, rice	Eden	0.4	oz.	0	1	0
	ribbons, sesame rice spirals	Eden	0.6	oz.	0	1	0
	ribbons, shells	Goya Conchas	0.4	oz.	0	1	0
	spaghetti	Eden	0.5	oz.	0	1	0
	spaghetti	Prince Square/Thin	0.5	oz.	0	1	0
	spaghetti, parsley-garlic	Eden	0.5	oz.	0	1	0

Category	Food	Brand	Amount	Unit			
Pasta, cooked	spaghetti, whole wheat	Eden	0.5	oz.	0	1	0
	tri-color	Mueller's	0.4	oz.	0	1	0
	vegetable rotini, spirals, shells	Eden/Herb's	0.5	oz.	0	1	0
	vegetable spirals, whole wheat	Eden	0.5	oz.	0	1	0
	plain		0.2	cup	0	1	0
	corn		0.3	cup	0	1	0
	spinach		0.2	cup	0	1	0
	whole wheat		0.3	cup	0	1	0
Pasta, refrigerated, plain	uncooked, w/egg		0.6	oz.	0	1	0
	uncooked, spinach w/egg		0.6	oz.	0	1	0
	cooked, w/egg		1.3	oz.	0	1	0
	cooked, spinach w/egg		1.3	oz.	0	1	0
Pata dishes, mix	cheese, cheddar	Lipton Pasta & Sauce	0.1	pkg., dry	0	1	0
	cheese, four, corkscrews	Noodle Roni	0.2	cup, prepared	1	1	0
	cheese, three	Lipton Pasta & Sauce	0.1	pkg., dry	0	1	0
	chicken, herb Parmesan	Golden Saute	0.1	pkg., dry	0	1	0
	chicken, primavera	Lipton Pasta & Sauce	0.1	pkg., dry	0	1	0
	chicken, stir-fry	Golden Saute	0.1	pkg., dry	0	1	0
	garlic, butter	Golden Saute	0.1	pkg., dry	0	1	0
	garlic, creamy	Lipton Pasta & Sauce	0.1	pkg., dry	0	1	0
	garlic, creamy, corkscrews	Noodle Roni	0.2	cup, prepared	2	1	0
	garlic, and herb	Spice Island Quick Meal	0.3	pkg.	0	1	0
	herb, tomato	Lipton Pasta & Sauce	0.1	pkg., dry	0	1	0
	mixed	Buckeye Oceans of	0.5	oz.	0	1	0
	primavera	Knorr Cup	0.3	pkg.	0	1	0
	primavera	Lipton Pasta & Sauce	0.1	pkg., dry	0	1	0
	primavera	Spice Island Quick Meal	0.3	pkg., dry	0	1	0
	salad	Buckeye Sunny Day	0.04	pkg.	0	1	0
	salad, Ceasar	Kraft	0.8	oz.	2	1	0
	salad, garlic primavera	Kraft	0.7	oz.	1	1	0
	salad, hearty	Buckeye	0.04	pkg., dry	0	1	0
	salad, Italian, light	Kraft	0.7	oz.	0	1	0
	salad, Italian herb	Fantastic	0.2	cup	0	1	0
	salad, Parmesan peppercorn	Kraft	0.9	oz.	3	1	0
	salad, ranch, classic, w/bacon	Kraft	0.8	oz.	2	1	0
	salad, seasoned	Buckeye Sunny	0.04	pkg.	0	1	0

FOOD ITEM	SPECIFICATIONS	BRAND NAME	QUANTITY	SIZE	PROTEIN BLOCKS	CARBOHYDRATE BLOCKS	FAT BLOCKS
	salad, spicy oriental	Fantastic	0.2	cup	0	1	0
	spinach and mushroom	Spice Island Quick Meal	0.3	pkg.	0	1	0
	tomato, creamy, basil	Spice Island Quick Meal	0.2	pkg.	0	1	0
	tomato, creamy, twists	Knorr Cup	0.2	pkg.	0	1	0
Pasta sauce, tomato		Campbell's	0.2	cup	0	1	0
		Campbell's Homestyle	0.3	cup	0	1	0
		Del Monte	0.4	cup	0	1	1
		Eden Organic	0.5	cup	0	1	1
		Eden Organic No Salt	0.5	cup	0	1	1
		Healthy Choice	0.6	cup	0	1	0
		Hunt's Homestyle	0.8	cup	0	1	1
		Hunt's Old Country	1.3	cup	1	1	2
		Hunt's Original	0.6	cup	0	1	1
		Paesana Casalinga	0.7	cup	0	1	2
		Patsy's Fileto di Pomodoro	0.8	cup	0	1	3
		Pomodoro Fresca Solo	0.8	cup	0	1	0
		Porino's	0.6	cup	0	1	4
		Prego	0.2	cup	0	1	1
		Prego Low Sodium	0.6	cup	0	1	2
		Prego Extra Chunky Supreme Tomato	0.3	cup	0	1	1
		Pritikin Original	0.8	cup	0	1	0
		Progresso	0.5	cup	0	1	1
	w/basil	Barilla	0.6	cup	0	1	1
	w/basil	Classico Di Napoli	0.7	cup	0	1	0
	w/basil	Del Monte	0.4	cup	0	1	0
	w/basil	Del Monte D'Italia	0.5	cup	0	1	1
	w/basil	Hunt's Classic	1.3	cup	1	1	2
	w/basil	Porino's	0.4	cup	0	1	1
	w/basil, zesty	Prego	0.04	cup	0	1	0
	w/beef, ground	Prego Extra Chunky	0.2	cup	0	1	0
	cheese, wine and herbs	Campbell's	0.3	cup	0	1	1
	beef or beef and pork	Porino's	0.2	cup	0	1	1
		Porino's	0.4	cup	0	1	2

Food	Brand	Amount	Unit			
cheese, four	Classico Di Parma	0.7	cup	2	1	0
cheese, four	Del Monte D'Italia	0.6	cup	1	1	0
cheese, three	Prego	0.3	cup	0	1	0
cheese and garlic, Italian	Hunt's	0.6	cup	1	1	0
fra diavolo	Patsy's	0.6	cup	2	1	0
garden	Porino's Chunky	0.3	cup	2	1	0
garden	Porino's Gardina Fresca	0.5	cup	1	1	1
garden	Pritikin Chunky	1.3	cup	0	1	0
garden, combination	Prego Extra Chunky	0.4	cup	0	1	0
garden, style	Del Monte	0.4	cup	0	1	0
garlic	Prego Extra Chunky Supreme	0.2	cup	1	1	0
garlic and cheese	Prego Extra Chunky	0.2	cup	0	1	0
garlic and herb	Del Monte	0.4	cup	0	1	0
garlic and herb	Healthy Choice	0.6	cup	2	1	0
garlic and herb	Hunt's Old Country	0.8	cup	0	1	1
garlic and onion	Del Monte	0.4	cup	0	1	0
garlic and onion	Healthy Choice Extra Chunky	0.6	cup	0	1	0
garlic and onion	Hunt's Chunky	0.4	cup	1	1	0
garlic and onion	Hunt's Classic	0.6	cup	0	1	0
garlic and onion, extra	Campbell's	0.5	cup	0	1	0
green pepper and mushroom	Del Monte	0.5	cup	1	1	0
hot	Pomodoro Fresca Cayenne	0.8	cup	0	1	0
Italian herb	Del Monte	0.4	cup	0	1	0
Italian spice	Aunt Millie's Family Style	0.3	cup	0	1	0
Italian style	Campbell's	0.2	cup	1	1	0
marinara	Aunt Millie's	0.6	cup	2	1	0
marinara	Barilla	0.6	cup	0	1	0
marinara	Campbell's	0.3	cup	0	1	0
marinara	Colavita	0.6	cup	1	1	0
marinara	Del Monte D'Italia Classic	0.5	cup	0	1	0
marinara	Hunt's Chunky	0.4	cup	3	1	0
marinara	Paesana	0.6	cup	2	1	0
marinara	Patsy's	0.6	cup	2	1	0
marinara	Prego	0.5	cup	0	1	0
marinara	Prince Chunky	0.4	cup	0	1	0
marinara	Prince Traditional	0.6	cup	0	1	0

CARBOHYDRATES

FOOD ITEM	SPECIFICATIONS	BRAND NAME	QUANTITY	SIZE	PROTEIN BLOCKS	CARBOHYDRATE BLOCKS	FAT BLOCKS
	marinara	Pritikin	2.5	cup	2	1	0
	marinara	Progresso	0.7	cup	0	1	2
	marinara	Progresso Authentic	1.3	cup	1	1	4
	marinara, w/pizza paste	Aunt Millie's	0.7	cup	0	1	1
	meat/meat flavor	Aunt Millie's	0.6	cup	0	1	1
	meat/meat flavor	Aunt Millie's Family Style	0.3	cup	0	1	1
	meat/meat flavor	Del Monte	0.5	cup	0	1	1
	meat/meat flavor	Healthy Choice	0.7	cup	0	1	0
	meat/meat flavor	Hunt's Homestyle	0.8	cup	0	1	0
	meat/meat flavor	Hunt's Old Country	1	cup	1	1	2
	meat/meat flavor	Hunt's Original	0.5	cup	0	1	1
	meat/meat flavor	Prego	0.3	cup	0	1	1
	meat/meat flavor	Prince Chunky	0.4	cup	0	1	1
	meat/meat flavor	Progresso	0.5	cup	0	1	2
	mushroom	Aunt Millie's	0.6	cup	0	1	1
	mushroom	Aunt Millie's Family Style	0.4	cup	0	1	0
	mushroom	Campbell's	0.2	cup	0	1	0
	mushroom	Del Monte	0.4	cup	0	1	0
	mushroom	Healthy Choice	0.6	cup	0	1	0
	mushroom	Healthy Choice Extra Chunky	0.6	cup	0	1	0
	mushroom	Hunt's Homestyle	0.8	cup	0	1	1
	mushroom	Hunt's Original	0.5	cup	0	1	1
	mushroom	Hunt's Old Country	1.3	cup	1	1	2
	mushroom	Prego	0.2	cup	0	1	1
	mushroom	Prego Extra Chunky Supreme	0.3	cup	0	1	1
	mushroom	Prince Chunky	0.4	cup	0	1	0
	mushroom	Progresso	0.6	cup	0	1	2
	mushroom	Weight Watchers	0.6	cup	0	1	0
	mushroom, and garlic	Barilla	1.3	cup	0	1	3
	mushroom, and garlic	Campbell's	0.3	cup	0	1	0
	mushroom, and garlic	Healthy Choice Super Chunky	0.7	cup	0	1	0
	mushroom, and green pepper	Prego Extra Chunky	0.4	cup	0	1	1
	mushroom, and onion	Prego Extra Chunky	0.3	cup	0	1	1

mushroom, Parmesan	Prego	0.3	cup	0	1	1
mushroom, and ripe olive	Classico Di Sicilia	0.7	cup	0	1	0
mushroom, and tomato	Prego Extra Chunky	0.3	cup	0	1	1
mushroom, w/spice, extra	Prego Extra Chunky	0.3	cup	0	1	1
mushroom, and sweet peppers	Healthy Choice Super Chunky	0.6	cup	0	1	0
olive, black, and mushrooms	Porino's	0.4	cup	0	1	1
olive, green and black	Barilla	0.7	cup	0	1	3
w/olives and mushrooms	Classico Di Sicilia	0.7	cup	0	1	0
onion and garlic	Classico Di Sorento	0.6	cup	0	1	2
onion and garlic	Porino's	0.4	cup	0	1	1
onion and garlic	Prego	0.3	cup	0	1	1
onion and garlic	Prego Extra Chunky	0.3	cup	0	1	1
oregano, zesty	Prego Extra Chunky	0.2	cup	0	1	0
w/Parmesan	Hunt's Classic	0.7	cup	0	1	1
w/Parmesan	Prego	0.3	cup	0	1	1
pepper, sweet or red, and garlic	Barilla	0.8	cup	0	1	2
pepper, sweet or red, and onion	Classico Di Salerno	0.8	cup	0	1	2
pepper, sweet or red, and onion	Porino's	0.4	cup	0	1	1
pepper, sweet or red, red	Del Monte D'Italia	0.5	cup	0	1	1
pepper, sweet or red, and Italian sausage	Aunt Millie's	0.7	cup	0	1	1
pepper, sweet or red, spicy	Barilla	0.7	cup	0	1	2
pepper, sweet or red, spicy	Classico Di Roma Arrabbiata	1.3	cup	1	1	2
w/pesto	Classico Di Genoa	0.6	cup	0	1	2
sausage, Italian	Hunt's	0.5	cup	0	1	1
sausage, Italian and fennel	Classico D'Abruzzi	0.8	cup	1	1	3
sausage and pepper	Prego Extra Chunky	0.2	cup	0	1	1
sausage and pepper and mushroom	Porino's	0.2	cup	0	1	1
spinach and cheese	Classico Di Firenze	0.7	cup	0	1	2
sun-dried tomato	Classico Di Capri	0.7	cup	0	1	2
w/vegetables	Hunt's Chunky	0.4	cup	0	1	0
w/vegetables	Prego Extra Chunky Supreme	0.4	cup	0	1	1

FOOD ITEM	SPECIFICATIONS	BRAND NAME	QUANTITY	SIZE	PROTEIN BLOCKS	CARBOHYDRATE BLOCKS	FAT BLOCKS
	w/vegetables, Italian	Healthy Choice Extra Chunky	0.6	cup	0	1	0
	w/vegetables, Italian	Hunt's Old Country	0.7	cup	0	1	1
	w/vegetables, primavera	Healthy Choice Super Chunky	0.6	cup	0	1	0
	zucchini and Parmesan	Classico Di Milano	0.6	cup	0	1	1
Pasta sauce, refrigerated, tomato	chunky tomato	Contadina Fat Free	0.6	cup	0	1	0
	marinara	Contadina	0.6	cup	0	1	2
	roasted garlic and artichoke	Monterey Pasta Company	0.7	cup	0	1	1
Pasta sauce mix		Knorr Parma Rosa	2.2	Tbsp.	0	1	1
		Lawry's	1.4	Tbsp.	0	1	0
	garlic and herb	Knorr	0.4	pkg.	0	1	2
	garlic and herb	Spice Islands	0.8	pkg.	0	1	3
	w/mushroom flavor	McCormick	1.7	Tbsp.	0	1	0
	primavera	Spice Islands Pouch	0.7	pkg.	0	1	2
	salad	Durkee Pouch	10	tsp.	1	1	0
	spaghetti	Durkee	0.8	cup, prepared	0	1	0
	spaghetti	Durkee Family	5	tsp.	0	1	0
	spaghetti, American style	Durkee	0.7	cup, prepared	0	1	0
	spaghetti, w/mushrooms	Durkee	1.3	cup, prepared	0	1	0
	spaghetti, zesty	Durkee	3.3	tsp.	0	1	0
Pastry shell	dough	Goya Discos	0.5	pc.	0	1	2
	patty	Pepperidge Farm	0.4	shell	0	1	2
	sheet, puff	Pepperidge Farm	0.2	sheet	0	1	3
	tart	Oronoque	0.8	3" shell	0	1	3
	tart	Pet-Ritz	0.8	3" shell	0	1	3
	tart	Pet-Ritz	0.3	of 6" shell	0	1	2
Pastry filling, canned	almond	Solo	0.9	Tbsp.	0	1	0
	apple, Dutch	Solo	1	Tbsp.	0	1	0
	apricot	Solo	1.1	Tbsp.	0	1	0
	blueberry, wild	Solo	1.1	Tbsp.	0	1	0
	cherry	Solo	1	Tbsp.	0	1	0
	date	Solo	0.8	Tbsp.	0	1	1
	nut, fancy	Solo	1	Tbsp.	0	1	1
	pecan	Solo	0.8	Tbsp.	0	1	1

Food	Description	Brand	Amount	Unit			
	pineapple	Solo	1	Tbsp.	○	—	○
	poppy seed	Solo	0.7	Tbsp.	○	—	○
	prune plum	Solo	1.1	Tbsp.	○	—	○
	raspberry, red	Solo	1	Tbsp.	○	—	○
	strawberry	Solo	1.1	Tbsp.	○	—	○
Peach	fresh		1.1	2 1/2" peach, 4 per lb.	○	—	○
	fresh, sliced		0.6	cup	○	—	○
	dried	Sonoma	0.4	oz.	○	—	○
	dried, sulfured, halves		0.1	oz.	○	—	○
	dried, sulfured, 10 halves		0.5	oz.	○	—	○
	dried, sun-dried	Del Monte	0.1	cup	○	—	○
	frozen, sliced, sweetened		0.2	cup	○	—	○
Peach, canned	w/cinnamon	Hunt's	0.2	oz.	○	—	○
	in juice, cling	S&W Ready-Cut California Sun	0.2	oz.	○	—	○
	in juice, cling	S&W Ready-Cut Tropical Sun	0.2	oz.	○	—	○
	in juice, cling	S&W Sweet Memory Ready-Cut Sun	0.2	oz.	○	—	○
	in juice or extra light syrup, diced	Del Monte Natural	0.3	oz.	○	—	○
		Libby's Lite	0.4	oz.	○	—	○
		S&W Natural	0.3	oz.	○	—	○
		Del Monte Naturals Snack Cup	2.7	oz.	○	—	○
	in extra light syrup, cling	Del Monte Lite	0.3	oz.	○	—	○
	in extra light syrup, freestone	Del Monte Lite	0.4	oz.	○	—	○
	in light syrup, diced	Del Monte Snack Cup	1.8	oz.	○	—	○
	in heavy syrup, cling	Del Monte/Del Monte Melba	0.2	oz.	○	—	○
	in heavy syrup, cling	S&W	0.2	oz.	○	—	○
	in heavy syrup, cling, diced	Del Monte Snack Cup	0.2	oz.	○	—	○
	in heavy syrup, freestone	Del Monte	0.2	oz.	○	—	○
	in heavy syrup, freestone	S&W	0.2	oz.	○	—	○
	raspberry flavor, cling, in heavy syrup	Del Monte	0.2	oz.	○	—	○
	spiced	Del Monte Natural Harvest	0.2	oz.	○	—	○
	spiced, in heavy syrup	Del Monte	0.2	oz.	○	—	○
	spiced, in heavy syrup	S&W	1.7	oz. pc.	○	—	○

FOOD ITEM	SPECIFICATIONS	BRAND NAME	QUANTITY	SIZE	PROTEIN BLOCKS	CARBOHYDRATE BLOCKS	FAT BLOCKS
Peach, frozen	sliced	Big Valley	0.6	cup	0	1	0
		Stilwell	0.8	cup	0	1	0
Peach butter		Smucker's	0.8	Tbsp.	0	1	0
Peach drink		After the Fall	2.7	fl. oz.	0	1	0
		Farmer's Market	2.4	fl. oz.	0	1	0
		Tree Top Quake	2.4	fl. oz.	0	1	0
Peach dumpling	frozen	Pepperidge Farm	0.2	pc.	0	1	1
Peach juice blend		Dole Orchard	2.1	fl. oz.	0	1	0
		Dole Orchard	2.1	fl. oz.	0	1	0
Peach nectar		Goya	2.2	fl. oz.	0	1	0
		Goya	2.1	fl. oz.	0	1	0
		Libby's	2	fl. oz.	0	1	0
		Libby's/Kern's	2	fl. oz.	0	1	0
		R.W. Knudsen	2.4	fl. oz.	0	1	0
Peanut butter caramel topping		Smucker's	0.9	Tbsp.	0	1	1
Peanut butter and jelly	graham	Smucker's Goober	1.3	Tbsp.	0	1	2
Peanut butter snack		Mr. P.B. Crisps	0.6	oz.	0	1	1
Pear	fresh w/ peel, sliced		0.4	cup	0	1	0
	dried		0.5	oz.	0	1	0
	dried, halves		0.1	cup	0	1	0
	dried	Sonoma	0.4	oz.	0	1	0
Pear, Asian, whole			1	medium, 2 1/4"x2 1/2" diam.	0	1	0
Pear, canned	in juice	S&W Ready Cut California Sun	0.2	cup halves or sliced	0	1	0
	in juice or extra light syrup	Libby's Lite	0.4	cup halves or sliced	0	1	0
	in extra lite syrup	Del Monte Natural/Lite	0.3	cup halves or sliced	0	1	0
	in light syrup, diced	Del Monte Snack Cup	2.8	cup	0	1	0
	in heavy syrup	Del Monte Snack Cup	1.8	oz.	0	1	0
	in heavy syrup, diced	Del Monte	0.2	cup halves or sliced	0	1	0
	Bartlett, in juice	Del Monte Snack Cup	1.9	oz.	0	1	0
		S&W Natural	0.2	cup halves or sliced	0	1	0

Food	Description	Brand	Amount	Unit			
Pear juice	Bartlett, in heavy syrup	S&W	0.2	cup halves or sliced	0	1	0
	ginger flavor	Del Monte Natural	0.2	cup halves or sliced	0	1	0
		After the Fall Harvest	3.3	fl. oz.	0	1	0
		After the Fall Rouge River	3	fl. oz.	0	1	0
		Heinke's	2.4	fl. oz.	0	1	0
Pear nectar	canned	R.W. Knudsen	2.4	fl. oz.	0	1	0
		Libby's	1.9	fl. oz.	0	1	0
		Libby's/Kern's	1.9	fl. oz.	0	1	0
		Santa Cruz	1.9	fl. oz.	0	1	0
Pear-Passion nectar	canned	Goya	2.4	fl. oz.	0	1	0
Peas, butter	frozen	Stilwell	2	cup	0	1	0
Peas, cream	canned	Allens/East Texas Fair	0.3	cup	1	1	0
Peas, chowder	canned	Allens/East Texas Fair/Homefolks	0.4	cup	1	1	0
	frozen	Stilwell	0.4	cup	1	1	0
Peas, edible-podded	fresh, raw		0.3	cup	0	1	0
	fresh, boiled, drained		1.3	cup	1	1	0
	fresh, sugar snap	Frieda's	1.3	oz.	0	1	0
	frozen, boiled, drained		2.5	cup	1	1	0
	frozen, sugar snap	Green Giant	1	cup	0	1	0
	frozen, sugar snap	Green Giant Harvest Fresh	1.9	cup	0	1	0
Peas, field	canned, fresh shell	Sunshine	0.8	cup	0	1	0
	canned, fresh shell, w/snaps	Allens/East Texas Fair/Homefolks	0.3	cup	1	1	0
	canned, fresh shell, w/snaps	Goya	0.3	cup	0	1	0
	canned, dry w/bacon	Trappey's	0.5	cup	1	1	0
	canned, dry w/snaps and bacon	Trappey's	0.5	cup	1	1	0
	frozen, w/snaps	Stilwell	0.3	cup	0	1	0
Peas, green, sweet, fresh	raw, in pod		0.3	cup	0	1	0
	raw, shelled		0.6	lb.	0	1	0
	boiled, drained		0.7	cup	1	1	0
Peas, green, canned		Del Monte	0.6	cup	0	1	0
		Del Monte No Salt	0.6	cup	0	1	0
		Goya	0.4	cup	0	1	0
		Goya Tender Sweet	0.5	cup	0	1	0
		S&W Petit Pois/Sweet	0.6	cup	0	1	0

CARBOHYDRATES

FOOD ITEM	SPECIFICATIONS	BRAND NAME	QUANTITY	SIZE	PROTEIN BLOCKS	CARBOHYDRATE BLOCKS	FAT BLOCKS
		Stokely	0.6	cup	1	1	0
		Stokely No Salt	0.6	cup	1	1	0
	early June	Sun-Vista	0.4	cup	1	1	0
	early June, dry	Crest Top	0.3	cup	0	1	0
	early or sweet	Green Giant	0.6	cup	1	1	0
	early or sweet	Green Giant Less Sodium	0.6	cup	1	1	0
	early or sweet	Green Giant LeSueur	0.5	cup	1	1	0
	early or sweet	Green Giant LeSueur Less Sodium	0.6	cup	0	1	0
	very young, small	Del Monte	0.7	cup	1	1	0
Peas, green, dried		Goya	0.1	cup	0	1	0
Peas, green, freezedried		Alpine Aire	0.3	cup	1	1	0
		Mountain House	0.6	cup	1	1	0
		Seabrook	0.7	cup	1	1	0
		Stilwell	0.7	cup	1	1	0
Peas, green, frozen	baby, early	Green Giant Harvest Fresh LeSueur	0.7	cup	0	1	0
	early June	Green Giant LeSueur	1	cup	1	1	0
	sweet	Green Giant	0.7	cup	1	1	0
	sweet	Green Giant Harvest Fresh	0.7	cup	0	1	0
	sweet, baby	Green Giant LeSueur	1	cup	1	1	0
	butter sauce, baby early	Green Giant LeSueur	0.6	cup	0	1	1
	butter sauce, sweet	Green Giant	0.6	cup	0	1	1
Peas, green, combinations	canned, w/mushrooms and onions	Green Giant LeSueur	0.5	cup	0	1	0
	canned, w/pearl onions	Green Giant	0.6	cup	1	1	0
	canned, w/pearl onions	S&W	0.6	cup	0	1	0
	canned, and carrots	Del Monte	0.5	cup	0	1	0
	canned, and carrots	Goya	0.6	cup	0	1	0
	canned, and carrots	Green Giant	0.6	cup	0	1	0
	canned, and carrots	S&W	0.6	cup	0	1	0
	canned, and carrots	Stokely	0.6	cup	0	1	0
	canned, and carrots	Stokely No Salt/Sugar	0.7	cup	0	1	0
	frozen, and carrots	Stilwell	0.7	cup	0	1	0
	frozen, mushrooms	Green Giant LeSueur	1.1	cup	1	1	0

Food	Description	Brand	Amount	Unit	P	C	F
Peas, lady	frozen, w/ pearl onions	Green Giant	0.7	cup	0	1	0
	frozen, w/ pearl onions	Green Giant Harvest Fresh	0.6	cup	0	1	0
	canned	Sunshine	0.4	cup	0	1	0
Peas, pepper	canned, w/ snaps	East Texas Fair	0.4	cup	1	1	0
Peas, purple hull	canned	Allens/East Texas Fair/Homefolks	0.3	cup	0	1	0
	canned	East Texas	0.3	cup	0	1	0
	frozen	Stilwell	0.3	cup	0	1	0
Peas, sprouted	raw		0.3	cup	0	1	0
	boiled, drained		1.7	oz.	0	1	0
Peas, white acre	canned	East Texas Fair	0.4	cup	0	1	0
Pecan topping	w/ syrup	Smucker's	0.8	Tbsp.	0	1	2
Penne dishes, mix, dry	Alfredo	Knorr	0.2	oz.	0	1	0
	herb and butter	Noodle Roni	0.2	cup, prepared	0	1	2
	herb and garlic	Golden Saute	0.1	pkg.	0	1	0
	w/ sun-dried tomato Parmesan	Knorr	0.1	cup	0	1	0
Pepper, seasoning	black, ground		10	tsp.	0	1	0
	black, whole		10	tsp.	0	1	0
	chili		10	tsp.	0	1	0
	white		5	tsp.	0	1	0
Pepper, banana	hot or mild	Vlasic	10	oz.	0	1	0
Pepper, cherry	hot	Trappey's	10	pcs.	0	1	0
	hot	Hebrew National	3.3	pcs.	0	1	0
	hot or mild	Progresso	3.3	pc.	0	1	0
	marinated, drained	Vlasic	5	oz.	0	1	0
	raw, green and red, w/ seeds	Progresso	20	Tbsp.	0	1	7
	raw, green and red, w/out seeds		2.5	medium, 1.6 oz.	0	1	0
Pepper, chili	chopped, w/liquid		0.7	cup	0	1	0
Pepper, chili, in jars	green, whole	Chi-Chi's	1.7	cup	0	1	0
	green, whole	Old El Paso	7.5	chili	0	1	0
	green, whole	Rosarita	10	chili	0	1	0
	green, diced	Chi-Chi's	12	oz.	0	1	0
	green, diced	Chi-Chi's	20	Tbsp.	0	1	0
	green, diced	Rosarita	10	Tbsp.	0	1	0

FOOD ITEM	SPECIFICATIONS	BRAND NAME	QUANTITY	SIZE	PROTEIN BLOCKS	CARBOHYDRATE BLOCKS	FAT BLOCKS
Pepper, chipotle	yellow, hot	Del Monte	13.3	pcs.	0	1	0
Pepper, jalapeno	spice sauce	Del Monte	6.7	Tbsp.	0	1	1
	whole	Goya	10	pcs.	0	1	0
	whole	Rosarita	12	oz.	0	1	0
	whole	Trappey's	6.7	pcs.	0	1	0
	whole, or wheels	Chi-Chi's	11	oz.	0	1	0
	diced	La Victoria	5.5	oz.	0	1	0
	diced	Rosarita	11	oz.	0	1	0
	hot	Vlasic	5.5	oz.	0	1	0
	marinated	La Victoria	5.5	oz.	0	1	0
	nacho, sliced	Rosarita	11	oz.	0	1	0
	pickled	La Victoria	5.5	oz.	0	1	0
	pickled	Old El Paso	20	pcs.	0	1	0
	pickled, whole	Del Monte	11	oz.	0	1	0
	pickled, sliced	Del Monte	10	oz.	0	1	0
	pickled, sliced	Old El Paso	5.5	oz.	0	1	0
	pickled, nacho, sliced	Del Monte	10	oz.	0	1	0
Pepper, nacho	pickled	Goya	70	slices	0	1	0
Pepper, stuffed	frozen	Stouffer's	3.8	oz.	0	1	1
Pepper, sweet	fresh, green and red, raw		2.5	medium, 3 3/4"x3"	0	1	0
	fresh, green and red, raw, chopped		1.7	cup	0	1	0
	fresh, green and red, boiled, drained		2.5	medium	0	1	0
	fresh, green and red, boiled, drained, chopped		1.3	cup	0	1	0
	fresh, yellow, raw		0.8	large	0	1	0
	fresh, yellow, raw		25	strips	0	1	0
	frozen, chopped		10	oz.	0	1	0
Pepper, sweet, in jars	filet		5	oz.	0	1	0
	fried, drained		10	Tbsp.	0	1	9

Food	Description	Brand	Amount	Unit	Protein	Fat	Carbohydrate
Pepper salad	rings		1.4	oz.	0	—	0
	roasted		5	pc.	0	—	0
	roasted, fire, w/garlic, oil	Paesana	10	Tbsp.	2	—	0
Peppercorn sauce mix		B&G	3.3	oz.	0	—	0
Pepperoncini		Knorr	6.7	tsp.	1	—	0
		Krinos	1.3	cup	0	—	1
		Nalley	10	oz.	0	—	0
		Zorba	25	pcs.	0	—	0
		Vlasic	10	oz.	0	—	0
Persimmon, fresh	salad		0.4	medium	0	—	0
Persimmon, dried	Japanese, fresh		0.6	oz.	0	—	0
	Japanese, dried		1.9	pcs.	0	—	0
Pesto sauce, mix	Japanese	Sonoma	0.5	oz.	0	—	1
	creamy	Knorr	1.7	pkg.	0	—	0
	red bell pepper	Spice Island	2.5	pkg.	2	—	1
	tomato	Knorr	0.7	pkg.	1	—	0
	tomato, sun-dried	Knorr	0.5	pkg.	0	—	0
		Spice Island	0.8	pkg.	0	—	0
		Knorr	0.4	pkg.	0	—	0
Picante sauce	all varieties	Pace	10	Tbsp.	0	—	0
	all varieties	Del Monte	10	Tbsp.	0	—	0
	black bean	Hunt's Homestyle	10	Tbsp.	0	—	0
	black-eyed pea	Arthur's	6.7	Tbsp.	0	—	0
	garlic, w/corn and honey	Arthur's	6.7	Tbsp.	0	—	0
	hot	Arthur's	6.7	Tbsp.	0	—	0
	hot	Chi-Chi's	10	Tbsp.	0	—	0
	hot	Old El Paso	10	Tbsp.	0	—	0
	hot, or mild	Sun-Vista	10	Tbsp.	0	—	0
	jalapeno, zesty, hot	Arthur's	10	Tbsp.	0	—	0
	jalapeno, zesty, medium	Rosarita	10	Tbsp.	0	—	0
	jalapeno, zesty, mild	Rosarita	10	Tbsp.	0	—	0
	medium	Rosarita	10	Tbsp.	0	—	0
	medium	Chi-Chi's	10	Tbsp.	0	—	0
	mesquite	Old El Paso	10	Tbsp.	0	—	0
	mild	Arthur's	10	Tbsp.	0	—	0
	mild	Chi-Chi's	10	Tbsp.	0	—	0

FOOD ITEM	SPECIFICATIONS	BRAND NAME	QUANTITY	SIZE	PROTEIN BLOCKS	CARBOHYDRATE BLOCKS	FAT BLOCKS
Pickle, cucumber	mild	Old El Paso	10	Tbsp.	0	1	0
	mild	Sun-Vista	10	Tbsp.	0	1	0
	bread and butter	Mrs. Fannings	1.4	oz.	0	1	0
	bread and butter	Shorr's	3.3	oz.	0	1	0
	bread and butter, chips	Claussen	2.5	oz.	0	1	0
	bread and butter, chunks	Nalley Banquet	1.4	oz.	0	1	0
	bread and butter, midgets	Vlasic Milwaukee	0.9	oz.	0	1	0
	bread and butter, sandwich	Claussen	1.8	oz.	0	1	0
	bread and butter, sandwich stackers	Vlasic	1.3	oz.	0	1	0
	bread and butter, slices	Nalley	1.4	oz.	0	1	0
	chips	Nalley Cucumber	1	oz.	0	1	0
	chips w/honey	Pickle Eater's	1.4	oz.	0	1	0
	dill	Nalley Banquet	10	oz.	0	1	0
	dill	Nalley Country	10	oz.	0	1	0
	dill	Nalley Dilliest	10	oz.	0	1	0
	dill	Vlasic Milwaukee	10	oz.	0	1	0
	dill, garlic	Nalley	10	oz.	0	1	0
	dill, hamburger chips/slices	Claussen	100	slices	0	1	0
	dill, onion	Nalley Walla Walla	10	oz.	0	1	0
	dill, tiny	Nalley Banquet	10	oz.	0	1	0
	dill, kosher	Claussen	10	oz.	0	1	0
	dill, kosher	Claussen Mini	8	oz. pc.	0	1	0
	dill, kosher	Hebrew National Barrel/Hot	2.5	pickle	0	1	0
	dill, kosher, sandwich stackers	Vlasic	10	oz.	0	1	0
	dill, kosher, slices	Claussen	11	oz.	0	1	0
	dill, kosher, snack chunks	Vlasic	10	oz.	0	1	0
	dill, kosher, spears	Claussen	12	oz.	0	1	0
	dill, kosher, spears	Pickle Eater's	10	oz.	0	1	0
	dill, kosher, spears	Vlasic	10	oz.	0	1	0
	dill, kosher, tiny	Del Monte	10	oz.	0	1	0
	dill, Polish, spears	Vlasic	10	oz.	0	1	0
	kosher	Shorr's Deli	10	oz.	0	1	0

Food	Type	Brand	Amount	Unit	Protein	Carbohydrate	Fat
Pickle dip, dill	kosher, whole	Rosoff/Shorr's	10	oz.	0	1	0
	kosher, halves	Hebrew National/Rosoff/Shorr's	10	oz.	0	1	0
	kosher, spears	Hebrew National/Shorr's	10	oz.	0	1	0
	sour	Claussen New York Deli	5	pickle	0	1	0
	sour, kosher	Hebrew National/Rosoff/ Shorr's New Half Sours	10	oz.	0	1	0
	sour, kosher, garlic	Hebrew National/Shorr's	10	oz.	0	1	0
	sour, kosher, spears	Rosoff/Shorr's Half Sour	10	oz.	0	1	0
	sweet	Nalley	1.1	oz.	0	1	0
	sweet, all varieties	Del Monte	0.9	oz.	0	1	0
	sweet, all varieties	Vlasic	0.9	oz.	0	1	0
	sweet, gherkins	Nalley	1.3	oz.	0	1	3
	sweet, midgets	Nalley	1.1	oz.	0	1	0
Pickle relish, cucumber	hamburger	Nalley	3.3	Tbsp.	0	1	0
	hamburger	Del Monte	1.4	Tbsp.	0	1	0
	hot dog	Nalley	3.3	Tbsp.	0	1	0
	hot dog	Del Monte	2.5	Tbsp.	0	1	0
	piccalilli, tomato	Nalley	3.3	Tbsp.	0	1	0
	red hot	Pickle Eater's	5	Tbsp.	0	1	0
	sweet	Ron's	2.5	Tbsp.	0	1	0
	sweet	Claussen	3.3	Tbsp.	0	1	0
	sweet	Del Monte	1.7	Tbsp.	0	1	0
	sweet	Hebrew National	2.5	Tbsp.	0	1	0
	sweet, honey	Pickle Eater's	2.5	Tbsp.	0	1	0
	sweet, regular or curry flavor	Vlasic	2.5	Tbsp.	0	1	0
Pickling spice		Tone's	10	tsp.	0	1	0
Pie	apple	Entenmann's Homestyle	0.04	pie	0	1	2
	coconut custard	Entenmann's	0.04	pie	0	1	1
	lemon	Entenmann's	0.03	pie	0	1	2
Pie, frozen	apple	Amy's	1.7	oz.	0	1	1
	apple	Banquet	0.05	pie	0	1	1
	apple	Mrs. Smith's 8"	0.04	pie	0	1	1
	apple	Mrs. Smith's 9"	0.03	pie	0	1	1
	apple	Mrs. Smith's 10"	0.02	pie	0	1	1
	apple	Mrs. Smith's Old Fashioned 9"	0.02	pie	0	1	1

FOOD ITEM	SPECIFICATIONS	BRAND NAME	QUANTITY	SIZE	PROTEIN BLOCKS	CARBOHYDRATE BLOCKS	FAT BLOCKS
	apple	Mrs. Smith's Reduced Fat	0.04	pie	0	1	1
	apple	Mrs. Smith's Reduced Fat No Sugar	0.05	pie	0	1	1
	apple, lattice	Mrs. Smith's	0.04	pie	0	1	1
	apple, Dutch	Mrs. Smith's 8"	0.03	pie	0	1	1
	apple, Dutch	Mrs. Smith's 9"	0.02	pie	0	1	1
	apple, Dutch	Mrs. Smith's 10"	0.02	pie	0	1	1
	apple, Dutch	Mrs. Smith's Old Fashioned	0.04	pie	0	1	1
	apple-cranberry	Mrs. Smith's	0.08	pie	0	1	2
	banana cream	Banquet	0.06	pie	0	1	1
	banana cream	Mrs. Smith's	0.06	pie	0	1	1
	banana cream	Pet-Ritz	0.03	pie	0	1	1
	berry	Mrs. Smith's	0.03	pie	0	1	1
	blackberry	Mrs. Smith's	0.04	pie	0	1	1
	blueberry	Mrs. Smith's	0.05	pie	0	1	1
	cherry	Banquet	0.04	pie	0	1	1
	cherry	Mrs. Smith's 8"	0.03	pie	0	1	1
	cherry	Mrs. Smith's 9"	0.02	pie	0	1	1
	cherry	Mrs. Smith's 10"	0.02	pie	0	1	1
	cherry	Mrs. Smith's Old Fashioned 9"	0.03	pie	0	1	1
	cherry	Mrs. Smith's Reduced Fat 8"	0.04	pie	0	1	1
	cherry	Mrs. Smith's Reduced Fat No Sugar 8"	0.04	pie	0	1	2
	cherry, lattice	Mrs. Smith's	0.08	pie	0	1	1
	chocolate cream	Banquet	0.05	pie	0	1	1
	chocolate cream	Mrs. Smith's	0.06	pie	0	1	1
	chocolate cream	Pet-Ritz	0.04	pie	0	1	2
	chocolate cream	Sara Lee	0.03	pie	0	1	1
	chocolate cream, French silk	Mrs. Smith's	0.08	pie	0	1	2
	coconut cream	Banquet	0.06	pie	0	1	1
	coconut cream	Mrs. Smith's	0.06	pie	0	1	1
	coconut cream	Pet-Ritz	0.05	pie	0	1	1
	coconut custard	Mrs. Smith's	0.06	pie	0	1	1
	fudge vanilla cream	Pet-Ritz	0.06	pie	0	1	1
	lemon cream	Banquet	0.07	pie	0	1	1

Food	Brand	Unit				
lemon cream	Mrs. Smith's	pie	0.06	0	1	1
lemon cream	Pet-Ritz	pie	0.06	0	1	1
lemon meringue	Mrs. Smith's	pie	0.03	0	1	0
lemon meringue	Sara Lee Homestyle	pie	0.03	0	1	1
mince/mincemeat	Banquet	pie	0.04	0	1	1
mince/mincemeat	Mrs. Smith	pie	0.03	0	1	1
peach	Banquet	pie	0.05	0	1	1
peach	Mrs. Smith 8"	pie	0.04	0	1	1
peach	Mrs. Smith 9"	pie	0.03	0	1	1
peanut butter chocolate cream	Pet-Ritz	pie	0.06	0	1	1
pecan	Mrs. Smith's 8"	pie	0.02	0	1	1
pecan	Mrs. Smith's 10"	pie	0.02	0	1	1
pumpkin	Banquet	pie	0.05	0	1	1
pumpkin, hearty	Mrs. Smith's 8"	pie	0.05	0	1	1
pumpkin, hearty	Mrs. Smith's 9"	pie	0.03	0	1	1
pumpkin cream	Pet-Ritz	pie	0.06	0	1	1
pumpkin custard	Mrs. Smith's 8"	pie	0.03	0	1	1
pumpkin custard	Mrs. Smith's 9"	pie	0.03	0	1	1
pumpkin custard	Mrs. Smith's 10"	pie	0.02	0	1	1
raspberry, red	Mrs. Smith's	pie	0.03	0	1	1
strawberry	Mrs. Smith's	pie	0.04	0	1	1
strawberry-rhubarb	Mrs. Smith's	pie	0.03	0	1	1
Pie, mix						
chocolate silk	Jell-O	pie, prepared	0.04	0	1	1
coconut cream	Jell-O	pie, prepared	0.04	0	1	2
Pie, snack						
apple	Tastykake Tastyklair	pie	0.18	0	1	1
apple	Aunt Fanny's	oz.	0.6	0	1	1
apple	Aunt Fanny's	oz.	0.6	0	1	1
apple	Drake's	cakes	0.3	0	1	1
apple	Hostess	pie	0.2	0	1	1
apple	McMillin's	oz.	0.7	0	1	1
apple	McMillin's	oz.	0.6	0	1	1
apple	Pet-Ritz	pie	0.2	0	1	1
apple, French	Tastykake	pie	0.2	0	1	1
apple, French	Hostess	pie	0.2	0	1	1
banana cream	Aunt Fanny's	pie	0.2	0	1	1

CARBOHYDRATES

FOOD ITEM	SPECIFICATIONS	BRAND NAME	QUANTITY	SIZE	PROTEIN BLOCKS	CARBOHYDRATE BLOCKS	FAT BLOCKS
	berry	Aunt Fanny's	0.7	oz.	0	1	1
	berry	Aunt Fanny's	0.7	oz.	0	1	1
	berry	McMillin's	0.7	oz.	0	1	1
	berry	McMillin's	0.7	oz.	0	1	1
	blackberry or blueberry	Hostess	0.2	pie	0	1	1
	blueberry	Pet-Ritz	0.2	pie	0	1	1
	blueberry	Tastykake	0.2	pie	0	1	1
	Boston creme	Aunt Fanny's	0.7	oz.	0	1	1
	Boston creme	Aunt Fanny's	0.7	oz.	0	1	1
	Boston creme	McMillin's	0.7	oz.	0	1	1
	Boston creme	McMillin's	0.7	oz.	0	1	1
	cherry	Aunt Fanny's	0.7	oz.	0	1	1
	cherry	Aunt Fanny's	0.7	oz.	0	1	1
	cherry	Drake's	0.6	oz.	0	1	1
	cherry	Hostess	0.5	oz.	0	1	1
	cherry	McMillin's	0.7	oz.	0	1	2
	cherry	McMillin's	0.7	oz.	0	1	2
	cherry	Pet-Ritz	0.2	pie	0	1	1
	cherry	Tastykake	0.2	pie	0	1	1
	chocolate creme	Aunt Fanny's	0.7	oz.	0	1	2
	chocolate creme	Aunt Fanny's	0.7	oz.	0	1	2
	chocolate pudding	McMillin's	0.7	oz.	0	1	1
	chocolate pudding	McMillin's	0.7	oz.	0	1	2
	coconut creme	Aunt Fanny's	0.7	oz.	0	1	1
	coconut creme	Aunt Fanny's	0.7	oz.	0	1	1
	coconut creme	Tastykake	0.2	pie	0	1	1
	coconut pudding	McMillin's	0.7	oz.	0	1	1
	coconut pudding	McMillin's	0.7	oz.	0	1	1
	lemon	Hostess	0.2	pie	0	1	1
	lemon	McMillin's	0.7	oz.	0	1	1
	lemon	McMillin's	0.7	oz.	0	1	1
	lemon	Pet-Ritz	0.1	pie	0	1	1
	lemon	Tastykake	0.2	pie	0	1	1

Food	Brand					
lemon creme	Aunt Fanny's	0.7	oz.	0	—	1
lemon creme	Aunt Fanny's	0.7	oz.	0	—	1
marshmallow, banana	Little Debbie	0.2	pie	0	—	1
marshmallow, chocolate	Little Debbie	0.2	pie	0	—	1
oatmeal creme	Little Debbie	0.2	pie	0	—	1
peach	Aunt Fanny's	0.7	oz.	0	—	1
peach	Aunt Fanny's	0.7	oz.	0	—	1
peach	Hostess	0.2	pie	0	—	1
peach	McMillin's	0.6	oz.	0	—	1
peach	McMillin's	0.6	oz.	0	—	1
peach	Tastykake	0.2	pie	0	—	1
peanut butter cream	McMillin's	0.2	pie	0	—	2
pineapple	Tastykake	0.2	pie	0	—	1
pineapple, cheese	Tastykake	0.2	pie	0	—	1
pumpkin	Aunt Fanny's	0.2	pie	0	—	1
pumpkin	McMillin's	0.2	pie	0	—	1
pumpkin	Tastykake	0.2	pie	0	—	1
raisin creme	Little Debbie	0.2	pie	0	—	1
strawberry	Aunt Fanny's	0.7	oz.	0	—	1
strawberry	Aunt Fanny's	0.7	oz.	0	—	1
strawberry	Hostess	0.2	pie	0	—	1
strawberry	McMillin's	0.7	oz.	0	—	1
strawberry	McMillin's	0.7	oz.	0	—	1
strawberry	Tastykake	0.2	pie	0	—	1
vanilla creme	Aunt Fanny's	0.7	oz.	0	—	1
vanilla creme	Aunt Fanny's	0.7	oz.	0	—	1
vanilla pudding	McMillin's	0.7	oz.	0	—	1
vanilla pudding	McMillin's	0.7	oz.	0	—	1

Pie crust

Food	Brand					
chocolate cookie	Ready Crust	0.1	crust	0	—	1
chocolate cookie	Oreo	0.1	crust	0	—	1
cookie crumbs	Nilla	1.4	oz.	0	—	1
cookie crumbs	Oreo	1.5	oz.	0	—	1
graham	Honey Maid	0.1	crust	0	—	1
graham, mini	Ready Crust	0.5	oz. crust	0	—	1
graham crumbs	Honey Maid	1.4	oz.	0	—	0
graham crumbs	Sunshine	1.4	oz.	0	—	1

FOOD ITEM	SPECIFICATIONS	BRAND NAME	QUANTITY	SIZE	PROTEIN BLOCKS	CARBOHYDRATE BLOCKS	FAT BLOCKS
Pie crust, frozen or refrigerated	shortbread	Ready Crust 9"	0.1	crust	0	1	1
	vanilla cookie	Nilla	0.1	crust	0	1	1
		Oronoque	0.2	crust	0	1	3
		Oronoque	0.3	of 6" crust	0	1	2
		Pet-Ritz 9"	0.1	crust	0	1	2
		Pet-Ritz 9 5/8"	0.1	crust	0	1	2
		Pillsbury	0.1	crust	0	1	2
	deep dish	Oronoque 9"	0.1	crust	0	1	3
	deep dish	Oronoque 10"	0.1	crust	0	1	2
	deep dish	Pet-Ritz	0.1	crust	0	1	2
	graham	Oronoque	0.1	crust	0	1	1
	graham	Pet-Ritz	0.1	crust	0	1	1
	vegetable shortening	Pet-Ritz	0.1	crust	0	1	2
	vegetable shortening, deep dish	Pet-Ritz	0.1	crust	0	1	2
Pie crust mix		Betty Crocker	0.1	of 9" crust	0	1	3
		Flako	0.2	cup, dry	0	1	2
		Pillsbury	0.1	of 9" crust	0	1	2
Pie filling, canned	apple	Lucky Leaf/Lucky Leaf Premium	0.2	cup	0	1	0
		Lucky Leaf Lite	0.2	cup	0	1	0
		Musselman's 21 oz.	0.2	cup	0	1	0
		Musselman's 24 oz.	0.1	cup	0	1	0
	apricot	Lucky Leaf	0.1	cup	0	1	0
	blackberry	Lucky Leaf	0.2	cup	0	1	0
	blueberry	Lucky Leaf	0.1	cup	0	1	0
	blueberry	Lucky Leaf Lite	0.2	cup	0	1	0
	blueberry	Lucky Leaf Premium	0.1	cup	0	1	0
	blueberry	Musselman's	0.1	cup	0	1	0
	cherry	Lucky Leaf/Musselman's	0.1	cup	0	1	0
	cherry	Lucky Leaf/Musselman's Lite	0.2	cup	0	1	0
	cherry, dark, sweet	Lucky Leaf/Musselman's	0.1	cup	0	1	0
	coconut creme	Lucky Leaf	0.1	cup	0	1	0
	lemon	Lucky Leaf/Musselman's 22 oz.	0.1	cup	0	1	0

Food	Brand	Amount	Unit	Pro	Carb	Fat
lemon	Musselman's 25 oz.	0.1	cup	0	1	0
lemon creme	Lucky Leaf	0.1	cup	0	1	0
mincemeat	Lucky Leaf	0.1	cup	0	1	0
mincemeat	None Such	0.1	cup	0	1	0
mincemeat	S&W	0.1	cup	0	1	0
mincemeat, w/brandy and rum	None Such	0.1	cup	0	1	0
mincemeat, condensed	None Such	1	tsp.	0	1	0
peach	Lucky Leaf	0.2	cup	0	1	0
pineapple	Lucky Leaf/Musselman's	0.1	cup	0	1	0
pumpkin, mix	Libby's	0.2	cup	0	1	0
pumpkin, mix	Stokely	0.1	cup	0	1	0
raisin	Lucky Leaf	0.1	cup	0	1	0
strawberry	Lucky Leaf/Musselman's	0.2	cup	0	1	0
strawberry-rhubarb	Lucky Leaf	0.1	cup	0	1	0
Pigeon peas						
fresh, raw		0.3	cup	0	1	0
fresh, boiled, drained		0.4	cup	0	1	0
dried		0.1	cup	0	1	0
dried, boiled		0.3	cup	0	1	0
canned, dried	Goya	0.3	cup	0	1	0
canned, green		0.5	cup	0	1	0
Pimiento	El Jib	2.5	pepper	0	1	0
	Tupi	7.5	oz.	0	1	0
	Goya	7.5	oz.	0	1	0
	S&W	7.5	oz.	0	1	0
Pina colada mixer						
bottled	Holland House/Mr. & Mrs. "T"	0.9	fl. oz.	1	1	0
canned	Goya	0.2	cup	0	1	0
frozen, prepared	Bacardi	2.2	fl. oz.	1	1	0
mix	Bar-Tenders	0.4	oz. pkt.	0	1	0
Pineapple						
fresh, baby, trimmed	Frieda's Sugarloaf	2.5	oz.	0	1	0
fresh, diced		0.5	cup	0	1	0
fresh, sliced	Dole	1	slices	0	1	0
canned, juice, all varieties except sliced	Del Monte	0.3	cup	0	1	0
canned, crushed	Dole	0.3	cup	0	1	0
canned, sliced	Del Monte	1.2	slices	0	1	0
canned, sliced	Dole	1.3	slices	0	1	0
canned, tidbits	Del Monte Snack	1.9	oz.	0	1	0

FOOD ITEM	SPECIFICATIONS	BRAND NAME	QUANTITY	SIZE	PROTEIN BLOCKS	CARBOHYDRATE BLOCKS	FAT BLOCKS
	canned, tidbits or chunks	Dole	0.3	cup	0	1	0
	canned, in light syrup	Del Monte Snack	1.8	oz.	0	1	0
	canned, in light syrup, all varieties except sliced	Dole	0.2	cup	0	1	0
	canned, in light syrup, sliced	Dole	2.4	oz.	0	1	0
	canned, in light syrup, w/mandarin orange	Dole	0.3	cup	0	1	0
	canned, in heavy syrup		1.6	oz.	0	1	0
	canned, in heavy syrup, all varieties, except sliced	Dole	0.2	cup	0	1	0
	canned, in heavy syrup, chunks, tidbits or crushed		0.2	cup	0	1	0
	canned, in heavy syrup, crushed or chunks	Del Monte	0.2	cup	0	1	0
	canned, in heavy syrup, sliced	Del Monte	0.8	slices	0	1	0
	canned, in heavy syrup, sliced	Dole	0.8	slices	0	1	0
	canned, in heavy syrup, sliced	S&W	0.2	cup	0	1	0
	canned, in extra heavy syrup, crushed		0.2	cup	0	1	0
	canned, in extra heavy syrup, cubed		0.1	cup	0	1	0
	dried	Sonoma	0.5	oz.	0	1	0
	frozen, chunks	Goya	0.2	pkg.	0	1	0
	frozen, unsweetened, chunks		0.2	cup	0	1	0
Pineapple, candied	assorted	Paradise/White Swan	2.5	pcs.	0	1	0
		Paradise/White Swan	0.4	oz.	0	1	0
	green	Paradise/White Swan	.3	pcs.	0	1	0
	red	Paradise/White Swan	3.1	pcs.	0	1	0
	slices, natural or color	S&W Glace	0.4	oz.	0	1	0
	wedges, natural or color	S&W Glace	2.2	pcs.	0	1	0

Food	Brand / Type	Description	Amount	Unit	P	C	F
Pineapple drink	Tropicana Punch 16 oz.		2.4	fl. oz.	0	1	0
Pineapple drink blends	Tropicana Punch		2.3	fl. oz.	0	1	0
	Farmer's Market	coconut	2.5	fl. oz.	0	1	0
	Kern's	coconut nectar	2.1	fl. oz.	0	1	1
	Kern's	coconut nectar	2.1	fl. oz.	0	1	1
	Dole	grapefruit, pink	2.1	fl. oz.	0	1	0
	Dole	grapefruit, pink	2.2	fl. oz.	0	1	0
	Goya	guava, nectar	2.1	fl. oz.	0	1	0
	Goya	passion fruit, nectar	2.1	fl. oz.	0	1	0
Pineapple juice	Del Monte		2.7	fl. oz.	0	1	0
	Del Monte		2.4	fl. oz.	0	1	0
	Del Monte Not from Concentrate		2.7	fl. oz.	0	1	0
	Dole Canned		2.5	fl. oz.	0	1	0
	Dole Chilled		2.5	fl. oz.	0	1	0
	Goya		2.4	fl. oz.	0	1	0
	Minute Maid		2.2	fl. oz.	0	1	0
	S&W		2.6	fl. oz.	0	1	0
	S&W		2.7	fl. oz.	0	1	0
	S&W		2.6	fl. oz.	0	1	0
Pineapple juice blends	Dole	frozen, prepared	2.4	fl. oz.	0	1	0
	R.W. Knudsen	coconut	2.2	fl. oz.	0	1	0
	Dole	grapefruit	2.2	fl. oz.	0	1	0
	Dole	grapefruit, frozen, prepared	2.5	fl. oz.	0	1	0
	Dole	orange	2.7	fl. oz.	0	1	0
	Dole	orange, frozen, prepared	2.5	fl. oz.	0	1	0
	Dole	orange-banana	2.5	fl. oz.	0	1	0
	Dole	orange-banana	2.3	fl. oz.	0	1	0
	Dole	orange-berry	2.2	fl. oz.	0	1	0
	Dole	orange-guava	2.5	fl. oz.	0	1	0
	Dole	orange-strawberry	2.2	fl. oz.	0	1	0
	Dole	passion fruit-banana	2.5	fl. oz.	0	1	0
	Dole	passion fruit-banana	2.3	fl. oz.	0	1	0
Pineapple topping	Kraft		0.6	Tbsp.	0	1	0
	Smucker's		0.6	Tbsp.	0	1	0
Pink beans	Goya	boiled	0.2	cup	0	1	0
	Goya	canned	0.4	cup	1	1	0
	Goya Guisadas	canned, in tomato sauce	0.4	cup	1	1	1

FOOD ITEM	SPECIFICATIONS	BRAND NAME	QUANTITY	SIZE	PROTEIN BLOCKS	CARBOHYDRATE BLOCKS	FAT BLOCKS
Pinquito beans	canned	S&W	0.3	cup	0	1	0
Pinto beans	dry	Arrowhead Mills	0.1	cup	0	1	0
	dry		0.6	cup	1	1	0
	boiled		0.3	cup	0	1	0
	canned, w/liquid		0.3	cup	0	1	0
	canned	Allens East Texas Fair/Brown Beauty	0.4	cup	0	1	0
	canned	Eden Organic	0.4	cup	0	1	0
	canned	Eden Organic Jars	0.3	cup	0	1	0
	canned	Gebhardt	0.4	cup	1	1	0
	canned	Goya	0.5	cup	1	1	0
	canned	Green Giant/Joan of Arc	0.3	cup	0	1	0
	canned	Old El Paso	0.4	cup	1	1	0
	canned	Progresso	0.4	cup	0	1	0
	canned	Stokely	0.3	cup	0	1	0
	canned	Sun-Vista	0.5	cup	0	1	0
	w/bacon	Trappey's	0.4	cup	0	1	0
	w/bacon	Trappey's Jalapinto	0.3	cup	0	1	0
	in tomato sauce	Goya Guisadas	0.4	cup	0	1	0
Pinto beans, sprouted	boiled, drained		10	oz.	1	1	0
Pitanga			10	medium	0	1	0
Pizza crust	refrigerated	Pillsbury	0.7	crust	0	1	1
	refrigerated	Totino's	0.1	crust	0	1	1
Pizza sauce		Contadina	0.8	cup	0	1	0
		Contadina Chunky	0.4	cup	0	1	0
		Contadina Pizza Squeeze	0.4	cup	0	1	1
		Pastorelli Italian Chef	0.6	cup	1	1	1
		Prince Traditional	0.8	cup	0	1	0
		Progresso	0.6	cup	0	1	1
		Ragu Quick	0.6	cup	0	1	0
	w/cheese, Italian	Contadina	0.8	cup	0	1	1
	w/cheese, Italian	Contadina Pizza Squeeze	0.4	cup	0	1	1
	w/cheese, three	Contadina Chunky	0.6	cup	0	1	1

Food	Description	Brand	Amount	Unit			
Pizza seasoning	mushroom	Contadina Chunky	0.6	cup	0	1	0
	pepperoni	Contadina	0.8	cup	1	1	0
		Tone's Presti's	7.5	tsp.	3	1	0
Plantain		Frieda's	1	oz.	0	1	0
	raw		0.2	medium	0	1	0
	raw, sliced		0.2	cup	0	1	0
	cooked, sliced		0.2	cup	0	1	0
	fried	Goya Tostone	0.8	pcs.	0	1	0
Plum	fresh, Japanese or hybrid		1	2 1/8" fruit	0	1	0
	fresh, sliced		0.5	cup	0	1	0
	canned, juice		0.3	cup	0	1	0
	canned, juice		2	plums and 2 Tbsp. liquid	0	1	0
	canned, light syrup		0.2	cup	0	1	0
	canned, light syrup		1.3	plums and 2 3/4 Tbsp. liquid	0	1	0
	canned, heavy syrup		0.2	cup	0	1	0
	canned, heavy syrup, whole		0.1	cup	0	1	0
Plum sauce		S&W	1	Tbsp.	0	1	0
		Ka-Me	1.4	Tbsp.	1	1	0
Poi		La Choy	0.1	cup	0	1	0
Poke greens		Allens	2.5	cup	1	1	1
Pokeberry shoots	raw		2.5	cup	1	1	1
	canned		5	cup	2	1	2
Polenta, refrigerated	boiled, drained	Frieda's	1	slices, 1/2"	2	1	1
	basil and garlic	San Gennaro's	1.3	slices, 1/2"	0	1	1
	sun-dried tomato	San Gennaro's	1.3	slices, 1/2"	0	1	1
Polenta mix		San Gennaro's	1.2	slices, 1/2"	0	1	1
Pomegranate		Fantastica	0.2	cup, prepared	0	1	0
			3.5	oz. fruit	0	1	0
Pomegranate juice		Frieda's	2	oz.	0	1	0
		R.W. Knudsen	2	fl. oz.	0	1	0
Popcorn		Arrowhead Mills	0.5	oz.	0	1	0
	hot air	Orville Redenbacher Original or White	1.1	Tbsp.	0	1	0
		Orville Redenbacher	1.1	Tbsp.	0	1	0
	microwave	Orville Redenbacher	1.3	Tbsp.	1	1	0

CARBOHYDRATES

FOOD ITEM	SPECIFICATIONS	BRAND NAME	QUANTITY	SIZE	PROTEIN BLOCKS	CARBOHYDRATE BLOCKS	FAT BLOCKS
	microwave	Redenbudders Movie Theater	1.5	Tbsp.	0	1	3
	microwave	Redenbudders Movie Theater Light	1.3	Tbsp.	0	1	1
	microwave	Smart Pop	1.3	Tbsp.	0	1	1
	microwave, butter	Orville Redenbacher	1.7	Tbsp.	0	1	4
	microwave, butter	Orville Redenbacher Light	1.3	Tbsp.	0	1	1
	microwave, caramel	Orville Redenbacher	0.9	Tbsp.	0	1	2
	microwave, cheddar	Orville Redenbacher	1.5	Tbsp.	0	1	3
	microwave, herb and garlic	Redenbudders	1.5	Tbsp.	0	1	2
	microwave, natural	Orville Redenbacher	1.3	Tbsp.	0	1	3
	micorwave, zesty	Redenbudders	1.5	Tbsp.	0	1	2
Popcorn, popped		Barrel O'Fun Canola	2.1	cups	0	1	2
		Barrel O'Fun Light	1.4	cups	0	1	0
		Chester's Triple Mix	0.8	cups	0	1	1
		Wise Choice	1.4	cups	0	1	1
	air-popped, white	Jolly Time	2.5	cups	0	1	0
	air-popped, yellow	Jolly Time	2.5	cups	0	1	0
	butter/butter flavor	Borden	0.8	oz.	0	1	3
	butter/butter flavor	Chester's	2.3	cups	0	1	3
	butter/butter flavor	Smarfood	1.9	cups	0	1	2
	butter/butter flavor	Smarfood Reduced Fat	1.8	cups	0	1	1
	butter/butter flavor	Wise Reduced Fat	1.7	cups	0	1	0
	caramel	Barrel O'Fun Fat Free	0.3	cup	0	1	0
	caramel	Chester's	0.3	cup	0	1	0
	caramel	Cracker Jack Fat Free	0.3	cup	0	1	0
	caramel	Smart Snackers	0.4	oz.	0	1	0
	caramel	Wise Fat Free	0.3	cup	0	1	1
	caramel, w/peanuts	Barrel O'Fun	0.3	cup	0	1	0
	caramel, w/peanuts	Cracker Jack	0.3	cup	0	1	0
	caramel, w/peanuts	Old Dutch	0.4	oz.	0	1	3
	cheddar, white	Barrel O'Fun	2.3	cups	0	1	3
	cheddar, white	Chester's	1.9	cups	0	1	3
	cheddar, white	Smarfood	1.2	cups	0	1	2
	cheddar, white	Smarfood Reduced Fat	1.7	cups	0	1	1

Category	Brand	Description	P	C	F	Amount	Unit
	Barrel O'Fun	cheese	0	1	3	1.9	cups
	Barrel O'Fun Low Fat	cheese	0	1	1	1.3	cups
	Jolly Time	microwave	0	1	3	3.1	cups
	Jolly Time Light	microwave	0	1	1	3.1	cups
	Pop Secret	microwave, nacho	0	1	2	3.3	cup
	Chester's	microwave, butter flavor	0	1	2	2.5	cups
	Jolly Time	microwave, butter flavor	0	1	2	3.1	cups
	Jolly Time Light	microwave, butter flavor	0	1	1	2.9	cups
	Cracker Jack Fat Free	toffee butter	0	1	0	0.3	cup
	Wise Fat Free	toffee butter	0	1	0	0.3	cup
	Cracker Jacks	toffee butter, w/peanuts	0	1	1	0.3	1.25 oz. box
	Cracker Jacks	toffee butter, w/pecans and almonds	0	1	1	0.5	oz.
Popcorn bar	Smartfood	toffee crunch	0	1	0	0.3	cup
	Franklin	toffee, w/nuts	0	1	0	0.2	cup
	Pop Secret	caramel	0	1	1	0.6	bar
	Pop Secret	chocolate	0	1	1	0.6	bar
Popcorn cakes	Mother's	apple cinnamon	0	1	0	1.1	cake
	Orville Redenbacher Mini	butter	0	1	0	0.5	oz.
	Orville Redenbacher	butter	0	1	0	1.4	cakes
	Orville Redenbacher Mini	butter	0	1	0	0.6	oz.
	Quaker Mini	caramel	0	1	0	4.6	cakes
	Orville Redenbacher	caramel or honey nut	0	1	0	1	cakes
	Orville Redenbacher Mini	cheddar, white	0	1	0	0.5	oz.
	Lundberg Mini	cheddar, white	0	1	0	4.5	cakes
	Orville Redenbacher	cheddar, white	0	1	0	1.4	cakes
	Orville Redenbacher Mini	cheddar, white	0	1	0	0.6	oz.
Pork gravy	Franco-American		3	1	0	1.3	cup
	Durkee	mix, prepared	0	1	7	0.8	cup
	French's	mix, prepared	0	1	0	0.8	cup
Pork seasoning mix	Durkee/French's Roasting Bag	barbeque glaze	0	1	1	0.3	pkg.
	Shake'n Bake Original Recipe	chops	0	1	0	0.1	pkg.
	Shake'n Bake		0	1	0	0.1	pkg.
	McCormick Bag' n Season		0	1	0	5	tsp. mix
	Oven Fry	extra crispy	0	1	0	0.1	pkg.
	Shake'n Bake	hot and spicy	0	1	0	0.1	pkg.

FOOD ITEM	SPECIFICATIONS	BRAND NAME	QUANTITY	SIZE	PROTEIN BLOCKS	CARBOHYDRATE BLOCKS	FAT BLOCKS
Pot roast seasoning mix	sparerib	Durkee Roasting Bag	0.2	pkg.	0	1	0
		Durkee Roasting Bag	0.6	pkg.	0	1	0
		French's Roasting Bag	0.4	pkg.	0	1	0
		Lawry's	10	tsp.	0	1	0
	onion	French's Roasting Bag	0.4	pkg.	0	1	0
	sauerbraten	Knorr	0.3	pkg.	0	1	1
Potato	raw, unpeeled		0.2	lb.	0	1	0
	raw, peeled		0.5	2.5" potato	0	1	0
	raw, peeled, diced		0.4	cup	0	1	0
	baked, in skin		0.2	4 3/4" x 2 1/3" in skin,	0	1	0
	baked, w/out skin		1.6	oz.	0	1	0
	baked, w/out skin		0.4	cup	0	1	0
	boiled, in skin, baby	Frieda's	1.8	oz.	0	1	0
	boiled, in skin, peeled		0.4	2.5" potato	0	1	0
	boiled, in skin, peeled		0.3	cup	0	1	0
	boiled, w/out skin		0.4	2.5" potato	0	1	0
	boiled, w/out skin		0.3	cup	0	1	0
	microwaved in skin		0.2	4 3/4" x 2 1/3" potato	0	1	0
	microwaved in skin, peeled		0.3	cup	0	1	0
	microwaved, skin only		1.1	oz.	0	1	0
	mashed, w/whole milk		0.3	cup	0	1	0
	mashed, w/whole milk, w/butter		0.3	cup	0	1	1
	mashed, w/whole milk, w/margarine		0.3	cup	0	1	1
Potato, canned	w/liquid		4.4	oz.	0	1	0
	drained		2	1.2 oz. potato	0	1	0
	whole	Butterfield/Sunshine	2.8	oz.	0	1	0
	whole	Stokely	5	oz.	0	1	0
	whole	Stokely No Salt	5	oz.	0	1	0
	whole, new	Del Monte	1.7	medium w/liquid	0	1	0

Food	Description	Brand / Product	Amount	Unit	Protein	Carbohydrate	Fat
Potato, frozen	whole, new	S&W	0.4	cup	0	1	0
	sliced	Butterfield	0.3	cup	0	1	0
	sliced	Del Monte	0.6	cup	0	1	0
	diced	Butterfield	0.3	cup	0	1	0
	mashed	Idahoan Real	0.2	cup	0	1	0
	mashed	Idahoan Complete	0.2	cup	0	1	0
	whole	Stilwell	2.3	pcs.	0	1	1
	fried or french-fried	Ore-Ida Deep Fried	1.4	oz.	0	1	1
	fried or french-fried	Ore-Ida Deep Fried Crinkle Cuts	1.3	oz.	0	1	1
	fried or french-fried	Ore-Ida Shoestring	1.4	oz.	0	1	1
	fried or french-fried	Ore-Ida Steak Fries	1.5	oz.	0	1	1
	fried or french-fried	Ore-Ida Crispers!	1.3	oz.	0	1	2
	fried or french-fried	Ore-Ida Crispy Crowns!	1.5	oz.	0	1	2
	fried or french-fried	Ore-Ida Crispy Crunchies!	1.5	oz.	0	1	1
	fried or french-fried	Ore-Ida Fast Fries	1.5	oz.	0	1	1
	fried or french-fried	Ore-Ida Golden Crinkles	1.3	oz.	0	1	1
	fried or french-fried	Ore-Ida Golden Fries	1.4	oz.	0	1	1
	fried or french-fried	Ore-Ida Golden Twirls	1.3	oz.	0	1	1
	fried or french-fried	Ore-Ida Golden Pixie Crinkles	1.4	oz.	0	1	1
	fried or french-fried	Ore-Ida Homestyle Wedges with Skin	1.6	oz.	0	1	2
	fried or french-fried	Ore-Ida Snackin' Fries	1.4	oz.	0	1	2
	fried or french-fried	Ore-Ida Texas Crispers!	1.5	oz.	0	1	1
	fried or french-fried	Ore-Ida Waffle Fries	1.4	oz.	0	1	1
	fried or french-fried	Ore-Ida Zesties	1.4	oz.	0	1	1
	fried or french-fried, cottage fries	Ore-Ida	1.1	oz.	0	1	1
	fried or french-fried, country fries	Ore-Ida	1.6	oz.	0	1	1
	fried or french-fried, crinkle cut	Empire Kosher	0.4	cup	0	1	0
	fried or french-fried, ranch flavor	Ore-Ida Fast Fries	1.4	oz.	0	1	1
	fried or french-fried, zesty	Ore-Ida Snackin' Fries	1.5	oz.	0	1	2
	hash brown	Ore-Ida Golden Patties	0.6	pc.	0	1	2
	hash brown	Ore-Ida Microwave	1.4	oz.	0	1	1
	hash brown, w/cheddar	Ore-Ida Cheddar Browns	0.7	pc.	0	1	1

FOOD ITEM	SPECIFICATIONS	BRAND NAME	QUANTITY	SIZE	PROTEIN BLOCKS	CARBOHYDRATE BLOCKS	FAT BLOCKS
	hash brown, country	Ore-Ida	0.7	cup	0	1	0
	hash brown, shredded	Ore-Ida	0.6	pc.	0	1	0
	hash brown, Southern style	Ore-Ida	0.4	cup	0	1	0
	hash brown, toaster	Ore-Ida	0.7	pcs.	0	1	1
	mashed	Ore-Ida	0.4	cup	0	1	0
	O'Brien	Ore-Ida	0.5	cup	0	1	0
	puffs	Hot Tots	2	oz.	0	1	1
	puffs	Tater Tots	1.9	oz.	0	1	1
	puffs	Tater Tots Microwave	1.4	oz.	0	1	1
Potato, mix, dry	au gratin	Betty Crocker Potato Buds	0.2	cup	0	1	0
	au gratin	Hungry Jack	0.2	cup	0	1	0
	cheddar and sour cream	Idahoan	0.1	cup	0	1	0
	French country	Betty Crocker	0.3	cup	0	1	0
	Italian, southern	Good Harvest	0.2	cup	0	1	0
	mashed	Good Harvest	0.1	cup	0	1	0
	mashed	Barbara's	0.2	cup	0	1	0
	mashed	Idahoan Flakes	0.2	cup	0	1	0
	mashed	Pillsbury Idaho	1	Tbsp.	0	1	0
	mashed, cheddar and bacon	Hungry Jack	0.2	cup	0	1	0
	mashed, cheese	Hungry Jack	0.2	cup	0	1	0
	scalloped	Betty Crocker	0.3	cup	0	1	0
	scalloped	Idahoan	0.2	cup	0	1	0
	scalloped, cheesy	Betty Crocker	0.3	cup	0	1	0
	scalloped, cheesy	Hungry Jack	0.2	cup	0	1	0
	scalloped, creamy	Hungry Jack	0.2	cup	0	1	0
	sour cream and chive	Hungry Jack	0.2	cup	0	1	0
	vegetable and herb	Good Harvest	0.2	cup	0	1	0
	Western	Idahoan	0.1	cup	0	1	0
Potato chips and crisps		Barbara's Regular/Ripple	0.6	oz.	0	1	2
		Barbara's No Salt	0.6	oz.	0	1	2
		Barrel O'Fun	0.6	oz.	0	1	2
		Barrel O'Fun Ripple	0.6	oz.	0	1	2
		Borden Lightly Salted	0.7	oz.	0	1	2

Descriptor	Food	Amount	Unit			
	Kettle Chips	0.6	oz.	0	1	2
	Kettle Crisps	0.5	oz.	0	1	0
	Lay's	0.6	oz.	0	1	2
	Lay's Baked	0.4	oz.	0	1	0
	Lay's Wavy	0.6	oz.	0	1	2
	Mr. Phipps Crisps	0.5	oz.	0	1	0
	Munchos	0.5	oz.	0	1	2
	New York Deli	0.7	oz.	0	1	0
	No Fries Original	0.4	oz.	0	1	2
	Old Dutch	0.6	oz.	0	1	0
	Old Dutch Ripl	0.6	oz.	0	1	2
	Ridgies Flat or Curlie	0.7	oz.	0	1	2
	Ridgies Super Crispy	0.7	oz.	0	1	2
	Ruffles	0.7	oz.	0	1	2
	Ruffles Reduced Fat	0.5	oz.	0	1	1
barbeque	Wise Ripple	0.7	oz.	0	1	2
barbeque	Barbara's	0.6	oz.	0	1	2
barbeque	Barrel O'Fun	0.6	oz.	0	1	2
barbeque	Borden	0.6	oz.	0	1	2
barbeque	Lay's Baked	0.4	oz.	0	1	0
barbeque	Lay's Hickory	0.6	oz.	0	1	2
barbeque	Lay's KC Masterpiece	0.6	oz.	0	1	2
barbeque	Mr. Phipps Crisps	0.5	oz.	0	1	1
barbeque	No Fries	0.4	oz.	0	1	0
barbeque	Munchos	0.6	oz.	0	1	2
barbeque	Old Dutch	0.6	oz.	0	1	2
barbeque	Old Dutch Ripl	0.6	oz.	0	1	2
barbeque, mesquite	Krunchers!	0.6	oz.	0	1	2
barbeque, mesquite	Old Dutch Kettle	0.5	oz.	0	1	1
barbeque, mesquite	Ruffles KC Masterpiece	0.6	oz.	0	1	2
Caribbean flavor	Borden Calypso	0.6	oz.	0	1	2
cheddar	Health Valley Puffs	0.5	oz.	0	1	0
cheddar, New York, w/herb	Kettle Chips	0.6	oz.	0	1	2
cheddar/sour cream	Barrel O'Fun Ripple	0.6	oz.	0	1	2
cheddar/sour cream	Old Dutch	0.6	oz.	0	1	2
cheddar/sour cream	Old Dutch Ripl	0.6	oz.	0	1	2

FOOD ITEM	SPECIFICATIONS	BRAND NAME	QUANTITY	SIZE	PROTEIN BLOCKS	CARBOHYDRATE BLOCKS	FAT BLOCKS
	cheddar/sour cream	Ruffles	0.6	oz.	0	1	2
	cheddar/sour cream	Wise Ripple	0.7	oz.	0	1	2
	cheddar/sour cream	Wise Super Crispy	0.6	oz.	0	1	2
	Dijon, golden	Ruffles	0.6	oz.	0	1	2
	dill pickle	Old Dutch	0.6	oz.	0	1	2
	honey barbeque	Kettle Crisps	0.5	oz.	0	1	0
	honey Dijon	Kettle Chips	0.6	oz.	0	1	2
	hot	Barrel O'Fun	0.6	oz.	0	1	2
	hot	Lay's Flamin'	0.6	oz.	0	1	2
	jalapeno	Krunchers!	0.6	oz.	0	1	2
	jalapeno jack	Kettle Chips	0.6	oz.	0	1	2
	jalapeno and cheddar	Old Dutch	0.6	oz.	0	1	1
	onion, French	Old Dutch Ripl	0.6	oz.	0	1	2
	onion, French	Ruffles	0.6	oz.	0	1	2
	onion and garlic	Barrel O'Fun	0.6	oz.	0	1	2
	onion and garlic	Borden	0.7	oz.	0	1	2
	onion and garlic	Lay's	0.6	oz.	0	1	2
	onion and garlic	Old Dutch	0.6	oz.	0	1	2
	pesto	Kettle Crisps	0.5	oz.	0	1	0
	ranch	Lay's Hidden Valley Wavy	0.7	oz.	0	1	3
	ranch	Ruffles	0.6	oz.	0	1	2
	ranch, puffs	Health Valley	0.5	oz.	0	1	0
	salsa and cheese	Lay's	0.5	oz.	0	1	2
	salsa w/mesquite	Kettle Chips	0.6	oz.	0	1	2
	salt and sour	Barrel O'Fun	0.6	oz.	0	1	2
	salt and vinegar	Borden	0.7	oz.	0	1	2
	salt and vinegar	Kettle Chips	0.6	oz.	0	1	2
	salt and vinegar	Lay's	0.6	oz.	0	1	2
	salt and vinegar	Old Dutch	0.5	oz.	0	1	1
	sour cream/onion	Barrel O'Fun	0.6	oz.	0	1	2
	sour cream/onion	Borden	0.7	oz.	0	1	2
	sour cream/onion	Lay's	0.6	oz.	0	1	2
	sour cream/onion	Lay's Baked	0.4	oz.	0	1	0

Item	Variety	Brand	Amount	Unit	Protein	Carbohydrate	Fat
	sour cream/onion	Mr. Phipps Crisps	0.5	oz.	0	1	1
	sour cream/onion	Old Dutch	0.6	oz.	0	1	2
	sour cream/onion	Ruffles Reduced Fat	0.5	oz.	0	1	1
	yogurt and green onion	Barbara's	0.6	oz.	0	1	2
	yogurt and green onion	Barbara's No Salt	0.6	oz.	0	1	2
	yogurt and green onion	Kettle Chips	0.6	oz.	0	1	2
Potato flour			0.1	cup	0	1	0
Potato pancake, frozen		Empire Kosher	2.5	oz. cake	0	1	1
	mini	Empire Kosher	1.8	cakes	0	1	1
Potato pancake mix		Knorr	1.1	Tbsp.	0	1	0
Potato seasoning mix		Potato Shakers	5	tsp.	0	1	0
	cheddar	Shake 'n Bake Perfect Potatoes	0.8	pkg.	1	1	4
	herb garlic	Shake 'n Bake Perfect Potatoes	0.3	pkg.	0	1	0
Potato sticks		Butterfield	0.6	oz.	0	1	2
		Butterfield	0.7	oz.	0	1	2
		Pik-Nik Fabulous Fries	0.4	cup	0	1	2
	hot	Chester's Fries Flamin'	0.6	oz.	0	1	2
	ketchup	Pik-Nik Ket'n Fries	0.5	oz.	0	1	1
	shoestring	French's	0.4	cup	0	1	2
	shoestring	Pik-Nik	0.6	cup	0	1	2
	shoestring	Pik-Nik	0.4	oz. can	0	1	2
	shoestring	Pik-Nik Less Salt	0.4	cup	0	1	2
	shoestring, BBQ	Pik-Nik	0.4	cup	0	1	2
	shoestring, sour cream/cheddar	Pik-Nik	0.4	cup	0	1	3
Poultry seasoning			10	tsp.	0	1	0
Pretzels		Barbara's Honeysweet	0.5	oz.	0	1	0
		Barrel O'Fun Mini	0.4	oz.	0	1	0
		Borden Tiny Thins/Mini	0.4	oz.	0	1	0
		Borden Thins/Ultra Thins	0.4	oz.	0	1	0
		Little Debbie	0.4	oz.	0	1	0
		Mister Salty Mini	0.4	oz.	0	1	0
		Old Dutch	0.4	oz.	0	1	0
		Pepperidge Farm Goldfish	18.8	pcs.	0	1	0
		Quinlan Beer	0.9	pcs.	0	1	0

FOOD ITEM	SPECIFICATIONS	BRAND NAME	QUANTITY	SIZE	PROTEIN BLOCKS	CARBOHYDRATE BLOCKS	FAT BLOCKS
		Quinlan Nuggets	0.4	oz.	0	1	0
		Quinlan Party Thins	0.4	oz.	0	1	0
		Quinlan Sticks	0.4	oz.	0	1	0
		Quinlan Thin	0.4	oz.	0	1	0
		Quinlan Tiny Thins/Mini	0.4	oz.	0	1	0
		Quinlan Ultra Thin	0.4	oz.	0	1	0
	bagel shaped	Manischewitz	0.4	oz.	0	1	0
	Bavarian	Barbara's	0.5	oz.	0	1	0
	Bavarian	Barbara's No Salt	0.5	oz.	0	1	0
	Bavarian	Rold Gold	0.5	oz.	0	1	0
	cheddar	Combos	0.5	oz.	0	1	1
	cheddar	Combos	0.5	oz.	0	1	1
	cheese	Handi-Snacks	0.9	oz.	0	1	2
	chips	Mr. Phipps	0.4	oz.	0	1	0
	chips	Mr. Phipps Fat Free	0.4	oz.	0	1	0
	chips	Mr. Phipps Lower Sodium	0.4	oz.	0	1	0
	chips	Mr. Salty	0.4	oz.	0	1	0
	chips	Mr. Salty Fat Free	0.4	oz.	0	1	0
	Dutch	Mister Salty	0.7	pcs.	0	1	0
	hard, plain		0.4	oz.	0	1	0
	honey, mustard-onion	Old Dutch	0.5	oz.	0	1	1
	honey, mustard-onion	Old Dutch	0.5	oz.	0	1	1
	mini	Barbara's	0.5	oz.	0	1	0
	mini	Barbara's No Salt	0.5	oz.	0	1	0
	mustard	Combos	0.5	oz.	0	1	1
	mustard	Combos	0.5	oz.	0	1	1
	nacho	Combos	0.5	oz.	0	1	1
	nacho	Combos	0.5	oz.	0	1	1
	9 grain	Barbara's	0.5	oz.	0	1	0
	oat bran nuggets	Smart Snackers	0.5	oz.	0	1	0
	pizza	Combos	0.5	oz.	0	1	1
	pizza	Combos	0.3	1.8 oz. bag	0	1	1
	rods	Old Dutch	1	pcs.	0	1	0

Food	Brand				Amount	Unit
rods	Rold Gold	0	1	0	1.3	pcs.
soft	Superpretzel	0	1	0	0.6	oz.
soft	Superpretzel Added Salt	0	1	0	0.6	oz.
soft, bites	Superpretzel	0	1	0	1.5	pcs.
soft, bites	Superpretzel Added Salt	0	1	0	1.5	pcs.
soft, cinnamon raisin	Superpretzel	0	1	0	0.5	pcs.
soft, cheese-filled, cheddar or pizza	Superpretzel Softstix	0	1	0	0.8	pcs.
soft, cheese-filled, nacho	Superpretzel Softstix	0	1	0	0.8	pcs.
sourdough	Quinlan	0	1	0	0.5	pc.
sourdough	Quinlan No Salt	0	1	0	0.5	pc.
sourdough, Bavarian or twists	Barbara's	0	1	0	0.4	oz.
sourdough, hard	Rold Gold	0	1	0	0.4	oz.
sticks	Bachman Stix	0	1	0	0.5	oz.
sticks	Mister Salty Fat Free	0	1	0	0.4	oz.
sticks	Old Dutch	0	1	0	0.4	oz.
sticks	Quinlan	0	1	0	0.4	oz.
sticks	Rold Gold Fat Free	0	1	0	0.4	oz.
sticks, sesame	Barbara's	0	1	0	0.6	oz.
thins	Old Dutch Fat Free	0	1	0	0.4	oz.
thins	Quinlan	0	1	0	0.4	oz.
thins	Rold Gold	0	1	0	0.4	oz.
thins	Rold Gold Fat Free	0	1	0	0.4	oz.
twists	Old Dutch	0	1	0	0.4	oz.
twists	Mister Salty	0	1	0	0.4	oz.
twists	Planters	0	1	0	0.4	oz.
twists	Planters	0	1	0	0.4	oz.
twists, tiny	Rold Gold Fat Free	0	1	0	0.4	oz.
Prickly pear	Frieda's	0	1	0	1.4	medium, 4.8 oz.
Prune						
canned, in heavy syrup, pitted		0	1	0	2.9	oz.
canned, in heavy syrup		0	1	0	1.3	oz.
canned, in heavy syrup		0	0	0	0.2	cup
canned, in heavy syrup		0	0	0	2.2	pcs, 2 Tbsp. liquid
canned, in heavy syrup	Sonoma	0	1	0	0.5	oz.

FOOD ITEM	SPECIFICATIONS	BRAND NAME	QUANTITY	SIZE	PROTEIN BLOCKS	CARBOHYDRATE BLOCKS	FAT BLOCKS
	canned, in heavy syrup, stewed	S&W	1.5	pcs.	0	1	0
	dehydrated, uncooked		0.1	cup	0	1	0
	dehydrated, cooked		0.1	cup	0	1	0
	dried		0.1	cup	0	1	0
	dried		0.5	oz.	0	1	0
	dried, w/pits		0.1	cup	0	1	0
	dried, pitted		1.9	prunes	0	1	0
	dried, pitted		0.1	cup	0	1	0
	dried, stewed, w/pits, unsweetened		0.2	cup	0	1	0
Prune juice		Del Monte	1.7	fl. oz.	0	1	0
		Goya	1.8	fl. oz.	0	1	0
		Lucky Leaf/Musselman's	1.8	fl. oz.	0	1	0
		R.W. Knudsen	1.6	fl. oz.	0	1	0
		S&W	1.8	fl. oz.	0	1	0
Pudding	banana	Del Monte Snack	1.5	oz.	0	1	0
	banana	Hunt's Snack Pack	1.4	oz.	0	1	1
	banana	Jell-O Snack	1.4	oz.	0	1	0
	banana, nondairy	Imagine	1.2	oz.	0	1	1
	butterscotch	Del Monte Snack	1.5	oz.	0	1	0
	butterscotch	Hunt's Snack Pack	1.5	oz.	0	1	1
	butterscotch	Rich's	1.4	oz.	0	1	1
	butterscotch	Swiss Miss	1.5	oz.	0	1	0
	butterscotch, nondairy	Imagine	1.2	oz.	0	1	1
	chocolate	Del Monte Snack	1.3	oz.	0	1	0
	chocolate	Del Monte Snack Fat Free	1.6	oz.	0	1	1
	chocolate	Hunts Snack Pack	1.4	oz.	0	1	0
	chocolate	Hunts Snack Pack Fat Free	1.7	oz.	0	1	0
	chocolate	Jell-O Snack	1.3	oz.	0	1	1
	chocolate	Jell-O Free Snack	1.5	oz.	0	1	0
	chocolate	Rich's	1.4	oz.	0	1	1
	chocolate	Swiss Miss	1.4	oz.	0	1	1

Food	Brand	Amount			
chocolate, or chocolate fudge	Swiss Miss Fat Free	1.5 oz.	0	1	0
chocolate, nondairy	Imagine	1 oz.	0	1	0
chocolate fudge	Del Monte Snack	1.3 oz.	0	1	0
chocolate fudge	Hunt's Snack Pack	1.4 oz.	0	1	1
chocolate fudge	Swiss Miss	1.3 oz.	0	1	1
chocolate fudge, parfait	Swiss Miss	1.4 oz.	0	1	0
chocolate marshmallow	Hunt's Snack Pack	1.5 oz.	0	1	1
chocolate vanilla parfait	Swiss Miss	1.4 oz.	0	1	1
chocolate swirl, caramel	Hunt's Snack Pack	1.4 oz.	0	1	1
chocolate swirl, caramel	Swiss Miss	1.4 oz.	0	1	1
chocolate swirl, caramel or vanilla	Jell-O Snack	1.3 oz.	0	1	1
chocolate swirl, caramel or vanilla	Jell-O Free Snack	1.5 oz.	0	1	0
chocolate swirl, milk	Hunt's Snack Pack	1.4 oz.	0	1	1
chocolate swirl, vanilla	Swiss Miss	1.4 oz.	0	1	1
lemon	Hunt's Snack Pack	1.1 oz.	0	1	0
lemon, nondairy	Imagine	1.1 oz.	0	1	0
S'mores swirl	Hunt's Snack Pack	1.4 oz.	0	1	0
tapioca	Del Monte Snack	1.5 oz.	0	1	1
tapioca	Hunt's Snack Pack	1.5 oz.	0	1	0
tapioca	Hunt's Snack Pack Fat Free	1.7 oz.	0	1	1
tapioca	Jell-O Snack	1.4 oz.	0	1	0
tapioca	Swiss Miss	1.5 oz.	0	1	0
tapioca	Swiss Miss Fat Free	1.7 oz.	0	1	0
vanilla	Del Monte Snack	1.5 oz.	0	1	0
vanilla	Del Monte Snack Fat Free	1.6 oz.	0	1	0
vanilla	Hunt's Snack Pack	1.4 oz.	0	1	0
vanilla	Hunt's Snack Pack Fat Free	1.7 oz.	0	1	0
vanilla	Jell-O Snack	1.4 oz.	0	1	1
vanilla	Jell-O Free Snack	1.5 oz.	0	1	0
vanilla	Rich's	1.4 oz.	0	1	1
vanilla	Swiss Miss	1.5 oz.	0	1	0
vanilla	Swiss Miss Fat Free	1.7 oz.	0	1	1
vanilla chocolate parfait	Swiss Miss	1.4 oz.	0	1	0
vanilla chocolate parfait	Swiss Miss Fat Free	1.5 oz.	0	1	0

FOOD ITEM	SPECIFICATIONS	BRAND NAME	QUANTITY	SIZE	PROTEIN BLOCKS	CARBOHYDRATE BLOCKS	FAT BLOCKS
Pudding mix	vanilla-chocolate swirl	Jell-O Snack	1.4	oz.	0	1	1
	vanilla-chocolate swirl	Jell-O Free Snack	1.5	oz.	0	1	0
	banana	Jell-O Sugar/Fat Free	0.4	cup, prepared	0	1	0
	banana cream	Jell-O	0.2	cup, prepared	0	1	0
	banana cream	Jell-O Instant	0.2	cup, prepared	0	1	0
	butter pecan	Jell-O Instant	0.2	cup, prepared	0	1	0
	butterscotch	Jell-O	0.2	cup, prepared	0	1	0
	butterscotch	Jell-O Instant	0.2	cup, prepared	0	1	0
	butterscotch	Jell-O Sugar/Fat Free	0.4	cup, prepared	0	1	0
	chocolate	D-Zerta	0.4	cup, prepared	0	1	0
	chocolate	Jell-O	0.2	cup, prepared	0	1	0
	chocolate	Jell-O Instant	0.1	cup, prepared	0	1	0
	chocolate	Jell-O Sugar Free	0.4	cup, prepared	0	1	0
	chocolate	Jell-O Sugar/Fat Free	0.3	cup, prepared	0	1	1
	chocolate	My*T*Fine	0.2	cup, prepared	0	1	0
	chocolate, milk	Jell-O	0.2	cup, prepared	0	1	0
	chocolate, milk	Jell-O Instant	0.1	cup, prepared	0	1	0
	chocolate fudge	Jell-O	0.2	cup, prepared	0	1	0
	chocolate fudge	Jell-O Instant	0.1	cup, prepared	0	1	0
	chocolate fudge	Jell-O Sugar/Fat Free	0.3	cup, prepared	0	1	0
	chocolate mousse, dry, dark	Alsa	2.2	Tbsp.	0	1	1
	chocolate mousse, dry, milk	Alsa	1.8	Tbsp.	0	1	1
	chocolate mousse, dry, white	Alsa	2.2	Tbsp.	0	1	1
	coconut cream	Jell-O	0.2	cup, prepared	0	1	0
	coconut cream	Jell-O Instant	0.2	cup, prepared	0	1	1
	custard	Jell-O Americana	0.2	cup, prepared	0	1	0
	custard, tropical	Goya Tembleque	0.2	cup, prepared	0	1	0
	flan	Alsa Creme Caramel	0.4	1 Tbsp. mix, caramel	0	1	0
	flan	Goya	0.2	cup, prepared	0	1	0
	flan	Jell-O	0.2	cup, prepared	0	1	0
	flan, w/caramel	Goya	0.2	cup, prepared	0	1	0
	lemon	Jell-O	0.2	cup, prepared	0	1	0

Food	Description	Brand	Amount	Unit			
	lemon	Jell-O Instant	0.2	cup, prepared	0	1	0
	pistachio	Jell-O Instant	0.2	cup, prepared	0	1	0
	pistachio	Jell-O Sugar/Fat Free	0.4	cup, prepared	0	1	0
	tapioca	Jell-O Americana	0.2	cup, prepared	0	1	0
	vanilla	Jell-O	0.2	cup, prepared	0	1	1
	vanilla	Jell-O Instant	0.2	cup, prepared	0	1	0
	vanilla	Jell-O Sugar Free	0.4	cup, prepared	0	1	0
	vanilla	Jell-O Sugar/Fat Free	0.4	cup, prepared	0	1	0
	vanilla, French	Jell-O Instant	0.2	cup, prepared	0	1	0
Pummelo	sections		0.2	medium, 5 1/2"	0	1	0
Pumpkin	fresh, pulp, raw, 1" cubes		0.6	cup	0	1	0
	fresh, pulp, boiled, drained, mashed		1.7	cup	0	1	0
	canned, w/ or w/out winter squash		0.8	cup	0	1	0
	canned	Libby's	0.7	cup	0	1	0
	canned	Stokely	0.4	cup	0	1	0
Pumpkin butter		Smucker's	0.7	Tbsp.	0	1	0
Pumpkin flower	raw		0.8	cup	0	1	0
	boiled, drained		5	cup	0	1	0
Pumpkin leaf	raw		2.5	cup	1	1	0
Pumpkin pie spice			5	tsp.	0	1	0
Purslane	raw		10	cup	0	1	0
	boiled, drained		5	cup	0	1	0
Quince	peeled, seeded	Frieda's	2.5	oz.	0	1	0
	pineapple, pulp	Eden	3.8	oz.	0	1	0
Quinoa		Arrowhead Mills	2.5	oz.	1	1	1
Quinoa seeds			2.5	oz.	1	1	1
Radish	sliced		0.1	cup	0	1	0
	raw		100	medium, 3/4"-1"	0	1	0
Radish, Oriental	sliced		5	cup	0	1	0
	raw, sliced		1.1	medium, 7"	0	1	0
	boiled, drained, sliced		5	cup	0	1	0
	dried		0.6	oz.	0	1	0

FOOD ITEM	SPECIFICATIONS	BRAND NAME	QUANTITY	SIZE	PROTEIN BLOCKS	CARBOHYDRATE BLOCKS	FAT BLOCKS
Rainbow baking morsels		Nestle	1	Tbsp.	0	1	1
Raisin	monukka/Thomson	Sonoma	0.1	cup	0	1	0
	golden seedless, not packed		0.1	cup	0	1	0
	golden seedless	Del Monte	0.1	cup	0	1	0
	golden seedless	S&W	0.1	cup	0	1	0
	golden seedless	Sun*Maid	0.1	cup	0	1	0
	muscat	Sun*Maid	0.1	cup	0	1	0
	seeded, not packed		0.1	cup	0	1	0
	seedless, not packed		0.1	cup	0	1	0
	seedless	Del Monte	0.1	cup	0	1	0
	seedless	Del Monte	0.4	oz.	0	1	0
	seedless	S&W	0.1	cup	0	1	0
	seedless	Sun*Maid	0.1	cup	0	1	0
Ranch dip mix	cracked pepper	Knorr	5	tsp.	0	1	0
Raspberry, red			0.6	pint	0	1	0
			1.7	cup	0	1	0
	frozen, sweetened		0.2	cup	0	1	0
	frozen, unsweetened		0.6	cup	0	1	0
Raspberry drink		Big Valley	2.4	fl. oz.	0	1	0
		Farmer's Market	3.1	fl. oz.	0	1	0
	hibiscus	R.W. Knudsen	2.5	fl. oz.	0	1	0
	lemon	Santa Cruz	2.4	fl. oz.	0	1	0
Raspberry juice		Heinke's	2.1	fl. oz.	0	1	0
	blend	Dole Country	2.4	fl. oz.	0	1	0
	cranberry	Apple & Eve	2.4	fl. oz.	0	1	0
		R.W. Knudsen	2.4	fl. oz.	0	1	0
	peach	R.W. Knudsen	2.8	fl. oz.	0	1	0
Raspberry nectar		Santa Cruz	0.1	cup	0	1	0
Raspberry syrup		R.W. Knudsen	0.8	oz.	0	1	1
Ravioli, frozen or refrigerated	cheddar-roasted garlic	Monterey Pasta Company Mediterranean	0.9	oz.	0	1	1
	cheese	Amy's	2.3	oz.	0	1	1
	cheese	Celentano	0.1	of 13-oz. pkg.	0	1	1

Item	Brand	Amount	Unit			
cheese	Celentano Great Choice	0.1	of 13-oz. pkg.	0	—	0
cheese	Stouffer's	2.3	oz.	1	—	0
cheese, four	Contadina	0.3	cup	1	—	0
cheese, four	Contadina Light	0.3	cup	0	—	0
cheese, mini	Celentano	0.9	oz.	0	—	0
cheese, mini, round	Celentano	0.9	oz.	0	—	0
crab, snow	Monterey Pasta Company	0.7	oz.	0	—	0
garden vegetable	Contadina Light	0.3	cup	1	—	0
garlic basil cheese	Monterey Pasta Company	0.8	oz.	1	—	0
gorgonzola roasted walnut	Monterey Pasta Company	0.9	oz.	1	—	0
Monterey Jack smoked	Monterey Pasta Company	0.9	oz.	0	—	0
parsley	Putney	0.2	cup	0	—	0
tofu	Tofutti	0.2	cup	0	—	0
Red beans dried	Goya Dominican	0.1	cup	0	—	1
canned	Allens	0.5	cup	0	—	0
canned	Green Giant/Joan of Arc	0.4	cup	0	—	0
canned	Stokely	0.3	cup	0	—	0
canned	Van Camp's	0.3	cup	0	—	0
canned, small	Hunt's	0.3	cup	0	—	0
Refried beans, canned	Allens	0.4	cup	1	—	1
	Chi-Chi's	0.4	cup	2	—	0
	Chi-Chi's Fat Free	0.4	cup	0	—	0
	Gebhardt	0.3	cup	1	—	0
	Gebhardt No Fat	0.3	cup	0	—	0
	Goya Dominican	0.3	cup	0	—	0
	Las Palmas	0.4	cup	1	—	0
	Las Palmas No Fat	0.4	cup	0	—	0
	Old El Paso	0.4	cup	1	—	0
	Old El Paso Fat Free	0.3	cup	0	—	1
bacon	Rosarita	0.3	cup	1	—	0
	Rosarita No Fat	0.3	cup	0	—	0
black beans	Rosarita	0.4	cup	1	—	1
black beans	Las Palmas	0.4	cup	0	—	1
black beans	Old El Paso	0.4	cup	1	—	1
w/cheese	Rosarita No Fat	0.3	cup	1	—	0
	Old El Paso	0.4	cup	0	—	1

FOOD ITEM	SPECIFICATIONS	BRAND NAME	QUANTITY	SIZE	PROTEIN BLOCKS	CARBOHYDRATE BLOCKS	FAT BLOCKS
	w/cheese, nacho	Rosarita	0.3	cup	0	1	1
	w/green chilies	Old El Paso	0.4	cup	0	1	0
	w/green chilies	Rosarita	0.3	cup	0	1	1
	w/green chilies, and lime	Rosarita No Fat	0.3	cup	1	1	0
	w/jalapeno	Gebhardt	0.4	cup	0	1	1
	w/onion	Rosarita	0.3	cup	1	1	0
	w/salsa, zesty	Rosarita No Fat	0.3	cup	1	1	0
	w/sausage	Old El Paso	0.7	cup	1	1	6
	spicy	Old El Paso	0.3	cup	1	1	6
	spicy	Rosarita	0.3	cup	0	1	0
	vegetarian	Chi-Chi's	0.4	cup	0	1	0
	vegetarian	Gebhardt	0.3	cup	1	1	1
	vegetarian	Old El Paso	0.5	cup	1	1	0
	vegetarian	Rosarita	0.3	cup	0	1	0
Refried beans, mix	vegetarian	Fantastic	0.3	cup	0	1	0
Remoulade sauce		Zararain's	0.3	cup	0	1	3
Rhubarb	fresh, diced	Junket	2.5	cup	1	1	0
	fresh, regular or hothouse	Frieda's	10	oz.	0	1	0
	frozen	Stilwell	3.3	cup	0	1	1
	frozen, cooked, sweetened		0.1	cup	0	1	0
Rice, dry	Arborio	Fantastic Foods	0.1	cup	0	1	0
	Arborio	Frieda's	0.1	cup	0	1	0
	Arborio, brown	Lundberg Nutra-Farmed	0.1	cup	0	1	0
	Arborio, white	Lundberg Nutra-Farmed	0.1	cup	0	1	0
	basmati, brown	Arrowhead Mills	0.1	cup	0	1	0
	basmati, brown	Fantastic Foods	0.1	cup	0	1	0
	basmati, brown	Lundberg Organic	0.1	cup	0	1	0
	basmati, brown	Lundberg Nutra-Farmed/Royal	0.1	cup	0	1	0
	basmati, white	Casbah	0.1	cup	0	1	0
	basmati, white	Fantastic Foods	0.1	cup	0	1	0
	basmati, white	Lundberg Organic	0.1	cup	0	1	0
	basmati, white	Lundberg Nutra-Farmed	0.1	cup	0	1	0
	blends	Lundberg Countrywild	0.1	cup	0	1	0

				○	—	○
blends	Lundberg Jubilee	0.1	cup			
blends	Lundberg Wild Blend	0.1	cup			
blends, field	Lundberg Japonica	0.1	cup			
brown	Carolina/Mahatma/River	0.1	cup			
brown	Lundberg Wehani	0.1	cup			
brown	Success	0.1	cup			
brown, long grain	Arrowhead Mills	0.1	cup			
brown, long grain	Lundberg Nutra-Farmed/Organic	0.1	cup			
brown, long grain	S&W	0.1	cup			
brown, long grain	Uncle Ben's Whole Grain	0.1	cup			
brown, long grain	Uncle Ben's Instant	0.1	cup			
brown, medium grain	Arrowhead Mills	0.1	cup			
brown, medium grain	Arrowhead Mills Quick	0.1	cup			
brown, quick	Lundberg	0.1	cup			
brown, short grain	Arrowhead Mills	0.1	cup			
brown, short grain	Lundberg Nutra-Farmed/Organic	0.1	cup			
brown, precooked	S&W Quick	0.1	cup			
glutinous or sweet		0.1	cup			
jasmine	Goya Fancy Blue Rose	0.1	cup			
jasmine, brown	Goya Valencia	0.1	cup			
sushi	Fantastic Foods	0.1	cup			
white, long grain	Fantastic Foods	0.1	cup			
white, long grain	Lundberg Organic	0.1	cup			
white, long grain	Canilla	0.1	cup			
white, long grain	Carolina	0.1	cup			
white, long grain	Mahatma	0.1	cup			
white, long grain	River/Water Maid	0.1	cup			
white, long grain	Success	0.1	cup			
white, long grain, extra	Goya	0.1	cup			
white, long grain, instant	Carolina	0.1	cup			
white, long grain, instant	Mahatma	0.1	cup			
white, long grain, instant	Minute	0.1	cup			
white, long grain, instant	Minute Premium	0.1	cup			
white, long grain, instant	Minute Boil in Bag	0.1	cup			
white, long grain, instant	Uncle Ben's	0.1	cup			

FOOD ITEM	SPECIFICATIONS	BRAND NAME	QUANTITY	SIZE	PROTEIN BLOCKS	CARBOHYDRATE BLOCKS	FAT BLOCKS
	white, long grain, parboiled	Uncle Bens Converted	0.1	cup	0	1	0
Rice bran	crude		0.4	cup	0	1	2
Rice cake	plain	Mother's Mini Unsalted	5.4	cakes	0	1	0
	all varieties	Lundberg	0.8	cake	0	1	0
	all varieties	Lundberg Unsalted	0.8	cake	0	1	0
	all varieties	Pritikin	1.3	cake	0	1	0
	all varieties	Pritikin Unsalted	1.3	cake	0	1	0
	all varieties, bars	Health Valley Crisp Fat Free	0.4	bars	0	1	0
	all varieties, except cheddar	Quaker Mini	3.8	cakes	0	1	0
	all varieties, except plain	Mother's Mini	3.8	cakes	0	1	0
	apple, cinnamon	Crispy Cakes	1.3	cake	0	1	0
	apple, cinnamon	Quaker	0.8	cake	0	1	0
	apple, crisp	Pritikin Mini	3.8	cakes	0	1	0
	brown	Lundberg Mini	3.8	cakes	0	1	0
	brown, toasted	Crispy Cakes	1.3	cake	0	1	0
	butter-flavored corn	Mother's	1.3	cake	0	1	0
	caramel nut	Pritikin Mini	0.8	cake	0	1	0
	cheese, cheddar	Crispy Cakes	1.3	cake	0	1	0
	cheese, cheddar, white	Quaker	1.1	cake	0	1	0
	cheese, cheddar, white	Quaker Mini	0.8	cake	0	1	0
	cheese, nacho	Lundberg Mini	4.2	cakes	0	1	0
	cheese, nacho corn	Quaker	1.1	cake	0	1	0
	cinnamon crunch	Quaker	0.8	cake	0	1	0
	dill, creamy	Lundberg	0.8	cake	0	1	0
	multigrain	Mother's	1.3	cake	0	1	0
	pizza or ranch	Crispy Cakes	1.3	cake	0	1	0
	vegetable, garden	Crispy Cakes	1.3	cake	0	1	0
	wheat	Mother's	1.3	cake	0	1	0
	wheat	Quaker	1.3	cake	0	1	0
Rice flour			1	Tbsp.	0	1	0
	brown	Goya	0.1	cup	0	1	0
	brown		0.1	cup	0	1	0

Item	Description	Brand	Amount	Unit			
Rice pudding mix	white	Goya	5	cup	5	—	7
	white	Jell-O Americana	0.1	cup	0	—	0
Rice seasoning mix	cinnamon and raisin	Uncle Ben's	0.2	cup, prepared	0	—	0
	cinnamon raisin or honey almond	Lundberg Elegant	0.2	cup, prepared	0	—	0
			0.4	oz.	0	—	0
	coconut	Lundberg Elegant	0.3	cup	0	—	1
	fried	Durkee	0.4	cup	1	—	0
	Mexican	Lawry's	1.3	pkg.	0	—	0
			1.5	Tbsp.	0	—	0
Rice syrup		Lundberg Nutra-Farmed/Organic	0.1	cup	0	—	1
Rigatoni dishes, mix		Noodle Roni	0.2	cup, prepared	0	—	0
Roll	cheddar and broccoli	Arnold Francisco 3"	0.5	roll	0	—	0
		Arnold Bran'nola Buns	0.4	roll	0	—	1
	assorted	Brownberry Hearth	0.4	roll	0	—	0
		Pepperidge Farm Hearth	1	rolls	0	—	0
		Roman Meal	0.7	rolls	0	—	0
	brown and serve	Pepperidge Farm	0.5	roll	0	—	0
	brown and serve	Pepperidge Farm 3	0.2	roll	0	—	0
	brown and serve, club	Pepperidge Farm 2	0.1	roll	0	—	0
	brown and serve, French	Arnold Francisco	0.6	roll	0	—	0
	brown and serve, French	Pepperidge Farm Heat & Serve	0.8	roll	0	—	1
	brown and serve, sourdough	Arnold 12 Pack	0.5	roll	0	—	0
	crescent, butter	Arnold 24 Pack	0.5	roll	0	—	0
	dinner	Arnold August Bros.	0.5	roll	0	—	0
	dinner	Arnold Bran'nola	0.8	roll	0	—	0
	dinner	Brownberry Francisco Intl.	0.4	roll	0	—	0
	dinner	Pepperidge Farm Country Style	1.3	rolls	0	—	0
	dinner	Roman Meal	0.7	rolls	0	—	1
	dinner, all varieties	Awrey's	1	rolls	0	—	0
	dinner, finger, poppy or sesame	Pepperidge Farm	1.4	rolls	0	—	1
	dinner, parker house	Pepperidge Farm	1.4	rolls	0	—	1
	dinner, potato	Arnold	0.9	rolls	0	—	0
	dinner, potato	Pepperidge Farm Deli Classic	0.8	roll	0	—	1
	dinner, sesame seed	Arnold	1	rolls	0	—	0

FOOD ITEM	SPECIFICATIONS	BRAND NAME	QUANTITY	SIZE	PROTEIN BLOCKS	CARBOHYDRATE BLOCKS	FAT BLOCKS
	dinner, wheat	Arnold August Bros.	0.5	roll	0	1	0
	dinner, white	Arnold August Bros.	0.5	roll	0	1	0
	egg, twist	Arnold Levy Old Country	0.3	roll	0	1	0
	French	Arnold 6"	0.3	roll	0	1	0
	French	Brownberry Francisco Intl. 6"	0.3	roll	0	1	0
	French	Pepperidge Farm	0.5	roll	0	1	0
	French, mini	Arnold Francisco	0.4	roll	0	1	0
	French, 7 grain	Pepperidge Farm	0.5	roll	0	1	0
	French, sourdough	Pepperidge Farm	0.5	roll	0	1	0
	golden twist	Pepperidge Farm Heat & Serve	0.8	roll	0	1	1
	hamburger	Arnold 8 Pack	0.4	roll	0	1	0
	hamburger	Arnold 12 Pack	0.4	roll	0	1	0
	hamburger	Arnold August Bros.	0.4	roll	0	1	0
	hamburger	Pepperidge Farm	0.4	roll	0	1	0
	hamburger	Roman Meal	0.5	roll	0	1	0
	hamburger, wheat	Arnold August Bros.	0.4	roll	0	1	0
	hoagie	Awrey's	0.2	roll	0	1	0
	hoagie	Pepperidge Farm Deli Classic	0.3	roll	0	1	0
	hoagie, multigrain	Pepperidge Farm	0.3	roll	0	1	0
	hot dog/frankfurter	Arnold 11 oz.	0.5	roll	0	1	0
	hot dog/frankfurter	Arnold 12 oz.	0.5	roll	0	1	0
	hot dog/frankfurter	Arnold 12 Pack	0.5	roll	0	1	0
	hot dog/frankfurter	Arnold Bran'nola	0.5	roll	0	1	0
	hot dog/frankfurter	Arnold New England	0.4	roll	0	1	0
	hot dog/frankfurter	Brownberry	0.4	roll	0	1	0
	hot dog/frankfurter	Pepperidge Farm	0.5	roll	0	1	0
	hot dog/frankfurter	Roman Meal	0.4	roll	0	1	0
	hot dog/frankfurter, Dijon	Pepperidge Farm	0.4	roll	0	1	0
	hot dog/frankfurter, potato	Arnold	0.5	roll	0	1	0
	hot dog/frankfurter, wheat	Brownberry	0.4	roll	0	1	0
	Italian	Arnold Savoni 8"	0.2	roll	0	1	0
	kaiser	Arnold August Bros.	0.3	roll	0	1	0
	kaiser	Arnold Francisco 6"	0.3	roll	0	1	0

Food	Brand	Amount	Unit	P	C	F
kaiser	Arnold Levy Old Country	0.3	roll	0	1	0
kaiser	Awrey's	0.3	roll	0	1	0
kaiser	Brownberry Hearth	0.3	roll	0	1	0
kaiser	Brownberry Francisco	0.3	roll	0	1	0
kaiser, sesame	Arnold Sandwich	0.4	roll	0	1	0
onion	Arnold Deli	0.3	roll	0	1	0
onion	Arnold August Bros.	0.3	roll	0	1	0
onion	Arnold Levy Old Country	0.3	roll	1	1	0
party	Pepperidge Farm 20	1.9	rolls	0	1	0
potato	Arnold	0.3	roll	0	1	0
potato, sesame	Arnold	0.3	roll	0	1	0
sandwich roll/bun	Pepperidge Farm Hearty	0.2	roll	0	1	0
sandwich roll/bun	Roman Meal	0.3	roll	0	1	0
sandwich roll/bun, multigrain	Pepperidge Farm	0.4	roll	0	1	0
sandwich roll/bun, onion	Pepperidge Farm	0.4	roll	0	1	0
sandwich roll/bun, potato	Brownberry	0.3	roll	1	1	0
sandwich roll/bun, potato	Pepperidge Farm	0.3	roll	0	1	0
sandwich roll/bun, sesame, soft	Arnold	0.4	roll	0	1	0
sandwich roll/bun, sesame seed	Pepperidge Farm	0.4	roll	0	1	0
sandwich roll/bun, soft	Arnold 8 Pack	0.4	roll	0	1	0
sandwich roll/bun, soft	Arnold 12 Pack	0.4	roll	0	1	0
sandwich roll/bun, sourdough	Pepperidge Farm	0.3	roll	0	1	0
sandwich roll/bun, wheat	Brownberry	0.4	roll	0	1	0
sandwich roll/bun, white	Brownberry	0.4	roll	0	1	0
sesame	Arnold August Bros.	0.3	roll	0	1	0
sourdough	Arnold Francisco	0.6	roll	0	1	0
steak	Arnold Premium	0.3	roll	0	1	0
steak	Arnold August Bros.	0.3	roll	0	1	0
steak	Arnold Francisco	0.3	roll	0	1	0
sub	Arnold August Bros.	0.3	roll	0	1	0
sub	Arnold Levy Old Country	0.3	roll	0	1	0
sub, super loaf	Arnold Francisco	0.7	oz.	0	1	0

FOOD ITEM	SPECIFICATIONS	BRAND NAME	QUANTITY	SIZE	PROTEIN BLOCKS	CARBOHYDRATE BLOCKS	FAT BLOCKS
Roll, frozen or refrigerated	butterflake	Rich's Homestyle	0.7	rolls	0	1	0
	crescent	Pillsbury	0.5	roll	0	1	1
		Pillsbury	0.8	rolls	0	1	2
	cheese	Pillsbury	0.4	roll	0	1	2
	garlic cheese	Pepperidge Farm	0.6	roll	0	1	1
Roll, mix	hot	Dromedary	0	pkg.	0	1	0
	hot	Pillsbury	0.1	cup	0	1	0
	hot	Pillsbury	0.03	pkg, prepared	1	1	0
Roman beans	dry	Goya	0.2	cup	0	1	0
	canned	Goya	0.2	cup	1	1	0
Roseapple			5	oz.	0	1	0
Roselle			1.3	cup	0	1	0
Rosemary	dried		10	tsp.	0	1	1
Rotini dishes, mix	mushroom sauce	Knorr	0.1	cup	0	1	0
	primavera	Lipton Pasta & Sauce	0.1	pkg.	0	1	0
Rum runner mixer	frozen, prepared	Barcardi	2.1	fl. oz.	0	1	0
Rutabaga	fresh, cubed, raw		1.3	cup	0	1	0
	fresh, cubed, boiled, drained		0.7	cup	0	1	0
	fresh, boiled, drained, mashed		0.6	cup	0	1	0
	canned	Sunshine	1.3	cup	0	1	0
Rye	whole grain		0.1	cup	0	1	0
Rye flakes	rolled	Arrowhead Mills	0.1	cup	0	1	0
Rye flour		Arrowhead Mills	0.2	cup	0	1	0
	dark	Arrowhead Mills	0.1	cup	0	1	0
	light		0.1	cup	0	1	0
	medium		0.1	cup	0	1	0
	medium	Pillsbury	0.1	cup	0	1	0
Rye-wheat flour		Pillsbury Bohemian Style	0.1	cup	0	1	0
Safflower kernels	dried		1	oz.	1	1	4
Safflower meal	partially defatted		0.8	oz.	1	1	0

Food	Variety	Brand	Amount	Unit	P	C	F
Saffron							
Salad blend mix, fresh	Caesar	Dole Salad-in-a-Minute	10	tsp	—	0	0
	classic	Dole	3.9	oz.	—	5	0
	French	Dole	11.7	oz.	—	1	0
	Italian	Dole	11.7	oz.	—	1	1
	Oriental	Dole Salad-in-a-Minute	17.5	oz.	—	2	0
	spinach	Dole Salad-in-a-Minute	3.2	oz.	—	2	0
Salad toppers	bacon cheddar or Caesar mix	Dole Salad-in-a-Minute	1.9	oz.	—	2	0
	cinnamon raisin	Pepperidge Farm	2.5	Tbsp.	—	2	0
	garlic Italian	Pepperidge Farm	2.5	Tbsp.	—	1	0
Salsa	all varieties	Del Monte Mexicana	20	Tbsp.	—	0	0
	all varieties	Del Monte Taquera	20	Tbsp.	—	0	0
	all varieties	Goya	10	Tbsp.	—	0	0
	all varieties	Kaukauna Extra Chunky	6.7	Tbsp.	—	0	1
	all varieties	La Victoria Ranchera	10	Tbsp.	—	0	0
	all varieties	La Victoria Victoria	20	Tbsp.	—	0	0
	all varieties	Marie's Tomato	10	Tbsp.	—	0	0
	all varieties	Pace Thick & Chunky	10	Tbsp.	—	0	0
	all varieties	Del Monte Traditional/Thick & Chunky/Fire Roasted	10	Tbsp.	—	0	1
	all varieties	Hunt's Alfresco Homestyle	10	Tbsp.	—	0	0
	all varieties	Hunt's Homestyle	3.3	Tbsp.	—	0	0
	all varieties	Old El Paso Chunky	10	Tbsp.	—	0	1
	all varieties	Old El Paso Homestyle	20	Tbsp.	—	0	0
	all varieties	Progresso	10	Tbsp.	—	0	0
	all varieties	Tostitos	10	Tbsp.	—	0	0
	cheese, w/chipotle or cilantro	S&W Ready-Cut	0.6	cup	—	0	0
	garlic	Del Monte	10	Tbsp.	—	0	0
	garlic, roasted	Marie's	10	Tbsp.	—	0	0
	green	Goya	10	Tbsp.	—	0	0
	green	La Victoria Jalapena	20	Tbsp.	—	0	1
	green chili	La Victoria	20	Tbsp.	—	0	0
	green chili, medium	Old El Paso	10	Tbsp.	—	0	0
	hot	Chi-Chi's	20	Tbsp.	—	0	0
	hot	Guiltless Gourmet	10	Tbsp.	—	0	0

FOOD ITEM	SPECIFICATIONS	BRAND NAME	QUANTITY	SIZE	PROTEIN BLOCKS	CARBOHYDRATE BLOCKS	FAT BLOCKS
	hot	La Victoria Thick N Chunky	20	Tbsp.	0	1	0
	hot	Las Palmas Mexicana	10	Tbsp.	0	1	0
	hot	Old El Paso Thick 'n Chunky	10	Tbsp.	0	1	0
	hot	Sun-Vista	10	Tbsp.	0	1	0
	hot or mild	Heluva Good Thick & Chunky	10	Tbsp.	1	1	0
	medium	Chi-Chi's	20	Tbsp.	0	1	0
	medium	La Victoria Suprema	20	Tbsp.	0	1	0
	medium	Las Palmas Mexicana	10	Tbsp.	0	1	0
	medium	Porino's	20	Tbsp.	0	1	0
	medium	Rosarita	10	Tbsp.	0	1	0
	medium	Rosarita Extra Chunky	20	Tbsp.	0	1	0
	medium, or mild	La Victoria Thick N Chunky	20	Tbsp.	0	1	0
	medium, or mild	Old El Paso Thick 'n Chunky	10	Tbsp.	0	1	0
	medium, or mild	S&W Ready-Cut	0.8	cup	0	1	0
	mild	Chi-Chi's	20	Tbsp.	0	1	0
	mild	La Victoria Suprema	10	Tbsp.	0	1	0
	mild	Las Palmas Mexicana	20	Tbsp.	0	1	0
	picante, see also "Picante sauce"	Old Dutch	10	Tbsp.	0	1	0
	picante	Old El Paso	10	Tbsp.	0	1	0
	picante, medium	La Victoria Suprema	20	Tbsp.	0	1	0
	picante, mild	La Victoria Suprema	20	Tbsp.	0	1	0
	pico de gallo	Chi-Chi's	10	Tbsp.	0	1	0
	pico de gallo	Old El Paso	10	Tbsp.	0	1	0
	red	La Victoria Jalapena	20	Tbsp.	0	1	0
	roasted	Rosarita	10	Tbsp.	0	1	0
	tomatillo, green	Rosarita	10	Tbsp.	0	1	0
	verde	Del Monte	10	Tbsp.	0	1	0
	verde	Old El Paso	10	Tbsp.	0	1	0
	verde, medium or mild	Chi-Chi's	6.7	Tbsp.	0	1	0
Salsify	raw, untrimmed		0.1	lb.	0	1	0
	raw, sliced		0.5	cup	0	1	0
	boiled, drained, sliced		0.6	cup	0	1	0

Food	Type/Flavor	Brand	Amount	Unit			
Sandwich dressing	bell pepper salsa	Vlasic Sandwich Zesters	5	Tbsp.	0	1	0
	garden onion	Vlasic Sandwich Zesters	5	Tbsp.	0	1	0
	Italian tomato	Vlasic Sandwich Zesters	6.7	Tbsp.	0	1	0
	jalapeno salsa	Vlasic Sandwich Zesters	5	Tbsp.	0	1	0
	mushroom and onion	Vlasic Sandwich Zesters	6.7	Tbsp.	0	1	0
Sandwich sauce		Durkee Famous	5	Tbsp.	1	1	10
		Manwich Original	0.4	cup	0	1	0
		Manwich Bold	0.2	cup	0	1	0
		Manwich Thick & Chunky	0.3	cup	0	1	0
	barbeque	Manwich	0.2	cup	0	1	0
	Mexican spice	Manwich	0.6	cup	0	1	0
	Sloppy Joe	Del Monte Original	0.2	cup	0	1	0
	Sloppy Joe	Green Giant	0.3	cup	0	1	0
	Sloppy Joe	Heinz	0.4	cup	0	1	0
	Sloppy Joe	Hormel Not-So-Sloppy Joe Sauce	0.2	cup	0	1	0
	Sloppy Joe	Libby's	0.3	cup	0	1	0
	Sloppy Joe, hickory flavor	Del Monte	0.2	cup	0	1	0
	Sloppy Joe, w/meat	Green Giant	0.3	cup	1	1	4
Sandwich sauce seasoning mix	Sloppy Joe	Lawry's	3.3	tsp.	0	1	0
Sapodilla			0.4	medium, 3"x2 1/2"	0	1	0
Sapote			0.3	cup	0	1	0
			0.1	medium, 11.2 oz.	0	1	0
	trimmed	Frieda's	1	oz.	0	1	0
Sauerkraut	white	Boar's Head	1	Tbsp.	0	1	0
		Claussen	33.3	cup	0	1	0
		Eden Organic	10	cup	2	1	0
		Frank's/Snowfloss	5	cup	0	1	0
		Hebrew National	20	Tbsp.	0	1	0
		Hebrew National/Shorr's New	1.3	cup	0	1	0
		Pickle Eater's Kozmic Kraut	0.4	cup	0	1	0
		Pickle Eater's Reduced Sodium	20	Tbsp.	0	1	0
		Rosoff Home Style	20	Tbsp.	0	1	0
			0.4	cup	0	1	0

FOOD ITEM	SPECIFICATIONS	BRAND NAME	QUANTITY	SIZE	PROTEIN BLOCKS	CARBOHYDRATE BLOCKS	FAT BLOCKS
		S&W 14 oz.	10	Tbsp.	0	1	0
		S&W 22oz.	10	Tbsp.	0	1	0
	Bavarian style	Stokely	2.5	cup	0	1	0
	Bavarian style	Del Monte	5	Tbsp.	0	1	0
	Bavarian style	Frank's/Snowfloss	6.7	Tbsp.	0	1	0
	Bavarian style	Stokely	20	Tbsp.	0	1	0
	sweet and sour	Stokely	1.3	cup	0	1	0
	sweet and sour	Stokely	5	Tbsp.	0	1	0
Sauerkraut juice		S&W	0.3	cup	0	1	0
		S&W	12.5	oz.	0	1	0
		Stokely	20	fl. oz.	0	1	0
Sausage biscuit, frozen		Hormel Quick Meal	0.3	pc.	0	1	2
	w/cheese	Weight Watchers	0.5	pc.	1	1	2
	w/egg	Hormel Quick Meal	0.3	pc.	0	1	3
	w/egg, cheese	Hormel Quick Meal	0.3	pc.	0	1	2
	w/egg, cheese	Swanson Great Starts	0.3	pc.	1	1	3
Sausage gravy mix		Durkee/French's	0.4	cup, prepared	0	1	1
Sausage seasoning	pork	Tone's	5	tsp.	0	1	1
Savory	ground		10	tsp.	0	1	0
Scallop squash	raw, sliced		5	cup	1	1	0
	boiled, drained, sliced		2.5	cup	1	1	0
	boiled, drained, mashed		1.7	cup	0	1	0
Scrapple		Jones Dairy Farm	2.5	oz.	1	1	3
Seafood sauce, cocktail		Bookbinder's Restaurant Style	0.2	cup	0	1	0
		Crosse & Blackwell	0.1	cup	0	1	0
		Del Monte	0.1	cup	0	1	0
		Heinz	0.2	cup	0	1	0
		Heluva Good Thick & Chunky	0.2	cup	0	1	0
		Maull's	1.8	Tbsp.	0	1	0
		Nalley	0.1	cup	0	1	0
		Sauceworks	0.2	cup	0	1	0
		S&W	1.7	tsp.	0	1	0
	hot and spicy	Bookbiner's	0.6	tsp.	0	1	0

Food	Description	Brand	Amount	Unit	Protein	Carbohydrate	Fat
Seasoning and coating mix	country	Shake'n Bake	0.2	pkt.	0	1	1
	glaze, honey mustard	Shake'n Bake	0.1	pkt.	0	1	0
	glaze, tangy honey	Shake'n Bake	0.1	pkt.	0	1	0
	Italian herb	Shake'n Bake	0.2	pkt.	0	1	0
Seaweed	agar, raw		5	oz.	0	1	0
	agar, dried	Eden	0.4	oz.	0	1	0
	hiziki		4.5	cup	0	1	0
	Irish moss, raw		9.1	oz.	0	1	0
	kelp, raw		3.3	oz.	0	1	0
	kombu	Eden	5	oz. of 7" pc.	0	1	0
	wakame, raw		3.3	oz.	0	1	0
	wakame, flakes	Eden	2.5	cup	0	1	0
Seitan mix	whole, grain	Arrowhead Mills	0.3	cup	1	1	0
Semolina	mix		0.1	cup	2	1	0
Semolina flour	partially defatted low fat	Arrowhead Mills	0.1	cup	0	1	0
			1.1	oz.	0	1	0
Shallot	fresh or stored, peeled		1	oz.	0	1	0
	fresh or stored, chopped		2	oz.	0	1	0
Shellie beans	canned, w/liquid		5	Tbsp.	1	1	0
	canned	Stokely	1.3	cup	1	1	0
Shells, pasta, mix	white cheddar	Noodle Roni	0.8	cup	1	1	0
Sherbert	orange	Carnation Cup	0.2	cup	0	1	0
	orange	Carnation Plastic	0.2	cup, prepared	0	1	0
	orange	Edy's	1.4	fl. oz.	0	1	0
	pink lemonade	Edy's	1.4	fl. oz.	0	1	0
	strawberry kiwi	Edy's	0.2	cup	0	1	0
	Swiss orange	Edy's	0.2	cup	0	1	0
	tangerine	Edy's	0.2	cup	0	1	0
	tropical	Edy's	0.2	cup	0	1	0
Shrimp entree, mix	creole	Luzianne	0.2	cup	0	1	0
Shrimp sauce		Crosse & Blackwell	0.1	pkg.	0	1	0
			0.1	cup	0	1	0
Snack bar	blueberry	Little Debbie Star Crunch	0.2	bar	0	1	0
	blueberry	Little Debbie Fruit Boosters	0.2	bar	0	1	1
	brownie	Sweet Rewards	0.3	bar	0	1	0
		Sweet Rewards	0.4	bar	0	1	0

FOOD ITEM	SPECIFICATIONS	BRAND NAME	QUANTITY	SIZE	PROTEIN BLOCKS	CARBOHYDRATE BLOCKS	FAT BLOCKS
	brownie	Sweet Success Chewy	0.5	bar	0	1	1
	chocolate chip	Sweet Success Chewy	0.5	bar	0	1	1
	chocolate raspberry or peanut butter	Sweet Success Chewy	0.5	bar	0	1	1
Snack chips and crisps	fig	Little Debbie Figaroos	0.2	bar	0	1	0
	strawberry	Little Debbie Fruit Boosters	0.2	bar	0	1	0
		Zing Chips	0.3	oz.	0	1	1
	apple cinnamon	Crunchwells Crumpet Chips	0.4	oz.	0	1	0
	cheddar	Old Dutch Multicrisps	0.5	oz.	1	1	1
	hot and spicy	Eden Wasabi	0.4	oz.	0	1	0
	mixed	Terra Chips	0.6	oz.	0	1	1
	onion	Funyons	0.5	oz.	0	1	1
	onion, French	Old Dutch Multicrisps	0.5	oz.	0	1	1
Snack mix		Cheez-It	0.3	cup	0	1	1
	cheddar	Chex Mix	0.3	cup	0	1	1
	cheddar, zesty	Chex Mix Bold n' Zesty	0.4	cup	0	1	2
	honey mustard and onion	Old Dutch Party Mix	0.3	cup	0	1	1
	nutty, extra	Pepperidge Farm Light Season	0.2	cup	0	1	1
		Pepperidge Farm Goldfish	0.2	cup	0	1	1
		Chex Mix	0.3	cup	0	1	2
		Pepperidge Farm Goldfish	0.3	cup	0	1	2
		Pepperidge Farm	0.3	cup	0	1	2
		Pepperidge Farm	0.3	cup	0	1	2
Snow pea sprouts		Jonathan's	1.7	cup	1	1	0
Soft drinks, carbonated	all varieties	R.W. Knudsen Spritzer Light	3.9	fl. oz.	0	1	0
	all varieties	R.W. Knudsen Fruit TeaZer	4.1	fl. oz.	0	1	0
	all varieties, sparkling	Santa Cruz	2.9	fl. oz.	0	1	0
	apple	R.W. Knudsen Spritzer	2.6	fl. oz.	0	1	0
	apple	Welch's Sparkling	1.9	fl. oz.	0	1	0
	apple, spiced	Natural Brew	2.6	fl. oz.	0	1	0
	amaretto almond	After the Fall Spritzer	3	fl. oz.	0	1	0
	berry	After the Fall Berrymeister Spritzer	2.7	fl. oz.	0	1	0
	birch beer	Canada Dry	2.7	fl. oz.	0	1	0

				P	C	F
boysenberry	R.W. Knudsen Spritzer	2.6	fl. oz.	0	1	0
café mocha	Natural Brew	3.2	fl. oz.	0	1	0
café mocha	Canada Dry Cactus Cooler	2.7	fl. oz.	0	1	0
café mocha	Canada Dry Hi-Spot	2.6	fl. oz.	0	1	0
cherry	After the Fall American Pie Spritzer	3.1	fl. oz.	0	1	0
cherry	Crush	2.1	fl. oz.	0	1	0
cherry	Sundrop	2.4	fl. oz.	0	1	0
cherry	Sunkist	2.1	fl. oz.	0	1	0
cherry, amaretto	Natural Brew	2.7	fl. oz.	0	1	0
cherry, black	After the Fall Spritzer	2.6	fl. oz.	0	1	0
cherry, black	Canada Dry	2.2	fl. oz.	0	1	0
cherry, black	R.W. Knudsen Spritzer	2.6	fl. oz.	0	1	0
cherry, black	Shasta	2.6	fl. oz.	0	1	0
cherry, French	Snapple	2.5	fl. oz.	0	1	0
cherry, spice	Slice	2.8	fl. oz.	0	1	0
cherry, wild	Canada Dry	2.6	fl. oz.	0	1	0
cherry-lime	Spree	2.4	fl. oz.	0	1	0
cherry-lime rickey	Snapple	2.7	fl. oz.	0	1	0
citrus	Canada Dry Half & Half	2.7	fl. oz.	0	1	0
citrus	Sunkist	2.9	fl. oz.	0	1	0
cola	Canada Dry Jamaica	2.7	fl. oz.	0	1	0
cola	Coca-Cola Classic	2.7	fl. oz.	0	1	0
cola	Juice Fizz Cooler	2.6	fl. oz.	0	1	0
cola	Pepsi/Crystal Pepsi	2.6	fl. oz.	0	1	0
cola	Shasta	2.6	fl. oz.	0	1	0
cola	Slice	2.5	fl. oz.	0	1	0
cola	Spree	2.6	fl. oz.	0	1	0
cola, cherry	R.W. Knudsen Spritzer	2.6	fl. oz.	0	1	0
cola, cherry	Shasta	2.5	fl. oz.	0	1	0
cola, cherry, wild	Pepsi	2.5	fl. oz.	0	1	0
cola, ginseng	Natural Brew	2.6	fl. oz.	0	1	0
collins mixer	Canada Dry	3.5	fl. oz.	0	1	0
collins mixer	Schweppes	2.9	fl. oz.	0	1	0
cranberry	After the Fall Tart 'n Sweet Spritzer	2.7	fl. oz.	0	1	0
cranberry	R.W. Knudsen Spritzer	2.4	fl. oz.	0	1	0
cranberry	Shasta	2.4	fl. oz.	0	1	0

FOOD ITEM	SPECIFICATIONS	BRAND NAME	QUANTITY	SIZE	PROTEIN BLOCKS	CARBOHYDRATE BLOCKS	FAT BLOCKS
	cran-orange	After the Fall Tart 'n Sweet Spritzer	2.7	fl. oz.	0	1	0
	cran-raspberry	After the Fall Tart 'n Sweet Spritzer	2.7	fl. oz.	0	1	0
	cream/creme	A&W	2.6	fl. oz.	0	1	0
	cream/creme	Hires	2.3	fl. oz.	0	1	0
	cream/creme	IBC	2.6	fl. oz.	0	1	0
	cream/creme	Mug	2.3	fl. oz.	0	1	0
	cream/creme	Shasta	2.3	fl. oz.	0	1	0
	cream/creme, vanilla	Canada Dry	2.4	fl. oz.	0	1	0
	cream/creme, vanilla	Crush	2.4	fl. oz.	0	1	0
	cream/creme, vanilla	Natural Brew	2.6	fl. oz.	0	1	0
	cream/creme, vanilla	R.W. Knudsen Spritzer	3.1	fl. oz.	0	1	0
	cream/creme, vanilla	Snapple	2.2	fl. oz.	0	1	0
	cream/creme, vanilla	Doc Shasta	2.8	fl. oz.	0	1	0
		Dr. Pepper	2.7	fl. oz.	0	1	0
		Dr. Slice	2.8	fl. oz.	0	1	0
	fruit punch/blend	Canada Dry Tahitian	2	fl. oz.	0	1	0
	fruit punch/blend	Juice Fizz	2.2	fl. oz.	0	1	0
	fruit punch/blend	Juice Fizz Maui Magic/Wild Red	2.4	fl. oz.	0	1	0
	fruit punch/blend	Shasta	2.1	fl. oz.	0	1	0
	fruit punch/blend	Slice	2.1	fl. oz.	0	1	0
	fruit punch/blend	Sunkist	2.2	fl. oz.	0	1	0
	fruit punch/blend	Welch's Sparkling	2	fl. oz.	0	1	0
	ginger ale	After the Fall Nantucket	3.1	fl. oz.	0	1	0
	ginger ale	Canada Dry	2.9	fl. oz.	0	1	0
	ginger ale	Canada Dry Golden	3	fl. oz.	0	1	0
	ginger ale	Natural Brew Outrageous	2.6	fl. oz.	0	1	0
	ginger ale	R.W. Knudsen Spritzer	2.7	fl. oz.	0	1	0
	ginger ale	Schwepps	3.3	fl. oz.	0	1	0
	ginger ale	Shasta	3.3	fl. oz.	0	1	0
	ginger ale, cherry	Canada Dry	2.7	fl. oz.	0	1	0
	ginger ale, cranberry	After the Fall	3.1	fl. oz.	0	1	0
	ginger ale, cranberry or lemon	Canada Dry	2.9	fl. oz.	0	1	0

ginger ale, grape, dry	Schweppes	2.9	fl. oz.	
ginger ale, grape, raspberry	After the Fall	3	fl. oz.	
ginger ale, raspberry	Schweppes	2.8	fl. oz.	
ginger beer	Goya	4	fl. oz.	
ginger beer	Schweppes	2.9	fl. oz.	
grape	After the Fall Concord Spritzer	2.4	fl. oz.	
grape	Canada Dry Concord	2.5	fl. oz.	
grape	Crush	2.1	fl. oz.	
grape	Juice Fizz Purple Thunder	2.1	fl. oz.	
grape	R.W. Knudsen Spritzer	2.6	fl. oz.	
grape	Schweppes	2.2	fl. oz.	
grape	Shasta	2.3	fl. oz.	
grape	Slice	2.1	fl. oz.	
grape	Welch's Sparkling	2.1	fl. oz.	
grapefruit	Schweppes	2.7	fl. oz.	
grapefruit	Shasta Ruby Red	2.3	fl. oz.	
grapefruit	Spree	2.6	fl. oz.	
grapefruit	Wink	2.4	fl. oz.	
grapefruit	Wink Diet	8.0	fl. oz.	
kiwi-lime	R.W. Knudsen Spritzer	2.7	fl. oz.	
kiwi-strawberry	After the Fall	2.7	fl. oz.	
kiwi-strawberry	Shasta	1.7	fl. oz.	
kiwi-strawberry	Snapple	3.2	fl. oz.	
lemon, bitter	Schweppes	2.8	fl. oz.	
lemon, sour	Canada Dry	3.5	fl. oz.	
lemon, sour	Schweppes	2.8	fl. oz.	
lemon, spicy	After the Fall Spritzer	2.9	fl. oz.	
lemonade	Country Time	2.8	fl. oz.	
lemonade	Sunkist	2.4	fl. oz.	
lemonade, Jamaica	R.W. Knudsen Spritzer	2.6	fl. oz.	
lemonade, tangerine, kiwi berry or raspberry	Country Time	2.7	fl. oz.	
lemon-lime	R.W. Knudsen Spritzer	2.6	fl. oz.	
lemon-lime	Schweppes	2.9	fl. oz.	
lemon-lime	Slice	2.7	fl. oz.	
lemon-lime	Spree	2.6	fl. oz.	

FOOD ITEM	SPECIFICATIONS	BRAND NAME	QUANTITY	SIZE	PROTEIN BLOCKS	CARBOHYDRATE BLOCKS	FAT BLOCKS
	lime	After the Fall Caribbean Spritzer	2.6	fl. oz.	0	1	0
	lime	Canada Dry Island	2.2	fl. oz.	0	1	0
	lime-lemon	Shasta Twist	2.9	fl. oz.	0	1	0
	mandarin-lime	R.W. Knudsen Spritzer	2.6	fl. oz.	0	1	0
	mandarin-lime	Spree	2.6	fl. oz.	0	1	0
	mandarin-pineapple	After the Fall Spritzer	2.9	fl. oz.	0	1	0
	mango	After the Fall Hawaiian Spritzer	2.4	fl. oz.	0	1	0
	mango	R.W. Knudsen Fandango Spritzer	2.4	fl. oz.	0	1	0
	mango ginger	After the Fall Spritzer	2.9	fl. oz.	0	1	0
		Mountain Dew	2.4	fl. oz.	0	1	0
	orange	After the Fall Icicle Spritzer	2.6	fl. oz.	0	1	0
	orange	After the Fall Zadachi Spritzer	2.7	fl. oz.	0	1	0
	orange	Canada Dry Sunripe	2.1	fl. oz.	0	1	0
	orange	Crush	2.1	fl. oz.	0	1	0
	orange	Orangina	3.2	fl. oz.	0	1	0
	orange	Shasta	2.2	fl. oz.	0	1	0
	orange	Sunkist	2.1	fl. oz.	0	1	0
	orange	Welch's Sparkling	2.1	fl. oz.	0	1	0
	orange	Slice	2.1	fl. oz.	0	1	0
	orange, mandarin	R.W. Knudsen Spritzer	2.7	fl. oz.	0	1	0
	orange passion fruit	Snapple	2.5	fl. oz.	0	1	0
	passion fruit	Canada Dry	2.4	fl. oz.	0	1	0
	peach	R.W. Knudsen Spritzer	2.9	fl. oz.	0	1	0
	peach	Shasta	2.5	fl. oz.	0	1	0
	peach	Snapple Melba	2.4	fl. oz.	0	1	0
	peach	Sunkist	2.4	fl. oz.	0	1	0
	peach	Welch's Sparkling	2.1	fl. oz.	0	1	0
	peach	After the Fall Spritzer	2.6	fl. oz.	0	1	0
	peach vanilla	Kristian Regale Swedish Sparkler	2.8	fl. oz.	0	1	0
	pear	Canada Dry	2.8	fl. oz.	0	1	0
	pineapple	Crush	2.1	fl. oz.	0	1	0
	pineapple	Shasta	2.1	fl. oz.	0	1	0
	pineapple	Slice	2.1	fl. oz.	0	1	0

Food	Brand	Amount	Protein	Carbohydrate	Fat
pineapple	Sunkist	2.1 fl. oz.	0	1	0
pineapple	Welch's Sparkling	2 fl. oz.	0	1	0
pineapple, orange	Shasta	2.4 fl. oz.	0	1	0
raspberry	After the Fall Spritzer	2.6 fl. oz.	0	1	0
raspberry	Snapple Royal	2.4 fl. oz.	0	1	0
raspberry, creme	Shasta	2.4 fl. oz.	0	1	0
raspberry, red	R.W. Knudsen Spritzer	2.6 fl. oz.	0	1	0
red	Shasta	2.5 fl. oz.	0	1	0
red	Slice	2.1 fl. oz.	0	1	0
root beer	A&W	3.6 fl. oz.	0	1	0
root beer	Hires	2.4 fl. oz.	0	1	0
root beer	IBC	2.6 fl. oz.	0	1	0
root beer	Mug	2.5 fl. oz.	0	1	0
root beer	Shasta	2.6 fl. oz.	0	1	0
root beer	Snapple Tru	2.5 fl. oz.	0	1	0
root beer	Spree	2.6 fl. oz.	0	1	0
	7Up	2.8 fl. oz.	0	1	0
	7Up Cherry	2.8 fl. oz.	0	1	0
sour mixer	Canada Dry	3.3 fl. oz.	0	1	0
strawberry	After the Fall Twist O' Spritzer	2.9 fl. oz.	0	1	0
strawberry	Canada Dry California	2.7 fl. oz.	0	1	0
strawberry	Crush	2.4 fl. oz.	0	1	0
strawberry	R.W. Knudsen Spritzer	2.6 fl. oz.	0	1	0
strawberry	Shasta	2.4 fl. oz.	0	1	0
strawberry	Slice	2.3 fl. oz.	0	1	0
strawberry	Sunkist	2.1 fl. oz.	0	1	0
strawberry	Welch's Sparkling	2.1 fl. oz.	0	1	0
strawberry, peach	Shasta	2.6 fl. oz.	0	1	0
strawberry, vanilla	After the Fall Spritzer	2.6 fl. oz.	0	1	0
	Sundrop	2.4 fl. oz.	0	1	0
tangerine spritzer	After the Fall	2.7 fl. oz.	0	1	0
tangerine spritzer	R.W. Knudsen	2.8 fl. oz.	0	1	0
tonic	Canada Dry	3 fl. oz.	0	1	0
tonic	Schweppes	3.3 fl. oz.	0	1	0
tonic	Shasta	2.6 fl. oz.	0	1	0
tonic, w/fruit flavors	Schweppes	3.6 fl. oz.	0	1	0

FOOD ITEM	SPECIFICATIONS	BRAND NAME	QUANTITY	SIZE	PROTEIN BLOCKS	CARBOHYDRATE BLOCKS	FAT BLOCKS
	tonic, w/lime	Canada Dry	3	fl. oz.	0	1	0
	vanilla bean	After the Fall Spritzer	2.6	fl. oz.	0	1	0
Sorbet	chocolate	Ben & Jerry's Doonesbury	0.1	cup	0	1	0
	chocolate	Haagen-Dazs	0.2	cup	0	1	0
	coffee	Tofutti	0.3	cup	0	1	0
	and cream, orange	Tofutti	0.2	cup	0	1	0
	and cream, orange	Haagen-Dazs	0.2	cup	0	1	1
	and cream, raspberry	Haagen-Dazs	0.1	cup	0	1	1
	lemon	Haagen-Dazs Zesty	0.2	cup	0	1	0
	lemon	Tofutti	0.2	cup	0	1	0
	lemonade, pink	Ben & Jerry's	0.1	cup	0	1	0
	mocha	Ben & Jerry's	0.2	cup	0	1	0
	orange-peach-mango	Tofutti	0.1	cup	0	1	0
	peach	Haagen-Dazs Orchard	0.1	cup	0	1	0
	pina colada	Ben & Jerry's	0.1	cup	0	1	0
	purple passion	Ben & Jerry's	0.2	cup	0	1	0
	raspberry	Haagen-Dazs	0.2	cup	0	1	0
	raspberry	Tofutti	0.1	cup	0	1	0
	strawberry	Haagen-Dazs	0.2	cup	0	1	0
	strawberry	Tofutti	0.2	cup	0	1	0
	strawberry, kiwi	Ben & Jerry's	0.4	cup	0	1	0
Sorbet bar	berry, wild	Haagen-Dazs	0.5	bar	0	1	0
	chocolate	Haagen-Dazs	0.4	bar	0	1	0
Sorbet-yogurt bar	chocolate and cherry	Haagen-Dazs Sorbet 'n Yogurt	0.04	bar	0	1	0
Sourghum syrup			1.4	cup	0	1	0
Soup mix, dry	barley, better	Aunt Patsy's Pantry	0.1	tbsp.	0	1	0
	barley, chowder	Buckeye Burgoo	0.4	pkg.	0	1	0
	barley, vegetable, hearty	Fantastic Cup	0.7	pkg.	0	1	0
	bean	Bean Cuisine Bouillabaisse	0.1	serving	0	1	0
	bean, black	Aunt Patsy's Pantry	0.6	pkg.	0	1	0
	bean, black	Bean Cuisine Island	0.3	serving	0	1	0
	bean, black	Knorr Cup	0.5	pkg.	0	1	0
	bean, black	Smart Soup		pkg.	0	1	0

CARBOHYDRATES

Food	Brand	Amount	Unit			
bean, black, hearty	Fantastic Jumpin' Cup	0.3	pkg.	0	1	0
bean, black, Santa Fe	Campbell's Soupsations	0.2	pkg.	0	1	0
bean, black, spicy, w/couscous	Health Valley	0.1	cup	0	1	0
bean, black, zesty, w/rice	Health Valley	0.2	cup	0	1	0
bean, 5, hearty	Fantastic Cup	0.3	pkg.	0	1	0
bean, many	Buckeye	0.05	pkg.	0	1	0
bean, many	Buckeye Northwest Bean	0.04	pkg.	0	1	0
bean, many	Buckeye	1.7	tbsp.	0	1	0
bean, navy	Knorr Cup	0.4	pkg.	0	1	0
bean, navy	Aunt Patsy's Pantry	1.4	tbsp.	0	1	1
bean, white	Bean Cuisine Provencale	0.7	serving	0	1	0
bean and ham	Hormel Micro Cup	0.4	pkg.	0	1	1
beef vegetable	Hormel Micro Cup	0.8	pkg.	0	1	0
broccoli, cream of	Knorr Chef's	2.5	tbsp.	0	1	1
broccoli-cheese, cheddar, creamy	Fantastic Cup	0.4	pkg.	0	1	0
broccoli-cheese, creamy	Cup-a-Soup	1.3	pkg.	0	1	1
broccoli-cheese, w/ham	Hormel Micro Cup	1	pkg.	0	1	4
broccoli-cheese, and rice	Uncle Ben's Hearty	0.4	pkg.	0	1	0
chicken	Campbell's Instant	0.4	pkg.	0	1	0
chicken, cream of	Cup-a-Soup	0.8	pkg.	0	1	1
chicken, hearty, supreme	Cup-a-Soup	0.7	pkg.	0	1	0
chicken noodle	Campbell's Soup/Recipe	1.6	tbsp.	0	1	1
chicken noodle	Cup-a-Soup	1.1	pkg.	0	1	0
chicken noodle, hearty	Cup-a-Soup	0.9	pkg.	0	1	0
chicken noodle	Hormel Micro Cup	0.8	pkg.	1	1	0
chicken, onion and rice	Kettle Creations	0.1	pkg.	0	1	0
chicken, pasta and beans	Kettle Creations	0.1	pkg.	0	1	0
chicken, rice	Hormel Micro Cup	0.6	pkg.	0	1	1
chicken, rice	Mrs. Grass	0.1	pkg.	0	1	0
chicken, thyme	Aunt Patsy's Pantry	1	tbsp.	0	1	1
chicken, vegetable	Smart Soup	0.4	pkg.	0	1	0
chili	Aunt Patsy's Pantry Cowgirl	1.4	tbsp.	0	1	0
chili, black bean	Aunt Patsy's Pantry	1.6	tbsp.	0	1	0
chili, chicken	Aunt Patsy's Pantry	1.2	tbsp.	0	1	0

FOOD ITEM	SPECIFICATIONS	BRAND NAME	QUANTITY	SIZE	PROTEIN BLOCKS	CARBOHYDRATE BLOCKS	FAT BLOCKS
	chili, chicken, white	Buckeye	0	pkg.	0	1	0
	chili, hearty	Fantastic Cha-Cha Cup	0.4	pkg.	1	1	0
	chili, lentil	Buckeye Rip Roar'n	1.5	tbsp.	1	1	0
	clam chowder, New England	Hormel Micro Cup	0.1	pkg.	1	1	1
	clam chowder, New England	Knorr Chef's	0.6	pkg.	0	1	1
	corn chowder	Knorr Cup	2.3	tbsp.	0	1	0
	corn chowder	Smart Soup	0.4	pkg.	0	1	0
	corn chowder and potato, creamy	Fantastic Cup	0.4	pkg.	0	1	0
	corn chowder w/tomatoes	Health Valley	0.3	cup	0	1	0
	couscous	Casbah Moroccan Stew Cup	0.3	pkg.	0	1	0
	couscous, w/lentil, hearty	Fantastic Cup	0.2	pkg.	0	1	0
	gumbo, New Orleans	Campbell's Soupsations	0.3	pkg.	0	1	1
	herb, fine	Knorr Box	1.4	tbsp.	0	1	0
	herb, golden, w/lemon	Lipton Recipe Secrets	2.5	tbsp.	0	1	0
	herb, Italian, w/tomato	Lipton Recipe Secrets	2	tbsp.	0	1	0
	herb w/garlic, savory	Lipton Recipe Secrets	1.4	tbsp.	0	1	1
	hot and sour	Knorr Box	2.2	tbsp.	0	1	0
	leek	Knorr Box	2	tbsp.	0	1	1
	lentil	Buckeye Great Lean 'n Lentils	1.4	tbsp.	1	1	0
	lentil, hearty	Smart Soup	0.3	pkg.	0	1	0
	lentil, hearty	Campbell's Soup/Recipe	0.3	pkg.	0	1	0
	lentil, hearty	Campbell's Soupsations	0.3	pkg.	0	1	0
	lentil, hearty	Fantastic Country Cup	0.3	pkg.	0	1	1
	lentil, red	Knorr Cup	0.3	pkg.	0	1	0
	lentil, w/couscous	Aunt's Patsy's Pantry	1.4	tbsp.	0	1	0
	minestrone	Health Valley	0.1	cup	0	1	0
	minestrone	Kettle Creations	0.1	pkg.	0	1	0
	minestrone	Smart Soup	0.4	pkg.	0	1	0
	minestrone, hearty	Fantastic Cup	0.4	pkg.	0	1	0

Food	Brand	Amount	Unit	Protein	Carbohydrate	Fat
minestrone, hearty	Knorr Cup	0.3	pkg.	0	1	0
mushroom, beefy	Lipton Recipe Secrets	2.5	tbsp.	0	1	0
mushroom, cream of	Cup-a-Soup	0.9	pkg.	0	1	1
mushroom, creamy	Fantastic Cup	0.4	pkg.	0	1	0
noodle	Nissin Top Ramen Damae	0.3	pkg.	0	1	1
noodle	Nissin Top Ramen Oriental	0.3	pkg.	0	1	1
noodle	Nissin Top Ramen Low Fat Oriental	0.3	pkg.	0	1	0
noodle, w/chicken broth	Mrs. Grass	0.2	pkg.	0	1	0
noodle, chicken free	Fantastic Cup	0.4	pkg.	0	1	0
noodle, extra	Lipton Soup Secrets	1.8	tbsp.	0	1	0
noodle, homestyle	Borden	0.2	pkg.	0	1	1
noodle, onion and Oriental	Sanwa Ramen	0.2	block	0	1	0
noodle, Oriental	Campbell's Ramen Low Fat	0.2	pkg.	0	1	0
noodle, Oriental	Campbell's Ramen Low Fat	0.2	block	0	1	0
noodle, Oriental	Sanwa Ramen	0.2	block	0	1	1
noodle, ring noodle	Cup-a-Soup	1	pkg.	0	1	0
noodle, beef	Campbell's Instant	0.4	pkg.	0	1	0
noodle, beef	Campbell's Ramen Fried Cup	0.2	pkg.	0	1	1
noodle, beef	Campbell's Ramen Low Fat	0.2	pkg.	0	1	1
noodle, beef	Campbell's Ramen Low Fat	0.2	block	0	1	0
noodle, beef	Campbell's/Sanwa Ramen	0.2	block	0	1	0
noodle, beef	Nissin Cup Noodles	0.2	pkg.	0	1	1
noodle, beef	Nissin Cup Noodles Twin	0.5	oz.	0	1	0
noodle, beef	Nissin Top Ramen	0.3	pkg.	0	1	1
noodle, beef	Nissin Top Ramen Low Fat	0.3	pkg.	0	1	1
noodle, beef, onion	Nissin Cup Noodles	0.2	pkg.	0	1	0
noodle, beef, spicy	Nissin Top Ramen	0.3	pkg.	0	1	0
noodle, chicken	Campbell's Ramen	0.2	pkg.	0	1	1
noodle, chicken	Campbell's Ramen Low Fat	0.2	pkg.	0	1	1
noodle, chicken	Campbell's Ramen Low Fat	0.2	block	0	1	1
noodle, chicken	Campbell's/Sanwa Ramen	0.2	pkg.	0	1	0
noodle, chicken	Knorr Box	1.1	tbsp.	0	1	1
noodle, chicken	Knorr Cup	0.5	pkg.	0	1	0
noodle, chicken	Lipton Soup Secrets	2.3	tbsp.	0	1	0
noodle, chicken	Lipton Soup Secrets Giggle Noodle	1.7	tbsp.	0	1	1
noodle, chicken	Lipton Soup Secrets Ring-O-Noodle	1.8	tbsp.	0	1	1

FOOD ITEM	SPECIFICATIONS	BRAND NAME	QUANTITY	SIZE	PROTEIN BLOCKS	CARBOHYDRATE BLOCKS	FAT BLOCKS
	noodle, chicken	Nissin Cup Noodles	0.2	pkg.	0	1	1
	noodle, chicken	Nissin Cup Noodles Twin	0.5	oz.	0	1	1
	noodle, chicken	Nissin Top Ramen	0.3	pkg.	0	1	0
	noodle, chicken	Nissin Top Ramen Low Fat	0.3	pkg.	0	1	1
	noodle, chicken	Sanwa Ramen Pride	0.2	block	0	1	1
	noodle, chicken, broth	Campbell's Instant	0.4	pkg.	0	1	0
	noodle, chicken, broth	Campbell's Soup/Recipe	0.1	cup	0	1	0
	noodle, chicken, broth	Lipton Soup Secrets	2	tbsp.	0	1	1
	noodle, chicken, curry	Mrs. Grass	0.2	pkg.	0	1	0
	noodle, chicken, curry	Campbell's/Sanwa Ramen	0.2	block	0	1	1
	noodle, chicken, curry	Sanwa Ramen Pride	0.2	pkg.	1	1	0
	noodle, chicken, hearty	Lipton Soup Secrets	0.2	cup	0	1	1
	noodle, chicken, mushroom	Nissin Cup Noodles	0.2	pkg.	0	1	1
	noodle, chicken, mushroom	Nissin Top Ramen	0.3	pkg.	0	1	0
	noodle, chicken, sesame	Nissin Top Ramen	0.3	pkg.	0	1	1
	noodle, chicken, spicy	Campbell's Ramen Low Fat	0.2	block	0	1	0
	noodle, chicken, spicy	Nissin Cup Noodles	0.3	pkg.	0	1	1
	noodle, chicken, spicy	Nissin Cup Noodles Twin	0.5	oz.	0	1	0
	noodle, chicken, w/vegetables	Health Valley	0.2	cup	0	1	0
	noodle, crab	Nissin Cup Noodles	0.2	pkg.	0	1	1
	noodle, lobster	Nissin Cup Noodles	0.2	pkg.	0	1	1
	noodle, pork	Campbell's Ramen Low Fat	0.2	pkg.	0	1	0
	noodle, pork	Campbell's Ramen Low Fat	0.2	block	0	1	0
	noodle, pork	Campbell's/Sanwa Oriental	0.2	block	0	1	1
	noodle, pork	Nissin Cup Noodles	0.2	pkg.	0	1	1
	noodle, pork	Nissin Top Ramen	0.3	pkg.	0	1	0
	noodle, shrimp	Campbell's Ramen	0.2	pkg.	1	1	1
	noodle, shrimp	Campbell's Ramen Low Fat	0.2	pkg.	0	1	0
	noodle, shrimp	Campbell's Ramen Low Fat	0.2	block	0	1	0
	noodle, shrimp	Nissin Cup Noodles	0.2	pkg.	0	1	1
	noodle, shrimp	Nissin Cup Noodles Twin	0.5	oz.	0	1	1
	noodle, shrimp	Nissin Top Ramen	0.3	pkg.	0	1	1

Food	Brand	Amount	Unit			
noodle, shrimp	Sanwa Ramen Pride	0.2	pkg.	1	1	1
noodle, shrimp, picante	Nissin Cup Noodles	0.2	pkg.	0	1	1
noodle, shrimp, Thai	Sanwa Ramen	0.2	block	0	1	1
noodle, shrimp, Thai	Sanwa Ramen Pride	0.2	pkg.	0	1	1
noodle, vegetable, beef	Mrs. Grass	0.2	pkg.	0	1	0
noodle, vegetable, beef	Sanwa Ramen Pride	0.2	pkg.	0	1	1
noodle, vegetable, curry	Fantastic Cup	0.4	pkg.	0	1	0
noodle, vegetable, egg, in broth	Campbell's Soupsations	0.4	pkg.	0	1	0
noodle, vegetable, garden	Nissin Cup Noodles	0.2	pkg.	0	1	1
noodle, vegetable, hearty	Campbell's Instant	0.3	pkg.	0	1	0
noodle, vegetable, hearty	Lipton Soup Secrets	2.5	tbsp.	0	1	1
noodle, vegetable, miso	Fantastic Cup	0.4	pkg.	0	1	0
noodle, vegetable, tomato	Campbell's/Sanwa Ramen Pride	0.2	pkg.	0	1	1
noodle, vegetable, tomato	Fantastic Cup	0.3	pkg.	1	1	0
onion	Campbell's Soup/Recipe	1.7	tbsp.	0	1	0
onion	Campbell's Soup/Recipe	2	tbsp.	0	1	0
onion	Knorr Box	2.2	tbsp.	0	1	0
onion	Lipton Recipe Secrets	2.5	tbsp.	0	1	0
onion	Mrs. Grass Soup/Recipe	0.4	pkg.	0	1	0
onion	Mrs. Grass Low Sodium	0.3	pkg.	0	1	0
onion, beefy	Lipton Recipe Secrets	1.7	tbsp.	0	1	0
onion, golden	Lipton Recipe Secrets	1.8	tbsp.	0	1	0
onion-mushroom	Lipton Recipe Secrets	2.9	tbsp.	0	1	0
onion-mushroom	Mrs. Grass Soup/Recipe	0.3	pkg.	0	1	0
orzo thyme	Buckeye	0.1	pkg.	0	1	0
oxtail	Knorr Box	2	tbsp.	0	1	1
pasta	Buckeye Many Mac	0	pkg.	0	1	0
pasta	Buckeye Starry	0.1	pkg.	0	1	0
pasta, Italiano	Health Valley Fat Free	0.2	cup	0	1	0
pasta, marinara, Parmesan, or Mediterranean	Health Valley Pasta Cup Fat Free	0.2	cup	0	1	0
pasta, ruffle	Lipton Soup Secrets	1.8	tbsp.	0	1	0
pasta and bean	Casbah Pasta Fasul	0.9	pkg.	1	1	1
pasta and bean	Kettle Creations	0.1	pkg.	0	1	0
pasta and bean	Bean Cuisine Ultima	0.5	serving	0	1	0

CARBOHYDRATES

FOOD ITEM	SPECIFICATIONS	BRAND NAME	QUANTITY	SIZE	PROTEIN BLOCKS	CARBOHYDRATE BLOCKS	FAT BLOCKS
	pasta and bean, white bean	Uncle Ben's Hearty	0.1	oz.	0	1	0
	pea, green	Cup-a-Soup	0.6	pkg.	0	1	1
	pea, snow, cream of	Knorr Chef's	2.7	tbsp.	0	1	1
	pea, split	Aunt's Patsy's Pantry	1.1	tbsp.	0	1	0
	pea, split	Bean Cuisine Thick as Fog	0.5	serving	0	1	0
	pea, split	Buckeye Country Pea Patchwork	0	pkg.	0	1	0
	pea, split	Knorr Cup	0.4	pkg.	0	1	0
	pea, split	Smart Soup	0.4	pkg.	0	1	0
	pea, split, hearty	Fantastic Cup	0.3	pkg.	0	1	0
	pea, split, w/carrots	Health Valley	0.2	cup	0	1	0
	potato, w/broccoli	Health Valley	0.2	cup	0	1	0
	potato cheese, w/ham	Hormel Micro Cup	0.6	pkg.	0	1	3
	potato leek	Knorr Cup	0.4	pkg.	0	1	0
	potato leek	Smart Soup	0.4	pkg.	0	1	0
	rice	Casbah Thai Yum	0.3	pkg.	0	1	0
	rice and beans	Casbah La Fiesta	0.3	pkg.	0	1	0
	rice and beans, black	Uncle Ben's Hearty	0.4	pkg.	0	1	0
	rice and beans, Cajun	Casbah Jambalaya	0.4	pkg.	0	1	0
	rice and beans, Cajun	Fantastic Cup	0.2	pkg.	0	1	0
	rice and beans, Caribbean	Fantastic Cup	0.2	pkg.	0	1	0
	rice and beans, curry, Bombay	Fantastic Cup	0.2	pkg.	0	1	0
	rice and beans, Mexican	Campbell's Soupsations	0.3	pkg.	0	1	0
	rice and beans, Northern Italian	Fantastic Cup	0.2	pkg.	0	1	0
	rice and beans, red	Smart Soup	0.3	pkg.	0	1	0
	rice and beans, Szechuan	Fantastic Cup	0.2	pkg.	0	1	0
	rice and beans, Tex-Mex	Fantastic Cup	0.2	pkg.	0	1	0
	spinach, cream of	Knorr Box	2	tbsp.	0	1	1
	tomato	Cup-a-Soup	0.5	pkg.	0	1	0
	tomato, basil	Knorr Box	1.3	tbsp.	0	1	0
	tomato, basil	Uncle Ben's Hearty	0.6	pkg.	0	1	0
	tomato, rice Parmesano	Fantastic Cup	0.2	pkg.	0	1	0

Food	Description	Brand	Amount	Unit	Protein	Carbohydrate	Fat
	tomato, vegetable	Campbell's Soupsations	0.4	pkg.	0	1	0
	vegetable	Campbell's Soup/Recipe	2.5	tbsp.	0	1	0
	vegetable	Knorr Box	3.3	tbsp.	0	1	0
	vegetable	Lipton Recipe Secrets	2.9	tbsp.	0	1	0
	vegetable, barley, hearty	Mrs. Grass Soup/Recipe	0.4	pkg.	0	1	0
	vegetable, beef	Fantastic Cup	0.4	pkg.	0	1	0
	vegetable, chicken flavor	Mrs. Grass	0.2	pkg.	0	1	0
	vegetable, chicken flavor	Cup-a-Soup	0.9	pkg.	0	1	0
	vegetable, chicken flavor	Knorr Cup	0.5	pkg.	0	1	0
	vegetable, chicken flavor, creamy	Cup-a-Soup	0.9	pkg.	0	1	1
Soup base	vegetable, w/rice and pasta	Ranco Natural	0.1	pkg.	0	1	0
Soup base, mix	vegetable, spring	Cup-a-Soup	1.1	pkg.	0	1	0
	vegetable, spring	Knorr	5	tbsp.	0	1	0
	bottled	Goya Sofrito	10	tsp.	0	1	0
	beef, ground, vegetable	Soup Starter	0.1	pkg.	0	1	0
	beef, ground, vegetable	Soup Starter Quick Cook	0.1	pkg.	0	1	0
	beef barley vegetable	Soup Starter	0.1	pkg.	0	1	0
	beef stew, hearty	Soup Starter	0.1	pkg.	0	1	0
	beef vegetable	Soup Starter	0.1	pkg.	0	1	0
	chicken noodle	Soup Starter	0.1	pkg.	0	1	0
	chicken noodle	Soup Starter Quick Cook	0.1	pkg.	0	1	0
	chicken and rice	Soup Starter	0.1	pkg.	0	1	0
	chicken and rice	Soup Starter Quick Cook	0.2	pkg.	0	1	0
	chicken vegetable	Soup Starter	0.1	pkg.	0	1	0
	chicken w/white and wild rice	Soup Starter	0.1	pkg.	0	1	0
Sour cream dip mix		Durkee	5	tsp.	0	1	1
Soursop			0.3	cup	0	1	0
Soy flour	stirred, full fat, raw	Arrowhead Mills	0.6	cup	2	1	3
	stirred, defatted		0.4	cup	1	1	2
	lowfat		0.4	cup	2	1	0
Soy sauce		Kikoman Light	10	tbsp.	2	1	0
		La Choy	10	tbsp.	1	1	0
		La Choy Lite	5	tbsp.	2	1	0

FOOD ITEM	SPECIFICATIONS	BRAND NAME	QUANTITY	SIZE	PROTEIN BLOCKS	CARBOHYDRATE BLOCKS	FAT BLOCKS
	dark	House of Tsang	10	tbsp.	0	1	0
	ginger flavor	House of Tsang	2.5	tbsp.	0	1	0
	ginger or mushroom flavor	House of Tsang Low Sodium	5	tbsp.	0	1	0
	hot	Try Me Dragon Sauce	10	tsp.	0	1	0
	tamari	Eden Domestic	5	tbsp.	1	1	0
	tamari	Eden Imported	5	tbsp.	1	1	0
	shoyu	Eden Imported	5	tbsp.	1	1	0
	shoyu	Eden Traditional	5	tbsp.	1	1	0
Spaghetti squash	baked or boiled, drained		1.3	cup	0	1	0
Spelt flakes		Arrowhead Mills	0.5	cup	0	1	0
Spelt flour		Arrowhead Mills	0.1	cup	0	1	0
Spinach	fresh, raw, chopped		2.5	cup	4	1	2
	fresh, boiled, drained		5	cup	3	1	1
	canned	Allens Popeye	1.7	cup	1	1	1
	canned	Allens Popeye Low Sodium	.5	cup	2	1	3
	canned	Del Monte	2.5	cup	1	1	3
	canned	Del Monte No Salt	2.5	cup	1	1	0
	canned	S&W	2.5	cup	2	1	0
	canned, chopped	Allen Popeye/Sunshine	2.5	cup	1	1	2
	frozen (see also "Spinach dishes")	Green Giant Harvest Fresh	5	cup	3	1	0
	frozen, in butter sauce	Green Giant	5	cup	2	1	5
Split peas, dried		Goya	0.1	cup	1	1	0
	boiled		0.4	cup	1	1	0
	green	Arrowhead Mills	0.1	cup	0	1	0
	yellow	Goya	0.1	cup	1	1	0
Sports drink	all flavors	Body Works	4.6	fl. oz.	0	1	0
	all flavors, except orange	Recharge	4	fl. oz.	0	1	0
	fruit punch	All Sport	3.3	fl. oz.	0	1	0
	grape	All Sport	3.6	fl. oz.	0	1	0
	lemon-lime or orange	All Sport	3.6	fl. oz.	0	1	0
	orange	Recharge	4	fl. oz.	0	1	0

Category	Description	Brand	Amount	Unit	Protein	Carbohydrate	Fat
Sprouts	bean, canned	La Choy	10	cup	1	1	0
	hot and spicy	Jonathan's	5	cup, 4 oz.	2	1	0
	mixed	Jonathan's Gourmet	10	cup, 3 oz.	3	1	0
Squash	lentil, adzuki, pea	Jonathan's	1.6	oz.	0	1	0
	canned	Stokely	0.7	cup	0	1	0
	frozen	Stilwell	5	cup	0	1	0
Steak sauce		A.1.	3.3	tbsp.	0	1	0
		A.1. Bold	1.7	tbsp.	0	1	0
		A.1. Thick and Hearty	1.4	tbsp.	0	1	0
		Alanna Irish	2.5	tbsp.	0	1	0
		Heinz 57	2.5	tbsp.	0	1	0
		HP	3.3	tbsp.	0	1	0
		Hunt's	5	tbsp.	0	1	0
		Maull's	1.7	tbsp.	0	1	0
		Texas Best	2.5	tbsp.	0	1	0
	and burger	Trappey's Great American	2.5	tbsp.	0	1	0
	Caribbean style	Try Me Bullfighter	2.5	tbsp.	0	1	0
	garlic peppercorn	Tabasco	2.5	tbsp.	0	1	0
	New Orleans style	Lea & Perrins	1.4	tbsp.	0	1	0
	New Orleans style	Tabasco	5	tbsp.	0	1	0
	sweet, mild	Trappey's Chef-Magic	5	tbsp.	1	1	0
	sweet, spicy	Maull's	2.5	tbsp.	0	1	0
		Lea & Perrins	1.4	tbsp.	0	1	0
		House of Tsang Classic	2.5	tbsp.	0	1	0
		House of Tsang Saigon Sizzle	1.1	tbsp.	0	1	0
		House of Tsang Szechuan Spicy	2.5	tbsp.	0	1	0
		Ka-Me	10	tbsp.	1	1	0
		Ken's Steak House	1.7	tbsp.	0	1	0
		Kikkoman	3.3	tbsp.	0	1	0
		Lawry's	2.5	tbsp.	0	1	0
		S&W Oriental	1.7	tbsp.	0	1	0
	honey	Ken's Steak House	1.7	tbsp.	0	1	0
Stir-fry sauce	mandarin soy	La Choy	0.3	cup	1	1	0
	and marinade	Mary Rose Halu	1.4	tbsp.	0	1	0
	and rib, garlic	Mi-Kee	0.9	tbsp.	0	1	0
	spicy	La Choy Szechuan	0.3	cup	0	1	0

Zone Food Blocks for Individual Food Ingredients 303

CARBOHYDRATES

FOOD ITEM	SPECIFICATIONS	BRAND NAME	QUANTITY	SIZE	PROTEIN BLOCKS	CARBOHYDRATE BLOCKS	FAT BLOCKS
	sweet and sour	House of Tsang	1.1	tbsp.	0	1	0
	sweet and sour, spicy	La Choy	0.1	cup	0	1	0
	teriyaki	La Choy	0.2	cup	0	1	0
Strawberry	fresh		0.6	pint	0	1	0
	fresh		1.3	cup	0	1	0
	canned in heavy syrup		0.2	cup	0	1	0
	frozen, unsweetened		0.8	cup	0	1	0
	frozen	Big Valley	0.6	cup	0	1	0
	frozen	Stilwell	0.6	cup	0	1	0
Strawberry drink		Capri Sun Cooler	2.3	fl. oz.	0	1	0
		Farmer's Market	2.4	fl. oz.	0	1	0
	nectar	Kern's	2	fl. oz.	0	1	0
	nectar	Libby's/Kern's	2	fl. oz.	0	1	0
Strawberry	banana	R.W. Knudsen	2.4	fl. oz.	0	1	0
drink blends	banana, cactus	R.W. Knudsen	2.5	fl. oz.	0	1	0
	banana, nectar	Kern's	2	fl. oz.	0	1	0
	guava	R.W. Knudsen	2.7	fl. oz.	0	1	0
	guava	Santa Cruz	3	fl. oz.	0	1	0
	kiwi	R.W. Knudsen	2.4	fl. oz.	0	1	0
	melon	R.W. Knudsen	2.5	fl. oz.	0	1	0
	orange banana	Veryfine Shivering Chillers	2.5	fl. oz.	0	1	0
Strawberry drink mix		Tree Top	2.9	fl. oz.	0	1	0
		Kool-Aid	4.4	fl. oz.	0	1	0
		Kool-Aid w/Sugar	2	fl. oz.	0	1	0
Strawberry juice		Veryfine Juice-Ups	2.4	fl. oz.	0	1	0
	nectar	R.W. Knudsen	0.3	cup	0	1	1
Strawberry milk	lowfat	Nestle Quik	0.3	cup	0	1	0
	lowfat	Nestle Quik	2.1	fl. oz.	0	1	0
	lowfat, banana	Nestle Quik	2.4	fl. oz.	0	1	1
	shake	Nestle Killer	2.2	oz.	0	1	1
	shake	Nestle Quik	2.2	oz.	0	1	1
Strawberry milk drink	canned	Sego	2.4	fl. oz.	0	1	0
	canned	Sego Lite	5	fl. oz.	1	1	1

Food	Type	Brand	Amount	Unit	P	C	F
Strawberry syrup	canned, creme	Carnation Instant Breakfast	2.6	fl. oz.	0	1	0
	mix, powder	Nestle Quik	0.8	tbsp.	0	1	0
	mix, powder, creme	Carnation Instant Breakfast	0.3	pkt.	0	1	0
	mix, powder, creme	Carnation Instant Breakfast No Sugar	0.8	pkt.	0	1	0
		Hershey's	0.7	tbsp.	0	1	0
		Knott's Berry Farm	0.6	tbsp.	0	1	0
		R.W. Knudsen	0.1	cup	0	1	0
		S&W Reduced Calorie	0.1	cup	0	1	0
Strawberry topping		Kraft	0.6	tbsp.	0	1	0
		Smucker's	0.7	tbsp.	0	1	0
	Melba	Dickinson's	0.8	tbsp.	1	1	1
Stroganoff gravy		Pepperidge Farm	0.6	cup	1	1	2
Stroganoff mix	vegetarian	Natural Touch	5	tbsp.	0	1	0
Stroganoff sauce	beef	Lawry's	1.7	tbsp.	0	1	0
Stroganoff seasoning mix		Durkee	0.4	pkg.	1	1	1
Strudel	apple	Entenmann's	0.1	strudel	0	1	0
Stuffing	apple and raisin	Arnold Unspiced	0.4	cup	0	1	0
	Cajun rice	Pepperidge Farm	0.1	cup	0	1	0
	chicken, classic	Good Harvest	0.2	cup	0	1	0
	corn bread	Pepperidge Farm	0.2	cup	0	1	0
	corn bread	Arnold	0.4	cup	0	1	0
	corn bread	Brownberry	0.4	cup	0	1	0
	corn bread, honey pecan	Pepperidge Farm	0.2	cup	0	1	0
	country style	Pepperidge Farm	0.2	cup	0	1	0
	cube	Pepperidge Farm	0.3	cup	1	1	1
	cube bread, unseasoned	Pepperidge Farm	0.3	cup	0	1	0
	garden and herb, country	Brownberry	0.4	cup	0	1	0
	herb seasoned	Pepperidge Farm	0.2	cup	0	1	0
	herb seasoned	Arnold	0.4	cup	1	1	1
	herb seasoned	Brownberry	0.2	cup	0	1	0
	sage and onion	Pepperidge Farm	0.2	cup	0	1	0
	sage and onion	Arnold	0.4	cup	0	1	0
	sage and onion	Brownberry 7 oz.	0.4	cup	0	1	0
	sage and onion	Brownberry 14 oz.	0.4	cup	0	1	0
	sage and onion	Pepperidge Farm	0.2	cup	0	1	0
	Santa Fe	Good Harvest	0.2	cup	0	1	0

FOOD ITEM	SPECIFICATIONS	BRAND NAME	QUANTITY	SIZE	PROTEIN BLOCKS	CARBOHYDRATE BLOCKS	FAT BLOCKS
	seasoned	Arnold	0.4	cups	0	1	0
	sourdough, San Francisco	Good Harvest	0.2	cup	0	1	0
	vegetable, harvest, and almond	Pepperidge Farm	0.2	cup	0	1	0
Stuffing mix	wild rice and mushroom	Pepperidge Farm	0.3	cup	0	1	1
	wild rice trio	Good Harvest	0.2	cup	0	1	0
	dry	Kellogg's Crouettes	0.4	cup	0	1	0
	dry, for beef	Stove Top	0.1	box	0	1	0
	dry, chicken flavor	Stove Top	0.1	box	0	1	0
	dry, chicken flavor	Stove Top Lower Sodium	0.1	box	0	1	0
	dry, chicken flavor	Stove Top Microwave	0.1	box	0	1	1
	prepared, chicken flavor w/rice	Rice-A-Roni	0.5	cup	0	1	1
	dry, corn bread	Stove Top	0.1	box	0	1	0
	dry, corn bread, homestyle	Stove Top Microwave	0.1	box	0	1	1
	prepared, corn bread, w/rice	Rice-A-Roni	0.4	cup	0	1	1
	dry, herb	Stove Top Flexible Serve	0.5	oz.	0	1	0
	prepared, herb and butter	Rice-A-Roni	0.5	cup	0	1	1
	dry, herbs, savory	Stove Top	0.1	box	0	1	0
	dry, long grain/wild rice	Stove Top	0.1	box	0	1	0
	dry, mushroom/onion	Stove Top	0.1	box	0	1	0
	dry, for pork	Stove Top	0.1	box	0	1	0
	dry, San Francisco style	Stove Top	0.1	box	0	1	0
	dry, for turkey	Stove Top	0.1	box	0	1	0
	prepared, w/wild rice	Rice-A-Roni	0.5	cup	0	1	1
Succotash	canned, kernel	S&W	0.3	cup	0	1	0
	canned, kernel	Stokely	0.4	cup	0	1	0
	frozen, boiled, drained		0.4	cup	0	1	0
Sugar, beet or cane	brown		0.3	oz.	0	1	0
	brown		0.1	cup, not packed	0	1	0
	brown		0.04	cup, packed	0	1	0
	granulated		0.3	oz.	0	1	0

Food	Description	Brand	Amount	Unit	Protein	Carbohydrate	Fat
Sugar, maple	granulated		0.05	cup	0	1	0
	granulated		0.8	tbsp.	0	1	0
	granulated		2.5	tsp.	0	1	0
	powdered or confectioner's		0.1	cup, sifted	0	1	0
	powdered or confectioner's		1.1	tbsp., unsifted	0	1	0
Sugar apple	medium		0.4	oz.	0	1	0
		Sweet 'n Low	10	pkt.	0	1	0
			3	oz.	0	1	1
Sunflower seed flour	partially defatted		0.2	cup	0	1	3
Swamp cabbage	raw, shoot		0.4	cup	0	1	1
	boiled, drained, chopped		60	oz.	0	1	0
Sweet potato	raw		5	cup	0	1	0
	baked in skin		0.3	5"x2"	0	1	0
	baked in skin, mashed		0.4	5"x2"	0	1	0
	boiled w/out skin		0.2	cup	0	1	0
	boiled w/out skin, mashed		1.5	oz.	0	1	0
Sweet potato, canned	in syrup, w/liquid		0.1	cup	0	1	0
	in syrup, drained		0.2	cup	0	1	0
	whole	Royal Prince/Trappey's	0.2	cup	0	1	0
	halves	Royal Prince	0.8	pcs. 5.7 oz.	0	1	0
	cut or pieces	Allens/Sugary Sam/Princella Yams	0.6	pcs. 5.7 oz.	0	1	0
	mashed	Princella/Sugary Sam	0.2	cup	0	1	0
	candied	Royal Prince	0.2	cup	0	1	0
	candied	S&W	0.1	cup	0	1	0
	orange-pineapple	Royal Prince	0.1	cup	0	1	0
Sweet potato, frozen	baked, cubed		0.3	cup	0	1	0
	candied	Mrs. Paul's	0.6	fl. oz.	0	1	0
	candied	Mrs. Paul's Sweets'n Apples	0.1	fl. oz.	0	1	0
	candied	Ore-Ida	1.2	pcs.	0	1	0
Sweet potato chips		Terra Chips	0.6	oz.	0	1	1
	cinnamon	Terra Chips	0.6	oz.	0	1	1
Sweet potato leaf	raw, chopped		5	cup	0	1	0
	steamed		2.5	cup	0	1	0
Sweet and sour drink mixer		Holland House/Mr. & Mrs. "T"/Rose's	1.5	fl. oz.	0	1	0

FOOD ITEM	SPECIFICATIONS	BRAND NAME	QUANTITY	SIZE	PROTEIN BLOCKS	CARBOHYDRATE BLOCKS	FAT BLOCKS
Sweet and sour dinner mix		La Choy	0.1	pkg.	0	1	0
Sweet and sour sauce		Contadina	2.2	tbsp.	0	1	0
		House of Tsang	2.5	tbsp.	0	1	0
		House of Tsang	1.3	oz. pkt.	0	1	0
		Kikkoman	2	tbsp.	0	1	0
		Kraft	1	tbsp.	0	1	0
		La Choy	1.3	tbsp.	0	1	0
		Sauceworks	1.3	tbsp.	0	1	0
		Woody's	1.1	tbsp.	0	1	0
	concentrate	House of Tsang	3.3	tsp.	0	1	0
	chicken	Gold's Dip'n Joy	1.3	tbsp.	0	1	0
	duck sauce	Ka-Me	0.9	tbsp.	0	1	0
	duck sauce	La Choy	1.2	tbsp.	0	1	0
	duck sauce, all varieties	Gold's	1.3	tbsp.	0	1	0
Swiss chard	raw, chopped		12.5	cup	1	1	0
	boiled, drained, chopped		2.5	cup	1	1	0
Swiss steak gravy mix	prepared	Durkee	0.6	cup	0	1	0
Swiss steak seasoning mix		Durkee/French's Roasting Bag	0.4	pkg.	0	1	0
Taco mix, dinner	cooking	Kylin Chili & Tomato	0.2	cup	0	1	0
		Lawry's	0.1	pkg.	0	1	1
		Old El Paso	1.1	tacos, prepared	0	1	2
		Pancho Villa	1.1	tacos, prepared	0	1	2
	vegetarian	Natural Touch	15	tbsp.	4	1	2
Taco sauce		Chi-Chi's Thick & Chunky	10	tbsp.	0	1	0
		Hunt's Manwich	0.4	cup	0	1	0
		Lawry's Chunky	10	tbsp.	0	1	0
		Lawry's Sauce'n Seasoner	6.7	tbsp.	0	1	0
		Pancho Villa	6.7	tbsp.	0	1	0
	green	La Victoria	10	tbsp.	0	1	0
	hot	Old El Paso	10	tbsp.	0	1	0
	medium	Old El Paso	10	tbsp.	0	1	0

Food	Type	Brand	Amount	Unit	P	C	F
Taco seasoning	mild	Old El Paso	10	tbsp.	0	1	0
Taco seasoning mix	mild or medium	Old El Paso Chunky	10	tbsp.	0	1	0
	red	La Victoria	10	tbsp.	0	1	0
		Tone's	6.7	tsp.	0	1	0
		Durkee Pouch	0.6	pkg.	0	1	0
		Durkee Pouch Family	0.3	pkg.	0	1	0
		Lawry's	1.7	tbsp.	0	1	0
		McCormick	6.7	tsp.	0	1	0
		Old El Paso	3.3	tsp.	0	1	0
		Old El Paso Less Salt	5	tsp.	0	1	0
		Pancho Villa	3.3	tsp.	0	1	0
	chicken	Lawry's	3.3	tsp.	0	1	0
	mild	Durkee Pouch	0.4	pkg.	0	1	0
	salad	Durkee Pouch	0.4	pkg.	0	1	0
	salad	Lawry's	3.3	tsp.	0	1	0
Taco shell		Gebhardt	1.9	shells	0	1	2
		Lawry's	1.5	shells	0	1	2
		Lawry's Super Size	0.9	shells	0	1	1
		Old El Paso	1.7	shells	0	1	2
		Old El Paso Super	1	shells	0	1	2
	mini	Pancho Villa	1.7	shells	0	1	2
	tostada	Rosarita	1.9	shells	0	1	2
	tostada	Old El Paso	3.9	shells	0	1	2
	tostada	Lawry's	1.5	shells	0	1	2
	tostaco	Rosarita	1.6	shells	0	1	1
		Old El Paso	1.1	shells	0	1	2
	white corn	Chi-Chi's	0.7	shell	0	1	1
	white corn	Old El Paso	0.9	shells	0	1	2
			1.7	shells	0	1	0
Tagliatelle	refrigerated, spinach	Contadina	0.3	cup	0	1	0
Tamarind			10	3"x1" fruit	0	1	0
	pulp	Goya	0.1	cup	0	1	0
	frozen, chunks	Goya	0.3	pkg.	0	1	0
Tamarind nectar	canned		1.9	fl. oz.	0	1	0
Tandoori paste	mild	Patak's	20	tbsp.	0	1	3

FOOD ITEM	SPECIFICATIONS	BRAND NAME	QUANTITY	SIZE	PROTEIN BLOCKS	CARBOHYDRATE BLOCKS	FAT BLOCKS
Tangerine	fresh		1.3	2 3/8", fruit	0	1	0
	fresh, sections w/out membrane		0.5	cup	0	1	0
	canned, in juice	S&W Mandarin	0.4	cup	0	1	0
	canned, in juice		0.4	cup	0	1	0
	canned, in light syrup	Del Monte	0.2	cup	0	1	0
	canned, in light syrup	S&W Mandarin	0.2	cup	0	1	0
	canned, in light syrup		0.3	cup	0	1	0
Tangerine juice	fresh		3	fl. oz.	0	1	0
	frozen, prepared	Minute Maid Beverage	2.4	fl. oz.	0	1	0
	blend	Dole Mandarin	2.1	fl. oz.	0	1	0
Tapioca	dry	Minute	2.5	tsp.	0	1	0
Taro	raw, sliced		0.4	cup	0	1	0
	cooked, sliced		0.2	cup	0	1	0
Taro chips	spiced	Terra	0.5	oz.	0	1	1
Taro leaf	raw		12.5	cup	2	1	1
Tarragon, dried	ground	McCormick	10	tsp.	0	1	0
Tea, iced	flavored, lemon, instant	Lipton	10	tsp.	0	1	0
		Schweppes	3.3	fl. oz.	0	1	0
		Snapple	4	fl. oz.	0	1	0
	all fruit flavors	Veryfine Chillers	3.8	fl. oz.	0	1	0
	all fruit flavors	Apple & Eve	2.9	fl. oz.	0	1	0
	all fruit flavors, herbal	Lipton Chilled	3.6	fl. oz.	0	1	0
		R.W. Knudsen Coolers	3.1	fl. oz.	0	1	0
	lemon	Snapple	2.9	fl. oz.	0	1	0
	lemon	Tropicana	2.9	fl. oz.	0	1	0
	lemon	Veryfine Chillers	3.1	fl. oz.	0	1	0
	mango or passion fruit	Snapple	2.7	fl. oz.	0	1	0
	mint	Snapple	2.5	fl. oz.	0	1	0
	peach	Snapple	2.9	fl. oz.	0	1	0
	peach	Tropicana	2.5	fl. oz.	0	1	0
	peach, raspberry, or strawberry	Snapple	2.8	fl. oz.	0	1	0

Food	Description	Brand	Amount	Unit	P	C	F
	peach-kiwi	Veryfine Chillers	4	fl. oz.	0	1	0
	raspberry	Snapple	2.8	fl. oz.	0	1	0
	raspberry	Tropicana	2.5	fl. oz.	0	1	0
	raspberry	Veryfine Chillers	3	fl. oz.	0	1	0
Tea, iced, mix	lemon flavor	Lipton	0.7	tbsp.	0	1	0
	w/out lemon	Lipton	0.8	tbsp.	0	1	0
Teff seed or flour		Arrowhead Mills	0.5	oz.	0	1	0
Teriyaki sauce		House of Tsang Korean Teriyaki	1.4	tbsp.	0	1	0
		La Choy	3.3	tbsp.	0	1	0
		La Choy Lite	2.5	tbsp.	0	1	0
		Mary Rose Sumi	1.3	tbsp.	0	1	0
	barbecue	Kikkoman	0.8	tbsp.	0	1	0
	baste and glaze	Kikkoman	0.5	tbsp.	0	1	1
	baste and glaze, w/honey and pineapple	S&W	1.7	tbsp.	0	1	0
	cooking and marinade	S&W Lite	1.7	tbsp.	0	1	1
	cooking and marinade	La Choy Chun King	3.3	tbsp.	0	1	0
	hot	Lawry's	1.7	tbsp.	0	1	0
	marinade	Kikkoman	5	tbsp.	0	1	0
	marinade	Lea & Perrins	2.5	tbsp.	0	1	0
	marinade and light	Kikkoman	3.3	tbsp.	0	1	0
	beef	Durkee	1.4	tbsp.	0	1	0
Thai sauce		World Harbors Nong Khai	1.7	tbsp.	0	1	0
Teriyaki seasoning mix	ground	McCormick	10	tsp.	1	1	0
Toaster muffins and pastries	apple	Toaster Strudel	0.3	pc.	0	1	0
	apple, cinnamon	Pop-Tarts	0.2	pc.	1	1	0
	apple, cinnamon	Thomas' Toast-r-Cakes	0.5	pc.	1	1	0
	banana nut	Thomas' Toast-r-Cakes	0.6	pc.	1	1	0
	blueberry	Pop-Tarts	0.3	pc.	1	1	0
	blueberry	Thomas' Toast-r-Cakes	0.5	pc.	1	1	0
	blueberry	Toaster Strudel	0.3	pc.	1	1	0
	blueberry, frosted	Pop-Tarts	0.3	pc.	0	1	0
	blueberry, frosted	Toastettes	0.3	pc.	0	1	0
	brown sugar-cinnamon	Pop-Tarts	0.3	pc.	1	1	0

FOOD ITEM	SPECIFICATIONS	BRAND NAME	QUANTITY	SIZE	PROTEIN BLOCKS	CARBOHYDRATE BLOCKS	FAT BLOCKS
	brown sugar-cinnamon, frosted	Pop-Tarts	0.3	pc.	0	1	1
	brown sugar-cinnamon, frosted	Toastettes	0.3	pc.	0	1	0
	cherry	Pop-Tarts	0.3	pc.	0	1	0
	cherry	Toaster Strudel	0.3	pc.	0	1	1
	cherry, frosted	Pop-Tarts	0.3	pc.	0	1	0
	cherry, frosted	Toastettes	0.3	pc.	0	1	0
	chocolate	Pop-Tarts Minis	0.3	pkt.	0	1	0
	chocolate fudge, frosted	Pop-Tarts	0.3	pc.	0	1	0
	chocolate graham	Pop-Tarts	0.3	pc.	0	1	1
	chocolate-vanilla creme, frosted	Pop-Tarts	0.3	pc.	0	1	0
	cinnamon	Toaster Strudel	0.3	pc.	0	1	1
	corn	Thomas' Toast-r-Cakes	0.5	pc.	0	1	1
	cream cheese	Toaster Strudel	0.4	pc.	0	1	1
	cream cheese, blueberry or strawberry	Toaster Strudel	0.4	pc.	0	1	1
	French toast style	Toaster Strudel	0.3	pc.	0	1	1
	fudge, frosted	Toastettes	0.3	pc.	0	1	0
	grape, frosted	Pop-Tarts	0.2	pc.	0	1	0
	grape, frosted	Pop-Tarts Minis	0.3	pkt.	0	1	0
	raisin bran	Thomas' Toast-r-Cakes	0.6	pc.	0	1	1
	raspberry	Toaster Strudel	0.3	pc.	0	1	1
	raspberry, frosted	Pop-Tarts	0.3	pc.	0	1	1
	S'mores	Pop-Tarts	0.3	pc.	0	1	0
	strawberry	Pop-Tarts	0.3	pc.	0	1	0
	strawberry	Pop-Tarts Minis	0.3	pkt.	0	1	0
	strawberry	Thomas' Toast-r-Cakes	0.5	pc.	0	1	1
	strawberry	Toaster Strudel	0.3	pc.	0	1	1
	strawberry	Toastettes	0.3	pc.	0	1	0
	strawberry, frosted	Pop-Tarts	0.2	pc.	0	1	0
	strawberry, frosted	Toastettes	0.3	pc.	0	1	0

CARBOHYDRATES

Food	Description	Brand	Amount	Unit	P	C	F
Tofu seasoning mix	breakfast scramble	Fantastic Classics	0.3	pkg.	0	1	0
	breakfast scramble	TofuMate	0.8	pkg.	0	1	0
	eggless salad	TofuMate	0.6	pkg.	0	1	0
	mandarin stir-fry	TofuMate	0.4	pkg.	0	1	0
	Mediterranean herb	TofuMate	0.8	pkg.	0	1	0
	Szechwan stir-fry	TofuMate	0.6	pkg.	0	1	0
	Texas taco	TofuMate	0.8	pkg.	0	1	0
Tom collins mixer	bottled	Holland House	0.7	fl. oz.	0	1	1
Tomatillo	1 5/8" diam.		5	med.	1	1	1
	chopped		1.7	cup	2	1	2
	in jars	La Victoria Entero	25	pcs.	2	1	2
	in jars, crushed	La Victoria	45	oz.	0	1	0
Tomato	raw		2	2 3/5"	0	1	0
	raw, chopped		1.3	cup	0	1	0
	boiled		0.8	cup	2	1	2
Tomato, canned	whole	Contadina Pasta Ready	1.3	cup	0	1	0
	whole	Contadina Recipe Ready	1.3	cup	0	1	0
	whole	Hunt's	0.8	cup	0	1	0
	whole	Del Monte	1.3	cup	0	1	0
	whole	Hunt's	6.7	pcs.	1	1	0
	whole	Hunt's No Salt	5	pcs.	0	1	0
	whole, Italian pear	Contadina	1.7	cup	0	1	0
	whole, Italian pear, w/basil	S&W	1.7	cup	0	1	0
	whole, pear	Hunt's	1.7	cup	0	1	0
	whole, peeled	Contadina	1.7	cup	0	1	0
	whole, peeled	Progresso	1.7	cup	0	1	0
	whole, peeled	S&W	1.7	cup	0	1	0
	whole, peeled	S&W No-Salt	1.7	cup	0	1	0
	whole, w/basil	Progresso	1.7	cup	0	1	0
	whole, w/basil	Progresso Imported	1.7	cup	0	1	0
	whole, w/green chilies	Ro*Tel	1.7	cup	1	1	1
	aspic	S&W	0.4	cup	0	1	0
	w/cheeses, three	Contadina Pasta Ready	0.6	cup	0	1	0
	chunky, chili	Del Monte	0.7	cup	0	1	0
	chunky, pasta	Del Monte	0.5	cup	0	1	0
	chunky, salsa	Del Monte	0.7	cup	0	1	0

FOOD ITEM	SPECIFICATIONS	BRAND NAME	QUANTITY	SIZE	PROTEIN BLOCKS	CARBOHYDRATE BLOCKS	FAT BLOCKS
	crushed	Contadina	0.8	cup	0	1	0
	crushed	Eden	2.5	cup	1	1	0
	crushed	Hunt's	0.8	cup	0	1	0
	crushed	Hunt's Angela Mia	1.3	cup	0	1	0
	crushed	Progresso	1.7	cup	0	1	0
	crushed	S&W	0.8	cup	0	1	0
	cut	Hunt's Choice Cut	1.3	cup	0	1	0
	cut, in juice	S&W Ready-Cut	1.7	cup	0	1	0
	cut, in juice	S&W Ready-Cut No-Salt	1.7	cup	0	1	0
	cut, in juice, Italian style	S&W Ready-Cut	1.7	cup	0	1	0
	cut, in puree	S&W Ready-Cut	1.3	cup	0	1	0
	diced	Del Monte	1.3	cup	0	1	0
	diced, w/basil, garlic, oregano	Del Monte	0.4	cup	0	1	0
	diced, w/onion, garlic	Del Monte	0.6	cup	0	1	0
	diced, w/roasted garlic	Hunt's Choice Cut	0.8	cup	0	1	0
	diced, Italian herb	Hunt's Choice Cut	0.8	cup	0	1	0
	w/green chilies, whole or diced	Ro*Tel	1.7	cup	0	1	0
	w/green chilies, diced	Chi-Chi's	0.6	cup	0	1	1
	w/mushrooms	Contadina Pasta Ready	0.6	cup	0	1	1
	w/olives	Contadina Pasta Ready	0.6	cup	0	1	1
	primavera	Contadina Pasta Ready	0.6	cup	0	1	1
	w/red pepper, crushed	Contadina Pasta Ready	0.6	cup	0	1	0
	stewed	Contadina	0.6	cup	0	1	0
	stewed	Del Monte	0.6	cup	0	1	0
	stewed	Del Monte No Salt	0.6	cup	0	1	0
	stewed	Green Giant Classic	0.8	cup	0	1	0
	stewed	Hunt's	0.8	cup	0	1	0
	stewed	S&W	0.8	cup	0	1	0
	stewed	S&W No-Salt	0.8	cup	0	1	0
	stewed, Cajun	Del Monte	0.6	cup	0	1	0

Item	Variety	Brand	Amount	Unit	P	C	F
	stewed, Italian	Contadina	0.6	cup	0	1	0
	stewed, Italian	Del Monte	0.7	cup	0	1	0
	stewed, Italian	Green Giant	0.8	cup	0	1	0
	stewed, Italian	S&W	0.8	cup	0	1	0
	stewed, Mexican	Contadina	0.6	cup	0	1	0
	stewed, Mexican	Del Monte	0.6	cup	0	1	0
	stewed, Mexican	Green Giant	0.8	cup	0	1	0
	wedges	Del Monte	0.6	cup	0	1	0
Tomato, dried			0.7	oz.	0	1	0
	bits		10	pc., 32 per cup	0	1	0
		Sonoma	0.4	cup	1	1	0
	flakes	Sonoma	10	tsp.	0	1	0
	halves	Christopher Ranch	2.5	tbsp.	1	1	0
	julienne	Sonoma	10	pcs.	1	1	0
	in oil, drained	Sonoma	35	strips	1	1	7
	pasta toss	Sonoma Spice Medley	5	tbsp.	0	1	0
	seasoning	Sonoma	0.5	cup	0	1	0
		Sonoma Season It	10	tsp.	0	1	0
Tomato, green			2	2 3/5"	0	1	0
Tomato, pickled		Claussen	10	oz.	0	1	0
Tomato juice		Campbell's	8.9	fl. oz.	0	1	0
		Campbell's Enhanced Flavor Low Sodium	8	fl. oz.	0	1	0
		Del Monte	8	fl. oz.	0	1	0
		Del Monte Not from Concentrate	10	fl. oz.	0	1	0
		Hunt's	13.3	fl. oz.	0	1	0
		Hunt's No Salt	13.3	fl. oz.	0	1	0
		R.W. Knudsen	5	fl. oz.	1	1	0
		Sacramento	13.3	fl. oz.	0	1	0
		S&W	10	fl. oz.	0	1	0
	garlic	R.W. Knudsen	5.7	fl. oz.	0	1	0
Tomato paste		Contadina	3.3	tbsp.	0	1	0
		Del Monte	3.3	tbsp.	0	1	0
		Goya	3.3	tbsp.	0	1	0
		Hunt's	5	tbsp.	0	1	0
		Hunt's No Salt	5	tbsp.	0	1	0

CARBOHYDRATES

FOOD ITEM	SPECIFICATIONS	BRAND NAME	QUANTITY	SIZE	PROTEIN BLOCKS	CARBOHYDRATE BLOCKS	FAT BLOCKS
		Progresso	3.3	tbsp.	0	1	0
		S&W	3.3	tbsp.	0	1	0
	w/garlic	Hunt's	5	tbsp.	0	1	0
	Italian	Contadina	2.9	tbsp.	0	1	0
	Italian	Hunt's	5	tbsp.	0	1	0
Tomato puree		Contadina	0.6	cup	0	1	0
		Hunt's	0.8	cup	0	1	0
		Progresso	0.6	cup	0	1	0
		Progresso	0.6	cup	0	1	0
Tomato sauce, canned	thick	Contadina	0.6	cup	0	1	0
(see also "Pasta sauce"		Contadina Thick & Zesty	1.3	cup	1	1	0
and "Tomato, canned"		Del Monte	0.6	cup	0	1	0
		Del Monte No Salt	0.6	cup	0	1	0
		Goya	0.8	cup	0	1	0
		Hunt's	1.3	cup	1	1	0
		Hunt's No Salt	1.3	cup	1	1	0
		Progresso	0.8	cup	0	1	0
		S&W	0.8	cup	0	1	0
	chili, chunky	Hunt's Ready Sauce	1.3	cup	1	1	0
	chunky	Hunt's Ready Sauce	1.3	cup	1	1	0
	chunky	Hunt's Ready Sauce Special	0.8	cup	0	1	0
	garden	S&W Original	0.8	cup	0	1	0
	garden, Italian herb	S&W	0.6	cup	0	1	0
	garden, mild Mexican	S&W	0.8	cup	0	1	0
	garlic	Hunt's Ready Sauce	1.3	cup	1	1	2
	garlic and herb	Hunt's Ready Sauce	1.3	cup	1	1	0
	herb	Hunt's	0.6	cup	0	1	1
	herb, country	Hunt's Ready Sauce	0.6	cup	0	1	1
	Italian	Contadina	0.6	cup	0	1	0
	Italian	Hunt's	0.6	cup	0	1	1
	Italian, chunky	Hunt's Ready Sauce	0.8	cup	0	1	1
	meatloaf	Hunt's Ready Sauce Meatloaf Fixin's	0.8	cup	0	1	0

Item	Description	Brand	Amount	Unit			
Tomato-beef cocktail	Mexican, chunky salsa	Hunt's Ready Sauce	0.8	cup	0	1	0
Tomato-chili cocktail	seasoned, lightly	Hunt's Ready Sauce	1.3	cup	0	1	1
		Eden	0.6	cup	0	1	0
		Beefamato	3.8	fl. oz.	0	1	0
		Snap-E-Tom	7.5	fl. oz.	0	1	0
Tomato-clam cocktail		Snap-E-Tom	8.3	fl. oz.	0	1	0
		Clamato	3	fl. oz.	0	1	0
	Caesar	Clamato	3	fl. oz.	0	1	0
Tortellini, frozen	cheese, three	Contadina	0.2	cup	1	1	0
or refrigerated	cheese, three, spinach	Contadina	0.2	cup	1	1	0
	mushroom	Contadina	0.2	cup	0	1	0
	spinach	Putney	0.2	cup	0	1	0
	tofu	Soy-Boy	0.3	cup	0	1	0
	tofu	Tofutti	0.2	cup	0	1	0
Tortilla	corn	Tyson	0.9	pcs.	0	1	0
	corn, white	Goya	0.8	pcs.	0	1	0
	flour	Goya	0.6	pc.	0	1	0
	flour	Mesa 6"	0.6	pc.	0	1	0
	flour	Old El Paso	0.3	pc.	0	1	0
	flour	Tyson	0.6	oz.	0	1	0
	flour	Tyson	0.6	oz.	0	1	0
	flour, small	Goya	0.8	pc.	1	1	0
	flour, heat pressed	Tyson	0.6	pcs.	0	1	0
	soft taco	Old El Paso	0.5	pcs.	0	1	0
Trail mix	Eden Fruit & Nuts		1.3	oz.	4	1	1
	California	Sonoma	0.1	cup	1	1	0
	California	Dole	0.5	oz.	0	1	0
	California	Dole	0.5	oz.	0	1	0
	California	Eden Harvest	0.8	oz.	2	1	0
	Hawaiian	Dole	0.5	oz.	0	1	0
	Hawaiian	Dole	0.5	oz.	0	1	0
	Sierra	Del Monte	0.6	oz.	1	1	0
	Sierra	Del Monte	0.6	oz.	0	1	0
	Sierra	Del Monte	0.1	cup	1	1	0
Tree fern	cooked, chopped		0.8	cup	1	1	0
Triticale	whole grain		0.1	cup	0	1	0

FOOD ITEM	SPECIFICATIONS	BRAND NAME	QUANTITY	SIZE	PROTEIN BLOCKS	CARBOHYDRATE BLOCKS	FAT BLOCKS
Triticale flour	whole grain		0.1	cup	0	1	0
Tuna entree mix, dry	broccoli, creamy	Tuna Helper	0.2	cup	0	1	0
	cheddar, garden	Tuna Helper	0.2	cup	0	1	0
	pasta, cheesy	Tuna Helper	0.2	cup	0	1	1
	pasta, creamy	Tuna Helper	0.2	cup	0	1	1
	pot pie	Tuna Helper	0.1	cup	1	1	2
Turkey gravy	roasted	Franco-American	0.8	cup	0	1	1
	seasoned, w/turkey	Heinz	0.8	cup	1	1	1
	mix, prepared	Pepperidge Farm	0.6	cup	1	1	1
	mix, prepared	Durkee/French's	0.6	cup	0	1	0
	mix, roasted, prepared	McCormick	0.6	cup	1	1	1
Turkey seasoning	w/gravy	Knorr	5	tsp.	0	1	0
	ground	McCormick Bag 'n Season	10	tsp.	1	1	1
Turnip	fresh or stored, raw, cubed		1.7	cup	0	1	0
	fresh or stored, boiled, cubed		2.5	cup	0	1	0
	fresh or stored, boiled, mashed		1.3	cup	0	1	0
Turnip greens	fresh, raw, untrimmed		0.8	lb.	0	1	0
	fresh, raw, chopped		5	cup	0	1	0
	fresh, boiled, chopped		5	cup	1	1	0
	canned, w/liquid	Allens/Sunshine	5	cup	2	1	0
	canned	Allens/Sunshine	5	cup	2	1	1
	canned, chopped, w/diced turnip		2.5	cup	1	1	2
Turnover, frozen or refrigerated	apple	Pepperidge Farm	0.2	pc.	0	1	1
	apple	Pillsbury	0.4	pcs.	0	1	1
	apple, iced	Pepperidge Farm	0.2	pc.	0	1	1
	apple, mini	Pepperidge Farm	0.6	pc.	0	1	2
	blueberry	Pepperidge Farm	0.2	pc.	0	1	1
	cherry	Pepperidge Farm	0.2	pc.	0	1	1
	cherry	Pillsbury	0.4	pcs.	0	1	1

Category	Item	Brand	Amount	Unit			
	cherry, iced	Pepperidge Farm	0.2	pc.	1	1	0
	cherry, mini	Pepperidge Farm	0.6	pc.	2	1	0
	peach	Pepperidge Farm	0.2	pc.	1	1	0
	peach, cobbler, mini	Pepperidge Farm	0.4	pc.	1	1	0
	raspberry	Pepperidge Farm	0.2	pc.	1	1	0
	raspberry, iced	Pepperidge Farm	0.2	pc.	1	1	0
	strawberry, mini	Pepperidge Farm	0.5	pc.	1	1	0
Vanilla flavor drink	canned	Sego	2.4	fl. oz.	0	1	0
	canned	Sego Lite	5	fl. oz.	1	1	1
	canned, creme	Sweet Success	2.8	fl. oz.	0	1	0
	canned, French	Sego Lite	5	fl. oz.	1	1	1
	mix, creamy	Sweet Success	0.6	pkt.	0	1	0
	mix, French	Carnation Instant Breakfast	0.3	pkt.	1	1	0
	mix, French	Carnation Instant Breakfast No Sugar	0.8	pkt.	0	1	0
Vanilla shake		Nestle Killer	2.1	oz.	0	1	0
		Nestle Quik	2.1	oz.	0	1	0
Vegetable antipasto		Paesana	12.5	oz.	1	1	1
Vegetable chips	50 chips	Eden	0.4	oz.	1	1	0
Vegetable dishes, frozen	mandarin	The Budget Gourmet Side Dish	4.6	oz.	13	1	1
	New England	The Budget Gourmet Side Dish	2.5	oz.	0	1	0
	samosa	Deep Indian Cuisine	1.3	pcs.	4	1	0
	spring, in cheese sauce	The Budget Gourmet Side Dish	6.1	oz.	2	1	0
Vegetable juice	low sodium	V-8 100%	8	fl. oz.	1	1	1
	low sodium	R.W. Knudsen Very Veggie	7.3	fl. oz.	4	1	0
	original, organic, or spicy	V-8	8	fl. oz.	0	1	0
	picante	R.W. Knudsen Very Veggie	7.3	fl. oz.	0	1	0
	spicy hot	V-8	8	fl. oz.	0	1	0
	tangy	V-8 100%	8	fl. oz.	0	1	0
		V-8 100%	7.3	fl. oz.	0	1	0
Vegetables, mixed, fresh	California style	Dole	10	oz.	0	1	1
	garden style	Dole	15	oz.	0	1	0
	New England	Dole	3.8	oz.	1	1	1
	Oriental style	Dole	1.5	oz.	0	1	0
Vegetables, mixed, canned		Del Monte	0.7	cup	0	1	0

FOOD ITEM	SPECIFICATIONS	BRAND NAME	QUANTITY	SIZE	PROTEIN BLOCKS	CARBOHYDRATE BLOCKS	FAT BLOCKS
		Del Monte No Salt	0.7	cup	0	1	0
		Goya	0.8	cup	0	1	0
		Green Giant	0.5	cup	0	1	0
		Green Giant Garden Medley	0.6	cup	0	1	0
		S&W	0.8	cup	0	1	0
		Stokely	0.8	cup	0	1	0
		Stokely No Salt	0.8	cup	0	1	0
	chop suey	La Choy	2.5	cup	1	1	0
	and sauce	House of Tsang Cantonese Classic	0.4	cup	0	1	0
	and sauce, hot and spicy	House of Tsang Szechuan	0.4	cup	0	1	0
	and sauce, sweet and sour	House of Tsang Hong King	0.1	cup	0	1	0
	and sauce, teriyaki	House of Tsang Tokyo	0.2	cup	0	1	0
	stew	Stokely	0.6	cup	0	1	0
Vegetables, mixed, frozen		Goya	0.7	cup	0	1	0
		Green Giant	0.8	cup	0	1	0
		Green Giant Harvest Fresh	0.8	cup	0	1	0
		Stilwell	0.5	cup	0	1	0
	butter sauce	Green Giant	0.8	cup	0	1	1
	California	Stilwell	2.5	cup	0	1	0
	Capri	Stilwell	1.7	cup	0	1	0
	English, cheddar	Green Giant	3.1	oz.	1	1	1
	French, garlic-Dijon	Green Giant	10	oz.	1	1	3
	Italian, Parmesan	Green Giant	6.7	oz.	1	1	1
	Japanese, teriyaki	Green Giant	5	oz.	0	1	1
	New England	Green Giant	0.6	cup	0	1	0
	Normandy, mushroom	Green Giant	4	oz.	0	1	0
	San Francisco	Green Giant	1.9	cup	1	1	0
	Santa Fe	Green Giant	3.8	cup	0	1	0
	stew	Ore-Ida	0.6	cup	0	1	0
	tropical	Goya Pasteles de Masa	0.5	pouch	0	1	3
	tropical	Goya Viando Sancocho	1.3	oz.	0	1	0
	tropical	Goya Yautia Malanga	0	pkg.	0	1	0
	Western	Green Giant	0.9	cup	0	1	1

Food	Description	Brand	Amount	Unit	Protein	Carbohydrate	Fat
Vine spinach	raw, untrimmed		0.8	lb.	0	1	0
Vinegar	balsamic	Pastorelli Italian Chef	5	tbsp.	0	1	0
Vodka sour mixer	instant	Bar-Tenders	0.7	pouches, 1.1 oz.	0	1	0
Waffle, frozen		Downyflake Butter & Syrup	0.6	pcs.	0	1	0
	apple cinnamon	Downyflake Crisp & Healthy	0.6	pcs.	0	1	0
	apple cinnamon	Downyflake Homestyle	1.3	pcs.	0	1	0
	blueberry	Downyflake Homestyle Jumbo	0.6	pcs.	0	1	0
	blueberry	Downyflake Hot 'n Buttery	0.7	pcs.	0	1	1
	blueberry	Eggo Homestyle	0.6	sets	0	1	1
	blueberry	Eggo Minis Homestyle	0.8	pcs.	0	1	0
	buttermilk	Nutri-Grain	0.7	pcs.	0	1	1
	buttermilk	Special K	0.6	pcs.	0	1	0
	buttermilk	Downyflake Crisp & Healthy	0.5	pcs.	0	1	0
	cinnamon	Eggo	0.5	pcs.	0	1	1
	cinnamon, toast	Aunt Jemima	0.6	pcs.	0	1	1
	multibran	Downyflake	0.5	sets	0	1	0
	nut and honey	Eggo	0.7	pcs.	0	1	1
	oat bran	Eggo Minis	0.7	pcs.	0	1	1
	oat bran w/fruit and nut	Aunt Jemima	0.7	pcs.	0	1	1
	oatmeal	Downyflake	0.6	pcs.	0	1	0
	raisin and bran	Eggo	0.7	sets	0	1	1
	strawberry	Aunt Jemima	0.6	pcs.	0	1	1
	whole grain	Eggo	0.7	pcs.	0	1	1
		Nutri-Grain	0.6	pcs.	0	1	0
		Eggo	0.7	pcs.	0	1	1
		Common Sense	0.6	pcs.	0	1	1
		Common Sense	0.7	pcs.	0	1	1
		Aunt Jemima	0.6	pcs.	0	1	0
		Nutri-Grain	0.6	pcs.	0	1	1
		Eggo	0.6	pcs.	0	1	1
		Aunt Jemima	0.8	pcs.	0	1	1
Walnut topping	syrup	Smucker's	0.8	tbsp.	0	1	0
Waterchestnuts, Chinese	fresh		5	med., 2"	0	1	0
	fresh, sliced		0.4	cup	0	1	0
	canned		13.3	med.	0	1	0
	canned, w/liquid, sliced		0.6	cup	0	1	0

FOOD ITEM	SPECIFICATIONS	BRAND NAME	QUANTITY	SIZE	PROTEIN BLOCKS	CARBOHYDRATE BLOCKS	FAT BLOCKS
	canned	La Choy	20	pcs.	0	1	0
	sliced	La Choy	10	tbsp.	0	1	0
	sliced	Sun Luck	0.8	cup	0	1	0
Watermelon	1" slice, 10" diam.		0.3	slice	0	1	0
	diced		0.8	cup	0	1	0
Watermelon drink		R.W. Knudsen Cooler	2.5	fl. oz.	0	1	0
Watermelon juice		After the Fall	3.3	fl. oz.	0	1	0
	canned	S&W	1.7	cup	0	1	0
	canned	Stokely	1.7	cup	0	1	0
	canned	Stokely No Salt	1.7	cup	0	1	0
	canned, golden	Del Monte	2.5	cup	1	1	0
	frozen	Seabrook	3.3	cup	1	1	1
Wax gourd	boiled, cubed		2.5	cup	0	1	0
Wheat, whole grain	hard red, spring	Arrowhead Mills	0.1	cup	0	1	0
	hard red, winter	Arrowhead Mills	0.1	cup	0	1	0
	hard red, winter	Shiloh Farms	0.1	cup	0	1	0
Wheat bran	crude		2.5	cup	3	1	2
	unprocessed		2.5	cup	3	1	0
	crude		10	tbsp.	1	1	1
	unprocessed	Quaker	1.1	cup	1	1	0
Wheat grass		Pines	10	servings	1	1	0
Wheat flakes		Arrowhead Mills	0.2	cup	0	1	0
Wheat flour	all-purpose, white	Goya	0.1	cup	0	1	0
	all-purpose, white	Pillsbury	0.1	cup	0	1	0
	all-purpose, white, bleached	Pillsbury	0.1	cup	0	1	0
	all-purpose, white, unbleached	Arrowhead Mills	0.1	cup	0	1	0
	all-purpose, white, unbleached, whole grain	Arrowhead Mills	0.1	cup	0	1	0
	cake, white		0.1	cup	0	1	0

Food	Description	Brand	Amount	Unit	P	C	F
	cake, white	Swan's Down	0.1	cup	0	1	0
	bread, white	Pillsbury	0.1	cup	0	1	0
	gluten	Arrowhead Mills	1.8	tbsp.	0	1	0
	pastry, soft, white, unbleached	Arrowhead Mills	0.1	cup	0	1	0
	pastry, soft, whole grain	Arrowhead Mills	0.2	cup	0	1	0
	presifted, white	Pillsbury Shake & Blend	0.1	cup	0	1	0
	self-rising, white	Pillsbury	0.1	cup	0	1	0
	self-rising, white, bleached or unbleached		0.1	cup	0	1	0
	whole grain	Arrowhead Mills	0.1	cup	0	1	0
	whole grain, stone ground	Pillsbury	0.1	cup	0	1	0
	whole wheat	Kretschmer	2.5	cup	0	1	0
Wheat germ	crude		5	tbsp.	0	1	1
	honey crunch	Kretschmer	0.8	oz.	0	1	1
	raw	Arrowhead Mills	2.1	tbsp.	0	1	1
	toasted		3.3	tbsp.	0	1	0
Wheat nuts		Sonoma	0.8	oz.	0	1	1
Wheat pilaf mix		Near East	2.5	tbsp.	0	1	0
Whey, fluid	acid		0.2	cup, prepared	0	1	0
	sweet		0.7	cup	0	1	0
Whiskey sour mixer	bottled	Holland House	0.7	cup	0	1	0
	bottled	Mr. & Mrs. "T"	1.1	fl. oz.	0	1	0
	mix	Bar-Tenders	1.5	fl. oz.	0	1	0
	mix	Bar-Tenders Lite	0.6	pkts.	0	1	0
	mix	Bar-Tenders Slightly Sour	15	pkts.	0	1	0
White bean	dried, boiled		0.6	pkts.	0	1	0
	dried, small, boiled		0.3	cup	0	1	0
	canned, w/liquid		0.2	cup	0	1	0
	canned	Goya	0.2	cup	0	1	0
	canned, small	S&W	0.4	cup	0	1	0
	canned, in tomato sauce	Goya Guisados	0.4	cup	0	1	0
			0.5	cup	0	1	0
White sauce mix		Knorr	0.6	oz. pkt.	0	1	2
			0.3	pkg.	0	1	1

FOOD ITEM	SPECIFICATIONS	BRAND NAME	QUANTITY	SIZE	PROTEIN BLOCKS	CARBOHYDRATE BLOCKS	FAT BLOCKS
Wild rice	raw		0.5	oz.	0	1	0
	raw		0.1	cup	0	1	0
	cooked	Fantastic Foods	0.3	cup	0	1	0
Wine	dessert or aperitif		3.3	fl. oz.	0	1	0
	dry or table		10	fl. oz.	0	1	0
	Marsala	Holland House	10	tbsp.	0	1	0
	red	Holland House	20	tbsp.	0	1	0
	sherry	Holland House	10	tbsp.	0	1	0
Wine cooler, pear	berry	Bartles & Jaymes	3.2	oz. bottle	0	1	0
	black cherry	Bartles & Jaymes	3.5	oz. bottle	0	1	0
	Fuzzy Navel	Bartles & Jaymes	2.6	oz. bottle	0	1	0
	iced tea, Long Island	Bartles & Jaymes	2.6	oz. bottle	0	1	0
	Mai Tai	Bartles & Jaymes	2.6	oz. bottle	0	1	0
	margarita	Bartles & Jaymes	2.4	oz. bottle	0	1	0
	original	Bartles & Jaymes	3.8	oz. bottle	0	1	0
	peach	Bartles & Jaymes	3.2	oz. bottle	0	1	0
	pina colada	Bartles & Jaymes	2.3	oz. bottle	0	1	0
	strawberry	Bartles & Jaymes	3.3	oz. bottle	0	1	0
	strawberry daiquiri	Bartles & Jaymes	3	oz. bottle	0	1	0
	tropical	Bartles & Jaymes	2.9	oz. bottle	0	1	0
Winged bean	dried, raw		0.2	cup	1	1	2
Wonton wrapper		Frieda's	2	pc.	0	1	0
		Nasoya	2.5	pcs.	0	1	0
Worcestershire sauce	wine and pepper	Lea & Perrins	10	tsp.	0	1	0
		Try Me	10	tsp.	0	1	0
Yam	baked or boiled		0.3	cup	0	1	0
Yard-long bean	dried, raw		0.1	cup	0	1	0
	dried, boiled		0.3	cup	0	1	0
	canned	Allens/Sunshine	1.7	cup	0	1	0
	frozen		0.1	cup	0	1	0
Yuca	fresh, raw, sliced	Goya	5	cup	1	1	0
Zucchini	fresh, boiled, drained, sliced		2.5	cup	1	1	0

fresh, boiled, drained, mashed		1.7	cup	0	1	0
canned, Italian style	Del Monte	0.7	cup	0	1	0
canned, Italian style	Progresso	0.8	cup	0	1	1
canned, Italian style, w/tomato juice		0.6	cup	0	1	0
frozen, sliced	Stilwell	6.7	cup	0	1	0
frozen	Empire	0.5	pc.	0	1	0

Zucchini, breaded

Fat Table

FOOD ITEM	SPECIFICATIONS	BRAND NAME	QUANTITY	SIZE	PROTEIN BLOCKS	CARBOHYDRATE BLOCKS	FAT BLOCKS
Almond, shelled	dried	Planters	0.2	oz.	0	0	1
	slivered	Planters	0.2	oz.	0	0	1
	slivered		0.04	cup	0	0	1
	dry-roasted, salted	Planters	0.2	oz.	0	0	1
	honey roasted		0.2	oz.	0	0	1
	oil roasted, salted		0.2	oz.	0	0	1
	slivered	Paradise, White Swan	0.04	cup	0	0	1
	slivered	Planters Gold Measure	0.2	oz.	0	0	1
	tamari-roasted	Eden	0.3	oz.	0	0	1
	toasted		0.2	oz.	0	0	1
Almond butter	Crunchy or creamy	Roaster Fresh	0.2	oz.	0	0	1
	salted		0.3	Tbsp.	0	0	1
Almond paste			0.4	oz.	0	0	1
		Solo	0.5	Tbsp.	0	1	1
Anchovy paste		Reese	1.3	Tbsp.	0	0	1
Avacado, California	1/2 medium trimmed		0.8	oz.	0	0	1
	pureed		0.6	oz.	0	0	1
Avacado dip			0.1	cup	0	0	1
		Kraft	1.5	Tbsp.	0	0	1
		Nalley	0.5	Tbsp.	0	0	1
Bacon bits	imitation	Hormel/Oscar Mayer	2	Tbsp.	1	0	1
	imitation	Bac*Os	2.9	Tbsp.	0	0	1
		McCormick	3	Tbsp.	1	0	1
Bacon dip	horseradish	Heluva Good	1	Tbsp.	0	0	1
		Kraft	1	Tbsp.	0	0	1
		Kraft Premium	1	Tbsp.	0	0	1
		Breakstone's	1	Tbsp.	0	0	1
	onion	Knudsen Premium	1.5	Tbsp.	0	0	1
		Kraft Premium	2	Tbsp.	0	0	1
		Nalley	0.5	Tbsp.	0	0	1
	cream cheese, all varieties	Tofutti Better Than Cream Cheese	0.3	oz.	0	0	1
Brazil nuts	shelled		0.2	oz.	0	0	1
Butter	regular, unsalted		0.1	oz.	0	0	1

Food	Item	Brand	Amount	Unit			
Butternuts	regular, unsalted		0.3	Tbsp.	0	0	1
	regular, unsalted		0.8	tsp.	0	0	1
	regular, salted		0.1	oz.	0	0	1
	regular, salted		0.3	Tbsp.	0	0	1
	regular, salted		0.8	tsp.	0	0	1
	whipped, unsalted		0.02	cup	0	0	1
	whipped, unsalted		0.4	Tbsp.	0	0	1
	whipped, unsalted		1.1	tsp.	0	0	1
	whipped, salted		0.02	cup	0	0	1
	whipped, salted		0.4	Tbsp.	0	0	1
	whipped, salted		1.1	tsp.	0	0	1
	dried, in shell		0.04	lb.	0	0	1
	dried, shelled		0.2	oz.	0	0	1
Cashew nuts	whole	Frito Lay	0.2	oz.	0	0	1
	dry roasted	Paradise/White Swan	0.2	oz.	0	0	1
	dry roasted, whole or halves		0.05	cup	0	0	1
	oil roasted		0.2	oz.	0	0	1
	oil roasted, whole or halves		0.05	cup	0	0	1
	oil roasted	Master Choice	0.2	oz.	0	0	1
	oil roasted	Planters	0.2	oz.	0	0	1
	oil roasted	Planters	0.2	oz.	0	0	1
	oil roasted	Planters Fancy	0.2	oz.	0	0	1
	oil roasted	Planters Fancy	0.2	oz.	0	0	1
	oil roasted	Planters Halves	0.2	oz.	0	0	1
	oil roasted	Planters Halves Lightly Salted	0.2	oz.	0	0	1
	oil roasted	Planters Munch 'N Go Singles	0.2	oz.	0	0	1
	honey roasted	Planters	0.3	oz.	0	0	1
	honey roasted	Planters/Planters Munch 'N Go	0.3	oz.	0	0	1
	honey roasted, and peanuts	Planters	0.3	oz.	0	0	1
Cashew butter		Roaster Fresh	0.2	oz.	0	0	1
Cheese, cream	cream cheese	Boar's Head	0.3	oz.	0	0	1
	cream cheese	Heluva Good	0.3	oz.	0	0	1

FOOD ITEM	SPECIFICATIONS	BRAND NAME	QUANTITY	SIZE	PROTEIN BLOCKS	CARBOHYDRATE BLOCKS	FAT BLOCKS
	cream cheese	Philadelphia Brand	0.3	oz.	0	0	1
	cream cheese	Weight Watchers Light	2.5	Tbsp.	0	0	1
	cream cheese	Western Creamy	0.9	Tbsp.	0	0	1
	cream cheese	Western Creamy Light	1.3	Tbsp.	0	0	1
	cream cheese, w/chive or pimiento	Philadelphia Brand	0.3	oz.	0	0	1
	cream cheese, soft, plain	Philadelphia Brand	0.6	Tbsp.	0	0	1
	cream cheese, soft, plain, light	Philadelphia Brand	1.2	Tbsp.	0	0	1
	cream cheese, soft, w/chives and onion	Philadelphia Brand	0.6	Tbsp.	0	0	1
	cream cheese, soft, w/herb and garlic	Philadelphia Brand	0.6	Tbsp.	0	0	1
	cream cheese, soft, w/olive and pimiento	Philadelphia Brand	0.7	Tbsp.	0	0	1
	cream cheese, soft, w/pineapple	Philadelphia Brand	0.7	Tbsp.	0	0	1
	cream cheese, soft, w/smoked salmon	Philadelphia Brand	0.7	Tbsp.	0	0	1
	cream cheese, soft, w/strawberries	Philadelphia Brand	0.7	Tbsp.	0	0	1
	cream cheese, whipped, plain	Breakstone's Temp-Tee	0.9	Tbsp.	0	0	1
	cream cheese, whipped, plain	Philadelphia Brand	0.8	Tbsp.	0	0	1
	cream cheese, whipped, w/smoked salmon	Philadelphia Brand	1	Tbsp.	0	0	1
Cheese dip	and bacon	Chi-Chi's Fiesta	2	Tbsp.	0	0	1
	blue	Nalley	0.5	Tbsp.	0	0	1
	cheddar, mild	Kraft Premium	1.5	Tbsp.	0	0	1
	cheddar, mild	Frito-Lay	2	Tbsp.	0	0	1
	cheddar, mild	Old Dutch	2	Tbsp.	0	0	1
	cheddar, and mustard	Heluva Good Pretzel	1	Tbsp.	0	0	1

Category	Descriptor	Brand	Amount	Unit	Protein	Carb	Fat
	chili	Fritos	2	Tbsp.	0	0	1
	hot	Price's Fiesta	0.9	Tbsp.	0	0	1
	nacho	Kraft Premium	1.2	Tbsp.	0	0	1
	nacho	Knudsen Premium	1.5	Tbsp.	0	0	1
	nacho	Nalley	0.5	Tbsp.	0	0	1
	nacho	Old Dutch	1.5	Tbsp.	0	0	1
	Parmesan garlic	Marie's	0.4	Tbsp.	0	0	1
	salsa	Heluva Good Cheese 'N Salsa	1.1	Tbsp.	0	0	1
	salsa	Old El Paso	2	Tbsp.	0	1	1
	salsa	Tostitos Con Queso	2.9	Tbsp.	0	2	1
	salsa	Tostitos Con Queso Low Fat	4	Tbsp.	0	0	1
Cheese sauce	all varieties	Kaukauna Micro Melt	1	Tbsp.	0	0	1
		Cheez Whiz Squeezable	0.7	Tbsp.	0	0	1
		Cheez Whiz Zap-A-Pack	0.7	Tbsp.	0	0	1
		Franco-American	0.4	cup	0	0	1
		Kaukauna	1	Tbsp.	0	0	1
	nacho	Cheez Whiz Zap-A-Pack	0.7	Tbsp.	1	0	1
	salsa	Durkee	0.5	pkg.	0	0	1
		French's	1.3	pkg.	0	0	1
		Knorr	0.3	pkg.	0	0	1
Cheese sauce mix	four	Durkee	0.3	pkg.	0	0	1
	nacho	Cheez Whiz	0.9	Tbsp.	0	0	1
		Squeez-A-Snak	0.7	Tbsp.	1	0	1
		Velveeta	0.5	oz.	1	0	1
		Velveeta Italiana	0.5	oz.	1	0	1
Cheese spread	American	Borden	0.5	oz.	0	0	1
	American	Easy Cheese	0.9	Tbsp.	1	0	1
	American	Harvest Moon	0.5	oz.	0	0	1
	American	Harvest Moon	0.5	oz.	0	0	1
	American	The Big!	0.5	slice	1	0	1
	w/bacon	Kraft	0.7	Tbsp.	0	0	1
	blue cheese	Kraft Roka	0.9	Tbsp.	1	0	1
	cheddar, sharp	Heluva Good	0.9	Tbsp.	0	0	1
	cheddar, w/bacon or horseradish	Heluva Good	0.9	Tbsp.	0	0	1
	cheddar, regular or bacon	Easy Cheese	0.9	Tbsp.	0	0	1

FAT

FOOD ITEM	SPECIFICATIONS	BRAND NAME	QUANTITY	SIZE	PROTEIN BLOCKS	CARBOHYDRATE BLOCKS	FAT BLOCKS
	cheddar, sharp	Easy Cheese	0.9	Tbsp.	0	0	1
	w/jalapenos	Cheez Whiz	0.7	Tbsp.	0	0	1
	w/jalapenos	Kraft	0.5	oz.	1	0	1
	w/jalapenos, hot	Velveeta Mexican	0.5	oz.	1	0	1
	w/jalapenos, mild	Velveeta Mexican	0.5	oz.	1	0	1
	limburger	Mohawk Valley	0.4	oz.	0	0	1
	nacho	Easy Cheese	0.9	Tbsp.	0	0	1
	nacho	The Big!	0.5	slice	1	0	1
	olive and pimiento	Kraft	1	Tbsp.	0	0	1
	Neufchatel, garden vegetable	Kaukauna	0.9	Tbsp.	0	0	1
	Neufchatel, garden cnd herb or ranch	Kaukauna	0.9	Tbsp.	0	0	1
	pimiento	Kraft	1	Tbsp.	0	0	1
	pimiento	Price's	0.9	Tbsp.	0	0	1
	pimiento	Price's Light	1.7	Tbsp.	1	0	1
	pineapple	Kraft	1.2	Tbsp.	0	0	1
	port wine	Heluva Good	0.9	Tbsp.	0	0	1
	salsa, hot	Cheez Whiz	0.9	Tbsp.	0	0	1
	salsa, mild	Cheez Whiz	0.9	Tbsp.	0	0	1
	sharp	Old English	0.7	Tbsp.	1	0	1
	slices	Velveeta	0.5	oz.	1	0	1
	slices	Velveeta	0.5	oz.	0	0	1
	slices	Velveeta	0.5	oz.	0	0	1
Clam dip	chunky, w/crackers	Red Devil Snackers	0.2	pkg.	0	0	1
	chunky, salad	Libby's Spreadables	0.1	cup	0	0	1
		Breakstone's Chesapeake	1.5	Tbsp.	0	0	1
		Heluva Good New England	1.3	Tbsp.	0	0	1
		Kraft	1.5	Tbsp.	0	0	1
		Kraft Premium	1.5	Tbsp.	0	0	1
		Nalley	0.6	Tbsp.	0	0	1
Clam sauce, canned	creamy	Progresso	0.3	cup	1	1	1
	red	Progresso	0.5	cup	1	1	1

Food	Description	Brand	Amount	Unit
Cream	white	Bookbinder's	0.1	cup
	white	Progresso	0.2	cup
	white	Progresso Authentic	0.2	cup
	half and half		0.1	cup
	half and half		1.7	Tbsp.
	light, coffee or table		0.1	cup
	light, coffee or table		1	Tbsp.
	medium (25% fat)		0.1	cup
	medium (25% fat)		0.8	Tbsp.
	whipping, light		0.04	cup
	whipping, light		0.7	Tbsp.
	whipping, heavy		0.03	cup
	whipping, heavy		0.5	Tbsp.
Cream, canned	light	Nestle Crema	1	Tbsp.
Cream, sour	half and half	Breakstone's	0.1	cup
		Heluva Good	1.2	Tbsp.
		Knudsen Hampshire	1.2	Tbsp.
		Sealtest	1	Tbsp.
	light	Breakstone's	1.2	Tbsp.
	light	Heluva Good	1.7	Tbsp.
	light	Knudsen Light	2.5	Tbsp.
		Sealtest Light	2.5	Tbsp.
		Sour Supreme	2.5	Tbsp.
Cream, whipped	nondairy, plain or flavored	Cool Whip Extra Creamy	1.2	Tbsp.
		Cool Whip Light	2.9	Tbsp.
		Cool Whip Nondairy	6.7	Tbsp.
		Kraft Real	4	Tbsp.
		Kraft Whipped Topping	4	Tbsp.
		La Crema Lite	4	Tbsp.
		Pet Whip	6.7	Tbsp.
		Rich's	2.9	Tbsp.
		Rich's	4	Tbsp.
	pressurized can		2.9	Tbsp.
	mix, prepared	D-Zerta	0.3	cup
	mix, prepared	Dream Whip	6.7	Tbsp.
	mix, prepared	Dream Whip	6.7	Tbsp.

FAT

FOOD ITEM	SPECIFICATIONS	BRAND NAME	QUANTITY	SIZE	PROTEIN BLOCKS	CARBOHYDRATE BLOCKS	FAT BLOCKS
Creamer, nondairy		Coffee-mate	3.3	Tbsp.	0	0	1
		Coffee-mate Lite	5	Tbsp.	0	0	1
		Rich's Coffee Rich	2	Tbsp.	0	0	1
		Rich's Coffee Rich Light	3.3	Tbsp.	0	0	1
		Rich's Farm Rich	2	Tbsp.	0	0	1
		Rich's Farm Rich Light	3.3	Tbsp.	0	0	1
	powder	Coffee-mate	5	tsp.	0	0	1
	powder	Cremora	3.3	tsp.	0	0	1
Creamer, nondairy, flavored	liquid	Coffee-mate all flavors	1.4	Tbsp.	0	1	1
	powdered	Coffee-mate all flavors	1	Tbsp.	0	1	1
Chicken fat	rendered	Empire Kosher	0.2	oz.	0	0	1
Coconut cream, canned			0.2	Tbsp.	0	0	1
			0.9	Tbsp.	0	0	1
Coconut milk		Goya	0.8	Tbsp.	0	0	1
Coconut milk, canned		Taste of Thai	0.6	Tbsp.	0	0	1
	light	Taste of Thai	0.1	cup	0	0	1
Coquito nuts	shelled	Frieda's	0.3	cup	0	0	1
			0.2	oz.	0	0	1
Dill dip		Bernstein's Zesty	0.5	Tbsp.	0	0	1
Filberts	dried		0.2	oz.	0	0	1
	dried, chopped		0	cup	0	0	1
	dried, blanched		0.2	oz.	0	0	1
	dry-roasted		0.2	oz.	0	0	1
	dry-roasted, salted		0.2	oz.	0	0	1
	oil-roasted		0.2	oz.	0	0	1
	oil-roasted, salted		0.2	oz.	0	0	1
	Italian, creamy	Marie's	0.3	Tbsp.	0	0	1
Flax seeds		Arrowhead Mills	0.9	Tbsp.	0	0	1
Garlic dip		Nalley	0.5	Tbsp.	0	0	1
Garlic spread		Lawry's Concentrate	1	tsp.	0	0	1
		Lawry's Ready-to-Spread	0.3	Tbsp.	0	0	1

Food	Brand	Description	Amount	Unit	P	C	F
Goose fat			0.1	oz.	0	0	1
Gorgonzola sauce	Monterey Pasta Company	refrigerated	0.3	oz.	0	0	1
Guacamole dip	Nalley		0.5	Tbsp.	0	0	1
Halvah	Joyva	chocolate	0.2	oz.	0	1	1
Ham salad spread	Libby's spreadable		0.2	cup	0	0	1
Ham spread	Cure 81		0.5	oz.	0	0	1
	Underwood	deviled	0.1	cup	0	0	1
	Red Devil Snackers	deviled w/crackers	0.1	pkg.	0	0	1
	Underwood	honey	0.05	cup	0	0	1
	Red Devil Snackers	honey w/crackers	0.1	pkg.	0	0	1
Hazelnut butter	Roaster Fresh		0.2	oz.	0	0	1
Hickory nut		dried, shelled	0.2	oz.	0	0	1
Hollandaise grilling sauce	Knorr Microwave		1.3	Tbsp.	0	0	1
Horseradish sauce	Heinz		1.3	tsp.	0	0	1
Hummus mix	Casbah		0.2	oz.	0	0	1
	Fantastic Foods	dip	2.9	Tbsp.	1	0	1
Jalapeno dip	Kraft	and cheddar	1.5	Tbsp.	0	0	1
	Old El Paso	and cheddar	6.7	Tbsp.	0	0	1
	Breakstone's	cheese	1.5	Tbsp.	0	0	1
	Frito-Lay		2	Tbsp.	0	0	1
	Kraft Premium		1.2	Tbsp.	0	0	1
Lard	Goya	pork	0.2	Tbsp.	0	0	1
	Progresso	pork	0.2	cup	0	0	1
Lobster sauce	Frieda's	rock	0.2	oz.	0	0	1
Macadamia nuts		raw	0.1	oz.	0	0	1
		dried, shelled	0.1	cup	0	0	1
		dried, shelled	0.03	oz.	0	0	1
		oil roasted	0.1	oz.	0	0	1
Margarine	Mazola		0.3	Tbsp.	0	0	1
	Mazola Light		0.5	Tbsp.	0	0	1
	Mazola Unsalted		0.3	Tbsp.	0	0	1
	Nucoa		0.3	Tbsp.	0	0	1
	Smart Beat Super Light/Trans Fat Free		1.4	Tbsp.	0	0	1
	Smart Beat Unsalted		1.3	Tbsp.	0	0	1

FAT

FOOD ITEM	SPECIFICATIONS	BRAND NAME	QUANTITY	SIZE	PROTEIN BLOCKS	CARBOHYDRATE BLOCKS	FAT BLOCKS
	soft	Chiffon Tub	0.3	Tbsp.	0	0	1
	soft	Parkay Tub	0.3	Tbsp.	0	0	1
	soft	Parkay Diet Tub	0.5	Tbsp.	0	0	1
	spread	Kraft Touch of Butter Stick	0.3	Tbsp.	0	0	1
	spread	Kraft Touch of Butter Tub	0.4	Tbsp.	0	0	1
	spread	Mazola Light	0.5	Tbsp.	0	0	1
	spread	Parkay Stick 53%	0.4	Tbsp.	0	0	1
	spread	Parkay Stick 70%	0.3	Tbsp.	0	0	1
	spread	Parkay Tub 50%	0.4	Tbsp.	0	0	1
	spread	Parkay Light Tub 40%	0.5	Tbsp.	0	0	1
	spread	Kraft Touch O Butter	0.3	Tbsp.	0	0	1
	squeeze	Parkay	0.3	Tbsp.	0	0	1
	squeeze	Chiffon Tub	0.4	Tbsp.	0	0	1
	whipped	Parkay Tub	0.4	Tbsp.	0	0	1
	whipped	Best Foods Real	0.3	Tbsp.	0	0	1
Mayonnaise		Blue Plate	0.3	Tbsp.	0	0	1
		Hellmann's Real	0.3	Tbsp.	0	0	1
		Hellmann's/Best Foods Light	0.6	Tbsp.	0	0	1
		Hellmann's/Best Foods Low Fat	3.3	Tbsp.	0	0	1
		Kraft Real	0.3	Tbsp.	0	0	1
		Master Choice	1.4	Tbsp.	0	0	1
		Nalley Real	0.3	Tbsp.	0	0	1
		Nalley Light	0.3	Tbsp.	0	0	1
		Smart Beat Super Light Reduced Fat	1	Tbsp.	0	0	1
		Weight Watchers Light	1.4	Tbsp.	0	0	1
		Weight Watchers Light Low Sodium	1.4	Tbsp.	0	0	1
	canola	Smart Beat Reduced Fat	1	Tbsp.	0	0	1
	dressing	Kraft Light	0.6	Tbsp.	0	0	1
	dressing	Miracle Whip Salad	0.4	Tbsp.	0	0	1
	dressing	Miracle Whip Light	1	Tbsp.	0	0	1
	dressing	Spin Blend	0.6	Tbsp.	0	0	1
	tofu	Nayonaise	1	Tbsp.	0	0	1
Nut topping		Planters	0.7	Tbsp.	0	0	1

Food	Brand			Amount	Unit
Nuts, mixed					
dry-roasted, w/peanuts		0	0	0.2	oz.
dry-roasted, w/peanuts, salted		0	0	0.2	oz.
dry-roasted	Planters	0	0	0.2	oz.
honey-roasted	Planters	0	0	0.2	oz.
oil-roasted, w/peanuts		0	0	0.2	oz.
oil-roasted, w/peanuts, salted		0	0	0.2	oz.
oil-roasted	Paradise/White Swan	0	0	0.2	oz.
oil-roasted	Planters	0	0	0.2	oz.
oil-roasted	Planters Deluxe	0	0	0.2	oz.
oil-roasted	Planters Lightly Salted	0	0	0.2	oz.
oil-roasted	Planters Unsalted	0	0	0.2	oz.
oil-roasted	Planters 3 1/2 oz.	0	0	0.2	oz.
oil-roasted, no Brazils	Planters Lightly Salted	0	0	0.2	oz.
oil-roasted, no Brazils	Paradise/White Swan Deluxe	0	0	0.2	oz.
oil-roasted, no Peanuts	Planters Select	0	0	0.2	oz.
cashews, w/almonds, macadamias		0	0	0.2	oz.
cashews, w/almonds, pecans	Planters Select	0	0	0.2	oz.
sesame, oil-roasted	Planters	0	0	0.3	oz.
tamari-roasted	Eden	0	0	0.3	oz.
all varieties and blends	Wesson	0		0.2	Tbsp.
almond, canola, cocoa butter, corn, cottonseed, hazelnut, nutmeg butter, oat, palm or poppyseed		0		0.2	Tbsp.
Oils					
avacado or mustard		0	0	0.2	Tbsp.
butter oil		0	0	0.2	Tbsp.
coconut		0	0	0.2	Tbsp.
cod liver		0	0	0.2	Tbsp.
corn, all varieties	Goya	0	0	0.2	Tbsp.
corn or canola/corn	Mazola	0	0	0.2	Tbsp.
herring		0	0	0.2	Tbsp.
olive, peanut, safflower, sesame, soybean, sun-		0	0	0.2	Tbsp.

FAT

FOOD ITEM	SPECIFICATIONS	BRAND NAME	QUANTITY	SIZE	PROTEIN BLOCKS	CARBOHYDRATE BLOCKS	FAT BLOCKS
	flower, vegetable or walnut Oriental cooking	House of Tsang Mongolian Fire/Saigon Sizzle	0.6	tsp.	0	0	1
	peanut or popcorn	Planters	0.2	Tbsp.	0	0	1
	popcorn, popping and topping	Orville Redenbacher	0.2	Tbsp.	0	0	1
	salmon		0.2	Tbsp.	0	0	1
	sardine		0.2	Tbsp.	0	0	1
	sesame, regular or hot pepper	Eden	0.2	Tbsp.	0	0	1
	sesame, regular or hot chili	House of Tsang	0.6	tsp.	0	0	1
	wok	House of Tsang	0.2	Tbsp.	0	0	1
Olives	Calamata	Krinos	2.3	pcs.	0	0	1
	Calamata	Zorba	1.7	pcs.	0	0	1
	green, w/pits		8.3	small	0	0	1
	green, w/pits		6.3	large	0	0	1
	green, w/pits		3.6	giant	0	0	1
	green, pitted		0.8	oz.	0	0	1
	green, cracked	Krinos	1.7	oz.	0	0	1
	green, queen/Spanish	S&W	2.9	pcs.	0	0	1
	green, queen/Spanish	Zorba	2.9	pcs.	0	0	1
	ripe, pitted, California	Vlasic	1.3	tsp. chopped, or 4-6 pcs.	0	0	1
	ripe, pitted	Lindsay	7.5	6 small, 5 medium, 4 large, or 1 1/3 tsp. chopped	0	0	1
	ripe, pitted	S&W	3.8	extra large	0	0	1
	ripe, pitted	S&W	4.3	jumbo	0	0	1
	ripe, pitted	Vlasic	5	large	0	0	1
	ripe, pitted	Vlasic	7.5	small	0	0	1

Description	Brand	Amount	Unit			
ripe, pitted, Spanish	Vlasic	11.4	small	0	0	—
ripe, w/pits	Lindsay	6.3	medium or 4 large	0	0	—
ripe, w/pits	S&W	2	super colossal	0	0	—
ripe, oil-cured	Krinos	0.3	oz.	0	0	—
ripe, oil-cured	Progresso	3	pcs.	0	0	—
ripe, Greek		4.3	medium	0	0	—
ripe, Greek		3.1	extra large	0	0	—
ripe, Greek, pitted		0.3	oz.	0	0	—
ripe, Greek	Krinos	0.5	oz.	0	0	—
ripe, Greek	Krinos Alfonso	0.5	oz.	0	0	—
ripe, Greek	Krinos Nafplion	1.7	oz.	0	0	—
ripe, Greek	Zorba	1.3	oz.	0	0	—
ripe, Greek	Krinos	0.6	oz.	0	0	—
royal		0.3	cup	0	1	—
salad	Goya	5.7	pcs.	0	0	—
stuffed, Manzanilla	Goya	6.3	pcs.	0	0	—
stuffed, Manzanilla	Lindsay	4.3	pcs.	0	0	—
stuffed, Manzanilla	S&W	4	pcs.	0	0	—
stuffed, queen	Goya	4	pcs.	0	0	—
stuffed, queen	Lindsay	4	pcs.	0	0	—
stuffed, queen	S&W, 4 3/4 oz.	4	pcs.	0	0	—
stuffed, queen	S&W, 7 oz.	3.3	pc.	0	0	—
stuffed, queen, stuffed w/tuna	S&W, 10 oz.	5	pcs.	0	0	—
Olive salad, drained						
Onion dip creamy	Progresso	2.5	Tbsp.	0	0	—
French	Kraft Premium	1.5	Tbsp.	0	0	—
French	Breakstone's	1.5	Tbsp.	0	0	—
French	Frito-Lay	1.2	Tbsp.	0	0	—
French	Heluva Good	1.2	Tbsp.	0	0	—
French	Heluva Good Light	2.9	Tbsp.	0	0	—
French	Knudsen Premium	1.5	Tbsp.	0	0	—
French	Kraft Premium	1.5	Tbsp.	0	0	—
French	Nalley	0.6	Tbsp.	0	0	—
French	Old Dutch	1.5	Tbsp.	0	0	—
French	Ruffles	1.2	Tbsp.	0	0	—
French	Ruffles Low Fat	6.7	Tbsp.	0	0	3

FAT

FOOD ITEM	SPECIFICATIONS	BRAND NAME	QUANTITY	SIZE	PROTEIN BLOCKS	CARBOHYDRATE BLOCKS	FAT BLOCKS
	French	Sealtest	1.5	Tbsp.	0	0	1
	green	Kraft	1.5	Tbsp.	0	0	1
	sour cream and	Lay's	6.7	Tbsp.	0	3	1
	toasted	Breakstone's	1.5	Tbsp.	0	0	1
Pate, canned							
	chicken liver		0.4	oz.	0	0	1
	chicken liver		0.8	Tbsp.	0	0	1
	goose liver, smoked		0.8	oz.	1	0	1
	goose liver, smoked		1.7	Tbsp.	0	0	1
	goose liver, smoked		0.2	oz.	0	0	1
	liver	Sells	0.5	Tbsp.	0	0	1
Pate, vegetarian		Bonavita Swiss	0.1	cup	0	0	1
Peanuts, shelled	unroasted		0.8	oz.	0	0	1
	boiled, salted		0.2	oz.	0	0	1
	dry-roasted		0.5	oz.	0	0	1
	dry-roasted	Little Debbie	0.04	cup	0	0	1
	dry-roasted	Planters	0.2	oz.	0	0	1
	dry-roasted	Planters Lightly Salted	0.2	oz.	0	0	1
	dry-roasted	Planters Unsalted	0.2	oz.	0	0	1
	honey-roasted	Frito Lay	0.04	cup	0	0	1
	honey-roasted	Planters	0.2	oz.	0	0	1
	honey-roasted, dry-roasted	Planters	0.3	oz.	0	0	1
	honey-roasted, oil-roasted	Planters Reduced Fat	0.4	oz.	0	0	1
	hot	Frito-Lay	0.04	cup	0	0	1
	hot and spicy	Planter's Heat	0.2	oz.	0	0	1
	oil-roasted		0.04	cup	0	0	1
	oil-roasted	Pennant	0.2	oz.	0	0	1
	oil-roasted	Planters	0.2	oz.	0	0	1
	oil-roasted	Planters Lightly Salted	0.2	oz.	0	0	1
	oil-roasted	Planters Munch 'N Go	0.2	oz.	0	0	1
	oil-roasted, cocktail	Planters	0.2	oz.	0	0	1
	oil-roasted, cocktail	Planters Lightly Salted	0.2	oz.	0	0	1

Peanut butter

Type	Brand	Amount	Unit			
oil-roasted, cocktail	Planters Unsalted	0.2	oz.	0	0	1
oil-roasted, fancy	Paradise/White Swan	0.2	oz.	0	0	1
oil-roasted, salted	Planters	0.2	oz.	0	0	1
Spanish	Planters	0.2	oz.	0	0	1
Spanish, raw	Planters	0.2	oz.	0	0	1
sweet	Planters Sweet N Crunchy	0.4	oz.	0	1	1
chunky or crunchy	Adams Natural	0.4	Tbsp.	0	0	1
chunky or crunchy	Adams Unsalted	0.4	Tbsp.	0	0	1
chunky or crunchy	Adams No-Stir	0.4	Tbsp.	0	0	1
chunky or crunchy	Peter Pan	0.4	Tbsp.	0	0	1
chunky or crunchy	Peter Pan Real	0.4	Tbsp.	0	0	1
chunky or crunchy	Peter Pan Whipped	0.5	Tbsp.	0	0	1
chunky or crunchy	Roasted Honey Nut Skippy Super Chunk	0.4	Tbsp.	0	0	1
chunky or crunchy	Skippy Super Chunk	0.4	Tbsp.	0	0	1
chunky or crunchy	Skippy Super Chunk Reduced Fat	0.5	Tbsp.	0	0	1
chunky or crunchy	Teddie Super	0.4	Tbsp.	0	0	1
chunky or crunchy, spread	Peter Pan Smart Choice	0.5	Tbsp.	0	0	1
chunky or creamy	Arrowhead Mills	0.4	Tbsp.	0	0	1
chunky or creamy	Peter Pan Very Low Sodium	0.3	Tbsp.	0	0	1
chunky or creamy	Roaster Fresh	0.4	Tbsp.	0	0	1
chunky or creamy	Roaster Fresh Unsalted	0.4	Tbsp.	0	0	1
chunky or creamy	Smucker's	0.4	Tbsp.	0	0	1
chunky or creamy	Smucker's Natural	0.4	Tbsp.	0	0	1
chunky or creamy	Smucker's Natural No Salt	0.4	Tbsp.	0	0	1
creamy or smooth	Adams Natural	0.4	Tbsp.	0	0	1
creamy or smooth	Adams Unsalted	0.4	Tbsp.	0	0	1
creamy or smooth	Adams No-Stir	0.4	Tbsp.	0	0	1
creamy or smooth	Peter Pan	0.4	Tbsp.	0	0	1
creamy or smooth	Peter Pan Real	0.4	Tbsp.	0	0	1
creamy or smooth	Peter Pan Whipped	0.5	Tbsp.	0	0	1
creamy or smooth	Roasted Honey Nut Skippy	0.4	Tbsp.	0	0	1
creamy or smooth	Skippy	0.4	Tbsp.	0	0	1
creamy or smooth	Skippy Reduced Fat	0.5	Tbsp.	0	1	1
creamy or smooth	Teddie	0.4	Tbsp.	0	0	1
creamy or smooth, spread	Peter Pan Smart Choice	0.5	Tbsp.	0	0	1

FAT

FOOD ITEM	SPECIFICATIONS	BRAND NAME	QUANTITY	SIZE	PROTEIN BLOCKS	CARBOHYDRATE BLOCKS	FAT BLOCKS
Peanut sauce	unsalted	Teddie	0.4	Tbsp.	0	0	1
	Oriental	House of Tsang Bangkok Padang	1.3	Tbsp.	0	0	1
	Oriental, cooking	Kylin Singapore Satay	0.3	cup	0	1	1
Pecans, shelled	chips	Planters	0.2	oz.	0	0	1
	halves	Planters Gold Measure	0.2	oz.	0	0	1
	halves	Planters	0.1	oz.	0	0	1
	halves	Paradise/White Swan	0.2	oz.	0	0	1
	pcs.	Planters	0.2	oz.	0	0	1
	dried		0.2	oz.	0	0	1
	dried, halves		0.04	cup	0	0	1
	dried, chopped		0.04	cup	0	0	1
	dry-roasted, salted		0.2	oz.	0	0	1
	honey-roasted		0.2	oz.	0	0	1
	oil-roasted, salted		0.1	oz.	0	0	1
Pesto sauce	in jars	Sonoma	0.1	cup	0	0	1
	refrigerated, basil	Contadina	0.03	cup	0	0	1
	refrigerated, sun-dried tomato	Contadina	0.03	cup	0	0	1
Pili nuts, dried	shelled		0.1	oz.	0	0	1
	shelled		0.03	cup	0	0	1
Pine nuts, dried	pignolia		0.2	oz.	0	0	1
	pignolia	Krinos	0.6	Tbsp.	0	0	1
	pignolia	Progresso	0.2	oz.	0	0	1
	pignolia		0.2	oz.	0	0	1
	pinyon		0.2	oz.	0	0	1
	pinyon		50	kernels	0	0	1
Pistachio nuts, shelled	dried, in shell	Dole	0.4	oz.	0	0	1
	dried		0.2	oz.	0	0	1
	dried	Dole	0.2	oz.	0	0	1
	dried	Sonoma	0.1	oz.	0	0	1
	dry-roasted, in shell, edible nuts	Planters	0.2	oz.	0	0	1
	dry-roasted		0.2	oz.	0	0	1

Food	Description	Brand	Amount	Unit			
Poppy seeds	dry-roasted		0.04	cup	0	0	—
	dry-roasted	Planters	0.2	oz.	0	0	—
	dry-roasted	Planters Munch 'N Go Singles	0.2	oz.	0	0	—
Pork fat	roasted		2.5	tsp.	0	0	—
Potato seasoning	cheddar, savory	Lipton Recipe Secrets	0.2	oz.	0	0	—
	garlic herb	Lipton Recipe Secrets	0.6	Tbsp.	0	0	—
	onion, California	Lipton Recipe Secrets	0.6	Tbsp.	0	0	—
Pumpkin seeds	roasted, shelled		0.6	Tbsp.	0	0	—
	roasted, shelled, salted		0.3	oz.	0	0	—
	tamari-roasted, spicy		0.3	oz.	0	0	—
Ranch dip		Eden	0.3	oz.	0	0	—
		Heluva Good Classic	1.2	Tbsp.	0	0	—
		Kraft	1.5	Tbsp.	0	0	—
		Marie's Creamy	0.3	Tbsp.	0	0	—
		Marie's Homestyle	0.4	Tbsp.	0	0	—
		Nalley	0.5	Tbsp.	0	0	—
		Old Dutch	4	Tbsp.	0	0	—
		Ruffles	1	Tbsp.	0	0	—
		Ruffles Low Fat	6.7	Tbsp.	3	0	—
		Marie's	0.4	Tbsp.	0	0	—
Salad dressing	bacon	Bernstein's	0.5	Tbsp.	0	0	—
	vegetable	Kraft	0.4	Tbsp.	0	0	—
	bacon and tomato	Kraft Deliciously Right	1.2	Tbsp.	0	0	—
	bacon and tomato	Knott's Berry Farm	4	Tbsp.	2	0	—
	berry vinaigrette	Bernstein's Dressing/Dip	0.3	Tbsp.	0	0	—
	blue cheese	Bernstein's Dressing/Dip Lite	0.7	Tbsp.	0	0	—
	blue cheese	Kraft Roka	0.9	Tbsp.	0	0	—
	blue cheese	Marie's Salad Bar Reduced Calorie	0.9	Tbsp.	0	0	—
	blue cheese	Bernstein's	0.5	Tbsp.	0	0	—
	blue cheese, creamy	Herb Magic	1.2	Tbsp.	1	0	—
	blue cheese, vinaigrette	Marie's	0.3	Tbsp.	0	0	—
	blue cheese, chunky	Marie's Reduced Calorie	0.9	Tbsp.	0	0	—
	blue cheese, chunky	Seven Seas	0.9	Tbsp.	0	0	—
	blue cheese, chunky	Wish-Bone	0.4	Tbsp.	0	0	—
	blue cheese, chunky	Wish-Bone Lite	0.9	Tbsp.	0	0	—
	Caesar	Bernstein's Dressing/Dip	0.6	Tbsp.	0	0	—

FAT

FOOD ITEM	SPECIFICATIONS	BRAND NAME	QUANTITY	SIZE	PROTEIN BLOCKS	CARBOHYDRATE BLOCKS	FAT BLOCKS
	Caesar	Bernstein's Extra Rich	0.5	Tbsp.	0	0	1
	Caesar	Kraft	0.5	Tbsp.	0	0	1
	Caesar	Kraft Deliciously Right	1.2	Tbsp.	0	0	1
	Caesar, cheese, 3	Salad Celebrations	2.9	Tbsp.	0	1	1
	Caesar, creamy	Seven Seas	0.4	Tbsp.	0	0	1
	Caesar, creamy	Seven Seas Viva	0.5	Tbsp.	0	0	1
	Caesar, creamy, w/cracked pepper	Lawry's	0.4	Tbsp.	0	0	1
	Caesar, garlic, roasted	Knott's Berry Farm	0.4	Tbsp.	0	0	1
	Caesar, olive oil	Wish-Bone	0.6	Tbsp.	0	0	1
	Caesar, olive oil	Wish-Bone Lite	1.2	Tbsp.	0	0	1
	Caesar, ranch	Kraft	0.4	Tbsp.	0	0	1
	cheese	Bernstein's Fantastico!	0.5	Tbsp.	0	0	1
	chicken salad, Oriental	Knott's Berry Farm	0.5	Tbsp.	0	0	1
	citrus vinaigrette	Knott's Berry Farm	6.7	Tbsp.	0	3	1
	coleslaw	Kraft	0.5	Tbsp.	0	0	1
	coleslaw	Marie's	0.5	Tbsp.	0	0	1
	Dijon vinaigrette	Wish-Bone Lite	1.2	Tbsp.	0	0	1
	dill, creamy	Nasoya Vegi-Dressing	1.2	Tbsp.	0	0	1
	French	Kraft	0.5	Tbsp.	0	0	1
	French	Kraft Deliciously Right	2	Tbsp.	0	1	1
	French	Kraft Deliciously Right Catalina	1.5	Tbsp.	0	1	1
	French	Nally	0.7	Tbsp.	0	0	1
	French	Wish-Bone	0.5	Tbsp.	0	0	1
	French, herbal, creamy	Bernstein's	0.5	Tbsp.	0	0	1
	French, w/honey	Kraft Catalina	0.5	Tbsp.	0	0	1
	French, style	Wish-Bone Lite	0.7	Tbsp.	0	0	1
	French, sweet 'n spicy	Wish-Bone	0.5	Tbsp.	0	0	1
	French, tangy	Marie's	0.5	Tbsp.	0	0	1
	French, vinaigrette, true	Herb Magic	0.3	Tbsp.	0	0	1
	fruit salad	Knott's Berry Farm	1.5	Tbsp.	0	1	1
	fruit vinaigrette	Knott's Berry Farm	6.7	Tbsp.	0	3	1
	garden, zesty	Kraft Salsa	1	Tbsp.	0	0	1

			Description	Brand	Amount	Unit
—	0	○	garlic, creamy	Kraft	0.5	Tbsp.
—	0	○	garlic, roasted, creamy	Wish-Bone	0.5	Tbsp.
—	0	○	green goddess	Seven Seas	0.5	Tbsp.
—	0	○	herb, garden	Nasoya Vegi-Dressing	1.2	Tbsp.
—	0	○	herbs and spices	Seven Seas	0.5	Tbsp.
—	0	○	honey Dijon	Kraft	0.4	Tbsp.
—	0	○	honey Dijon	Wish-Bone	0.6	Tbsp.
—	0	○	honey mustard	Bernstein's Dressing/Dip	0.5	Tbsp.
—	0	○	honey mustard	Knott's Berry Farm	0.5	Tbsp.
—	0	○	honey mustard	Marie's	0.4	Tbsp.
—	1	○	honey mustard	Nalley	0.5	Tbsp.
—	0	○	Italian	Bernstein's	0.4	Tbsp.
—	0	○	Italian	Bernstein's Reduced Calorie	4	Tbsp.
—	0	○	Italian	Bernstein's Restaurant	1.5	Tbsp.
—	0	○	Italian	Bernstein's Wine Country	0.5	Tbsp.
—	0	○	Italian	Kraft Deliciously Right	0.9	Tbsp.
—	0	○	Italian	Kraft House	0.5	Tbsp.
—	0	○	Italian	Kraft Presto	0.4	Tbsp.
—	0	○	Italian	Ott's Zesty	0.6	Tbsp.
—	0	○	Italian	Seven Seas Viva	0.5	Tbsp.
—	0	○	Italian	Seven Seas Viva Reduced Calorie	1.5	Tbsp.
—	0	○	Italian	Wish-Bone	0.7	Tbsp.
—	0	○	Italian	Wish-Bone Classic House	0.4	Tbsp.
—	0	○	Italian	Wish-Bone Lite	10	Tbsp.
—	0	○	Italian	Wish-Bone Robusto	0.6	Tbsp.
—	0	○	Italian, cheese, 2	Seven Seas	0.9	Tbsp.
—	0	○	Italian, cheese and garlic	Bernstein's	0.5	Tbsp.
—	0	○	Italian, creamy	Kraft	0.5	Tbsp.
—	0	○	Italian, creamy	Kraft Deliciously Right	1.2	Tbsp.
—	0	○	Italian, creamy	Nasoya Vegi-Dressing	1.2	Tbsp.
—	0	○	Italian, creamy	Seven Seas	0.5	Tbsp.
—	1	○	Italian, creamy	Seven Seas Reduced Calorie	1.2	Tbsp.
—	0	○	Italian, creamy	Wish-Bone	0.6	Tbsp.
—	0	○	Italian, creamy	Wish-Bone Lite	1.7	Tbsp.
—	0	○	Italian, garlic, creamy	Marie's	0.3	Tbsp.
—	0	○	Italian, garlic, creamy	Marie's Reduced Calorie	0.9	Tbsp.

FAT

FOOD ITEM	SPECIFICATIONS	BRAND NAME	QUANTITY	SIZE	PROTEIN BLOCKS	CARBOHYDRATE BLOCKS	FAT BLOCKS
	Italian, herb, and garlic, creamy	Bernstein's	0.5	Tbsp.	0	0	1
	Italian, olive oil	Seven Seas Reduced Calorie	1.2	Tbsp.	0	0	1
	Italian, olive oil	Wish-Bone	1	Tbsp.	0	0	1
	Italian, zesty	Kraft	0.5	Tbsp.	0	0	1
	olive oil vinaigrette	Wish-Bone	1.2	Tbsp.	0	0	1
		Ott's Famous Original	1	Tbsp.	0	1	1
		Ott's Famous Reduced Calorie	2	Tbsp.	0	1	1
	Peppercorn, ground	Knott's Berry Farm	0.4	Tbsp.	0	0	1
	poppyseed	Herb Magic	0.4	Tbsp.	0	0	1
	poppyseed	Knott's Berry Farm	0.7	Tbsp.	0	0	1
	poppyseed	Marie's	0.5	Tbsp.	0	0	1
	poppyseed	Ott's Reduced Calorie	0.9	Tbsp.	0	0	1
	potato salad	Best Foods/Hellmann's One Step	0.4	Tbsp.	0	0	1
	potato salad	Best Foods/Hellmann's One Step 1/3 Less Fat	0.5	Tbsp.	0	0	1
	ranch	Bernstein's Dressing/Dip	0.5	Tbsp.	0	0	1
	ranch	Bernstein's Dressing/Dip Lite	1	Tbsp.	0	0	1
	ranch	Kraft	0.3	Tbsp.	0	0	1
	ranch	Kraft Deliciously Right	0.5	Tbsp.	0	0	1
	ranch	Kraft Salsa	0.5	Tbsp.	0	0	1
	ranch	Marie's Salad Bar Reduced Calorie	0.9	Tbsp.	0	0	1
	ranch	Nalley	0.7	Tbsp.	0	0	1
	ranch	Ott's Buttermilk	0.4	Tbsp.	0	0	1
	ranch	Seven Seas	0.4	Tbsp.	0	0	1
	ranch	Seven Seas Reduced Calorie	0.7	Tbsp.	0	0	1
	ranch	Wish-Bone	0.4	Tbsp.	0	0	1
	ranch	Wish-Bone Lite	0.7	Tbsp.	0	0	1
	ranch, buttermilk	Kraft	0.4	Tbsp.	0	0	1
	ranch, buttermilk	Marie's	0.3	Tbsp.	0	0	1
	ranch, creamy	Marie's Reduced Calorie	0.7	Tbsp.	0	0	1
	ranch, cucumber	Kraft	0.4	Tbsp.	0	0	1
	ranch, cucumber	Kraft Deliciously Right	1.2	Tbsp.	0	0	1

Food	Brand	Amount	Unit			
ranch, Parmesan	Marie's	0.4	Tbsp.	0	0	1
ranch, Parmesan garlic	Bernstein's	0.5	Tbsp.	0	0	1
ranch, peppercorn	Kraft	0.3	Tbsp.	0	0	1
ranch, sour cream and onion	Kraft	0.3	Tbsp.	0	0	1
raspberry vinaigrette	Knott's Berry Farm	2.9	Tbsp.	0	1	1
red wine vinegar, and oil	Seven Seas	0.5	Tbsp.	0	0	1
red wine vinegar, and oil	Seven Seas Reduced Calorie	1.2	Tbsp.	0	0	1
Roquefort	Bernstein's Dressing/Dip	0.4	Tbsp.	0	0	1
Russian	Kraft	0.6	Tbsp.	0	0	1
Russian	Salad Celebrations	4	Tbsp.	0	2	1
Russian	Seven Seas Viva	0.4	Tbsp.	0	0	1
Russian	Wish-Bone	1	Tbsp.	0	1	1
salsa and sour cream	Bernstein's Dressing/Dip	0.7	Tbsp.	0	0	1
Santa Fe	Wish-Bone	0.4	Tbsp.	0	0	1
sesame garlic	Nasoya Vegi-Dressing	1.2	Tbsp.	0	0	1
Sierra	Wish-Bone	0.4	Tbsp.	0	0	1
sour cream and dill	Marie's	0.3	Tbsp.	0	0	1
Thousand Island	Bernstein's Dressing/Dip	0.5	Tbsp.	0	0	1
Thousand Island	Kraft	0.6	Tbsp.	0	1	1
Thousand Island	Kraft Deliciously Right	1.5	Tbsp.	0	0	1
Thousand Island	Marie's	0.3	Tbsp.	0	0	1
Thousand Island	Marie's Salad Bar	0.4	Tbsp.	0	0	1
Thousand Island	Nalley	0.5	Tbsp.	0	0	1
Thousand Island	Nasoya Vegi-Dressing	1.5	Tbsp.	0	1	1
Thousand Island	Salad Celebrations	4	Tbsp.	0	2	1
Thousand Island	Wish-Bone	0.5	Tbsp.	0	0	1
Thousand Island Lite	Wish-Bone	1.2	Tbsp.	0	1	1
Thousand Island, w/bacon	Kraft	0.5	Tbsp.	0	0	1
tomato, sun-dried, vinaigrette	Knott's Berry Farm	0.7	Tbsp.	0	0	1
tuna salad	Best Foods/Hellmann's One Step	0.4	Tbsp.	0	0	1
buttermilk, farm	Good Seasons	0.5	Tbsp.	0	0	1
Caesar, gourmet	Good Seasons	0.4	Tbsp.	0	0	1
cheese garlic	Good Seasons	0.4	Tbsp.	0	0	1
garlic and herbs	Good Seasons	0.4	Tbsp.	0	0	1

FOOD ITEM	SPECIFICATIONS	BRAND NAME	QUANTITY	SIZE	PROTEIN BLOCKS	CARBOHYDRATE BLOCKS	FAT BLOCKS
	honey mustard	Good Seasons	0.4	Tbsp.	0	0	1
	Italian	Good Seasons	0.4	Tbsp.	0	0	1
	Italian	Good Seasons Reduced Calorie	1.2	Tbsp.	0	0	1
	Italian, mild	Good Seasons	0.4	Tbsp.	0	0	1
	Italian, zesty	Good Seasons	0.4	Tbsp.	0	0	1
	Italian, zesty	Good Seasons Reduced Calorie	1.2	Tbsp.	0	0	1
	Mexican spice	Good Seasons	0.4	Tbsp.	0	0	1
	Oriental sesame	Good Seasons	0.4	Tbsp.	0	0	1
	ranch	Good Seasons	0.5	Tbsp.	0	0	1
	ranch	Good Seasons Reduced Calorie	1.2	Tbsp.	0	0	1
	cream cheese	Vita	0.04	cup	0	0	1
Salt pork	raw		0.1	oz.	0	0	1
Sandwich spread		Blue Plate	0.4	Tbsp.	0	0	1
		Hellmann's	0.6	Tbsp.	0	0	1
		Kraft Spread & Burger Sauce	0.6	Tbsp.	0	0	1
		Loma Linda	0.2	cup	0	0	1
		Roaster Fresh	0.2	oz.	0	0	1
Sesame butter	partially defatted		0.2	oz.	0	0	1
Sesame meal	from whole seeds		0.4	Tbsp.	1	0	1
Sesame paste	whole, brown		0.04	cup	0	0	1
Sesame seeds	whole, roasted, toasted	Arrowhead Mills	0.2	oz.	0	0	1
	kernels, decorticated		0.04	cup	0	0	1
	kernels, decorticated, dried	Arrowhead Mills	2	tsp.	0	0	1
	kernels, decorticated, toasted		0.2	oz.	0	0	1
Shortening	lard or vegetable oil		0.2	Tbsp.	0	0	1
	vegetable, regular/butter flavor	Crisco	0.3	Tbsp.	0	0	1
Spinach dip		Marie's	0.4	Tbsp.	0	0	1
Sunflower seeds	dried, in shell	Arrowhead Mills	0.2	cup	0	0	1
	dry-roasted, in shell	Planters	0.4	oz. bag	0	0	1
	dry-roasted, in shell	Planters	0.2	cup	0	0	1
	dry-roasted, in shell	Planters Original	0.2	cup	0	0	1

FAT

Food	Description	Brand	Amount	Unit	P	C	F
Sunflower seed	dry-roasted, in shell	Planters Munch 'N Go	0.2	oz. edible	0	0	1
Sunflower seed	dry-roasted, kernels, salted	Planters	0.2	oz.	0	0	1
Sunflower seed	dry-roasted, kernels	Planters	0.04	cup	0	0	1
Sunflower seed	honey-roasted, kernels	Planters	0.2	oz.	0	0	1
Sunflower seed	oil-roasted, kernels	Planters	0.2	oz.	0	0	1
Sunflower seed	oil-roasted, kernels	Planters Munch 'N Go	0.04	cup	0	0	1
Sunflower seed	oil-roasted, kernels	Planters	0.2	oz.	0	0	1
Sunflower seed	barbecued kernels	Planters Munch 'N Go	0.7	Tbsp.	0	0	1
Sunflower seed	barbecued kernels	Planters	0.2	oz.	0	0	1
Sunflower seed	salted kernels		0.3	oz.	0	0	1
Sunflower seed	tamari-roasted	Eden	0.4	Tbsp.	0	0	1
Sunflower seed butter			0.2	oz.	0	0	1
Tahini		Roaster Fresh	0.2	oz.	0	0	1
Tahini		Arrowhead Mills	0.2	oz.	0	0	1
Tahini		Joyva	0.3	Tbsp.	0	0	1
Tahini		Krinos	0.3	Tbsp.	0	0	1
Tahini sauce mix		Casbah	0.2	oz.	0	0	1
Tartar sauce		Bookbinder's	0.5	Tbsp.	0	0	1
Tartar sauce		Hellmann's/Best Foods	0.4	Tbsp.	0	0	1
Tartar sauce		Hellmann's/Best Foods Low Fat	4	Tbsp.	0	2	1
Tartar sauce		Nalley	0.3	Tbsp.	0	0	1
Tartar sauce		Sauceworks	0.6	Tbsp.	0	0	1
Tartar sauce		Sauceworks	0.4	Tbsp.	0	0	1
Tartar sauce	lemon herb flavor	Marie's	0.2	Tbsp.	0	0	1
Tomato dip	sun-dried	Paradise/Wild Swan	0.04	cup	0	0	1
Turkey fat			0.2	oz. pkg.	0	0	1
Walnut, dried	black		0.2	oz.	0	0	1
Walnut, dried	black, shelled		0.04	cup	0	0	1
Walnut, dried	black, chopped		0.2	oz.	0	0	1
Walnut, dried	English or Persian, shelled		0.04	cup	0	0	1
Walnut, dried	English or Persian, pcs.	Planters	0.05	cup	0	0	1
Walnut, dried	English or Persian, halves	Planters	0.05	cup	0	0	1
Walnut, dried	halves	Planters Gold Measure	0.2	oz. pkg.	0	0	1
Walnut, dried	pieces	Planters	0.04	cup	0	0	1

PART III

Zone Food Blocks for Prepared Meals

If time is of the essence, then prepared (either frozen or in cans) meals can be a godsend. However, be aware that many of these prepared meals can take you quickly out of the Zone if they aren't balanced with regard to Zone Food Blocks.

PREPARED MEAL ITEM	SPECIFICATIONS	BRAND NAME	SERVING SIZE	PROTEIN BLOCKS	CARBOHYDRATE BLOCKS	FAT BLOCKS
Alfredo Sauce		Ragu	1/4 cup	0	0	3
		Progresso	1/4 cup	1	0	5
	three cheese	Lawry's	3 Tbs.	0	0	1
	refrigerated	Contadina	1/4 cup	1	0	6
	refrigerated	Contadina Light	1/4 cup	1	1	2
Alfredo Sauce mix		Knorr	1/3 pkg.	0	1	1
		Spice Island	1/2 pkg.	0	1	1
Amaranth entree	canned	Health Valley Fast Menu	1 cup	1	3	0
Angel Hair pasta entree	frozen	Lean Cuisine	1 pkg.	1	3	1
	frozen	Smart Ones	1 pkg.	1	3	1
	frozen w/sausage	Marie Callender's	1 pkg.	2	4	5
Angel Hair pasta mix	chicken	Golden Saute	1/2 pkg. dry	1	5	1
	w/herbs	Noodle Roni	1 cup prepared	1	4	4
	parmesan	Golden Saute	1/2 cup, dry	1	4	2
		Noodle Roni Parmesano	1 cup prepared	1	4	5
Apple Fritters	frozen	Mrs. Paul's	2 pcs.	1	4	4
Apple Pastry	frozen, dumpling	Pepperidge Farm	1 pc.	0	5	4
	pocket	Tastykake	1 pc.	0	4	8
	puffs	Entenmann's	1 pc.	0	4	4
	frozen, squares	Pepperidge Farm	1 pc.	0	3	3
Bean Dishes, mix	Italian	Knorr Cup	1 pkg.	1	5	1
Bean Entree, frozen	white Parisian	Weight Watchers	9.87 oz.	2	1	3
Bean Loaf	frozen,	Natural Touch	1" slice	1	1	3
Bean Salad	deli style	S&W	1/2 cup	1	2	0
	marinated	S&W	1/2 cup	0	1	0
	three bean	Green Giant	1/2 cup	0	1	0
	three bean	Hanover	1/3 cup	0	2	0
Beans and Franks		Campbell's	1 cup	3	3	4
		Hormel	7 1/2 oz.	2	3	4
		Kid's Kitchen	7 1/2 oz.	2	3	4
		Libby's Diner	7 3/4 oz.	2	3	5
		Van Camp's Beanie Weenee	1 cup	2	3	5
	baked	Van Camp's Beanie Weenee	1 cup	3	5	5

Category	Item	Brand	Serving			
Beef Dinner, frozen	barbeque	Van Camp's Beanie Weenee	1 cup	2	4	3
	chili	Van Camp's Beanie Weenee	1 can	2	2	4
	and broccoli	Swanson	1 pkg	2	5	3
	and broccoli	Swanson Hungry Man	1 pkg	4	7	5
	chicken fried steak	Banquet	1 pkg	4	7	15
	chicken fried steak	Marie Callender's	1 pkg	3	7	10
	chicken fried steak w/gravy	Swanson	1 pkg	5	5	8
	and gravy	Swanson	1 pkg	2	4	2
	and peppers Cantonese	Healthy Choice	1 pkg	2	1	2
	pot roast, Yankee	The Budget Gourmet Light & Healthy	1 pkg	3	3	2
	pot roast, Yankee	Healthy Choice	1 pkg	3	4	2
	pot roast, Yankee	Swanson	1 pkg	1	3	2
	pot roast, Yankee	Swanson Hungry Man	1 pkg	2	5	4
	roast beef sandwich, smothered	Swanson	1 pkg	2	5	4
	Salisbury steak	Banquet	1 pkg	4	5	15
	Salisbury steak	The Budget Gourmet Light & Healthy	1 pkg	3	3	3
	Salisbury steak	Healthy Choice	1 pkg	3	5	2
	Salisbury steak	Swanson	1 pkg	4	4	7
	Salisbury steak	Swanson Hungry Man	1 pkg	7	4	11
	Salisbury steak, con queso	Patio	1 pkg	3	3	7
	sirloin	The Budget Gourmet Light & Healthy Special Recipe	1 pkg	3	4	2
	sirloin, chopped w/gravy	Swanson	1 pkg	2	3	3
	sirloin, meatballs and gravy	The Budget Gourmet Light & Healthy	1 pkg	3	4	3
	sirloin, tips	Swanson Hungry Man	1 pkg	4	4	5
	sirloin, tips, w/noodles	Swanson	1 pkg	2	3	3
	sirloin, in wine sauce	The Budget Gourmet Light & Healthy	1 pkg	3	3	2
	Stroganoff	Healthy Choice	1 pkg	3	5	2
	teriyaki	The Budget Gourmet Light & Healthy	1 pkg	3	4	2
	tips	Healthy Choice	1 pkg	3	3	2
	tips, sauce	Healthy Choice	1 pkg	3	4	2
	chow mein	La Choy Bi-Pack	1 pkg	1	2	1
Beef Entree, canned	goulash	Hormel	7 1/2 oz. can	2	2	4
	pepper (steak)	La Choy	1/5 pkg	0	1	0
	pepper steak, Oriental	La Choy Bi-Pack	1 cup	2	1	1

PREPARED MEALS

PREPARED MEAL ITEM	SPECIFICATIONS	BRAND NAME	SERVING SIZE	PROTEIN BLOCKS	CARBOHYDRATE BLOCKS	FAT BLOCKS
	pepper steak, Oriental, w/noodles	La Choy Bi-Pack	1 cup	3	2	1
	pot roast	Dinty Moore American Classics	10 oz.	4	2	1
	roast, w/mashed potato	Dinty Moore American Classics	10 oz.	3	3	2
	Salisbury steak	Dinty Moore American Classics	10 oz.	3	2	5
	stew	Dinty Moore	1 cup	2	2	5
	stew	Dinty Moore, Can	7 1/2 oz.	2	1	3
	stew	Dinty Moore, Cup	7 1/2 oz.	2	1	3
	stew	Dinty Moore American Classics	10 oz.	2	2	4
	stew	Hormel Micro cup	7 1/2 oz.	2	1	3
	stew	Hunts Homestyle	1 cup	2	2	2
	stew	Libby's Diner	7 3/4 oz.	2	2	7
	stew	Nally's	7 1/2 oz.	1	2	3
	stew	Nally's Big Chunk	1 cup	2	2	4
	stew, burger	Dinty Moore Hearty Cup	7 1/2 oz.	2	2	4
Beef Entree, freeze dried	w/peppers, onions, rice	Mountain House	1 cup	2	3	2
	stew	Mountain House	1 cup	1	2	1
	Stroganoff, w/noodles	Mountain House	1 cup	1	3	3
Beef Entree, frozen	teriyaki, w/rice	Mountain House	1 cup	2	4	1
	barbeque, mesquite	Healthy Choice	1 pkg.	3	4	1
	broccoli, Beijing	Healthy Choice	1 pkg.	3	6	1
	Cantonese	The Budget Gourmet	1 pkg.	2	4	3
	chipped	Banquet Topper	4 oz.	1	1	1
	chipped, creamed	Stouffer's	4.4 oz.	1	1	4
	ground, w/rice	Goya	1 pkg.	4	12	12
	mesquite, w/rice	Lean Cuisine Café Classics	1 pkg.	2	4	2
	Oriental	The Budget Gourmet, Light & Healthy	1 pkg.	2	4	3
	Oriental	Lean Cuisine Café Classics	1 pkg.	2	3	3
	Oriental	Stouffer's Lunch Express	1 pkg.	2	4	3
	patty	Swanson Fun Feast	1 pkg.	4	5	6
	patty, charbroiled, gravy and	Morton	1 pkg.	2	2	5
	patty, gravy and	Banquet	1 pkg.	2	2	7

patty, mushroom, gravy and	Banquet	1 patty	1	1	4
patty, onion gravy and	Banquet	1 patty	1	1	5
pepper steak	The Budget Gourmet	1 pkg.	3	4	3
pepper steak	Stouffer's	1 pkg.	2	5	3
pepper steak	Weight Watchers	1 pkg.	3	3	2
pepper steak, Oriental	Healthy Choice	1 pkg.	3	3	1
pie or pot pie	Banquet	1 pkg.	1	4	5
pie or pot pie	Stouffer's	1 pkg.	3	4	9
pie or pot pie	Swanson	1 pkg.	5	4	8
pie or pot pie	Swanson Hungry Man	1 pkg.	8	7	13
pot pie, Yankee	Marie Callender's	1 pkg.	2	6	15
pot roast, w/potatoes	Lean Cuisine	1 pkg.	2	2	2
pot roast, w/potatoes	Stouffer's Homestyle	1 pkg.	3	2	3
roast	Healthy Choice Hearty Handfuls	6.1 oz.	2	5	2
roast, open face	The Budget Gourmet	1 pkg.	2	3	6
Salisbury steak	Banquet	1 pkg.	2	3	5
Salisbury steak	Healthy Choice	1 pkg.	3	3	2
Salisbury steak	Lean Cuisine	1 pkg.	3	3	3
Salisbury steak	Stouffer's Homestyle	1 pkg.	3	3	6
Salisbury steak, gravy and	Banquet	1 patty	2	1	5
Salisbury steak, gravy and	Banquet Toppers	5 oz	1	1	5
Salisbury steak, gravy and	Morton	1 pkg.	1	2	3
Salisbury steak, gravy, mashed potato	Swanson	1 pkg.	4	2	6
Salisbury steak, grilled	Weight Watchers	1 pkg.	3	2	3
Salisbury steak, sirloin	The Budget Gourmet Light & Healthy	1 pkg.	3	3	2
shredded, w/rice	Goya	1 pkg.	5	13	8
sirloin, cheddar melt	The Budget Gourmet	1 pkg.	2	3	7
sirloin in herb sauce	The Budget Gourmet Light & Healthy	1 pkg.	3	3	2
sirloin, peppercorn	Lean Cuisine Café Classics	1 pkg.	2	2	2
sirloin, roast supreme	The Budget Gourmet	1 pkg.	2	2	4
sirloin tips, and noodles	Swanson	1 pkg.	2	2	3
sirloin tips, w/vegetables	The Budget Gourmet	1 pkg.	2	2	4
sliced	Banquet Country	2 slices	4	2	2
sliced, gravy and	Banquet	2 slices	2	1	1
sliced, gravy and	Banquet Topper	4 oz.	1	0	1

PREPARED MEAL ITEM	SPECIFICATIONS	BRAND NAME	SERVING SIZE	PROTEIN BLOCKS	CARBOHYDRATE BLOCKS	FAT BLOCKS
	steak, chicken fried	Banquet, Country	1 pkg.	2	4	7
	Philly	Healthy Choice Hearty Handfuls	6.1 oz.	2	5	2
	stew	Banquet	1 cup	2	1	1
	stew w/rice	Goya	1 pkg.	5	13	6
	stir-fry	Tyson Kit	1 cup	2	3	1
	Stroganoff	The Budget Gourmet Light & Healthy	1 pkg.	3	3	2
	Stroganoff	Stouffer's	1 pkg.	3	3	7
	tips, Francais	Healthy Choice	1 pkg.	3	4	2
Beef Hash, canned		Broadcast Morning Classics Original	1 cup	1	2	4
		Castleberry's	1 cup	3	2	9
	corned beef	Dinty Moore Cup	7 1/2 oz.	3	2	7
		Goya	1 cup	2	2	10
		Libby's	1 cup	3	2	12
		Mary Kitchen	1 cup	3	2	8
		Nalley	1 cup	3	2	11
	roast beef	Libby's	1 cup	3	2	11
		Mary Kitchen	1 cup	3	2	8
Beef Sandwich, frozen	sausage flavor	Broadcast Morning Classics	1 cup	1	2	4
	barbeque	Hormel Quick Meal	1 pc.	2	6	2
	barbeque	Hot Pockets	1 pc.	2	6	1
	broccoli	Lean Pockets	1 pc.	1	5	1
	cheddar	Hot Pockets	1 pc.	2	5	2
	cheeseburger	Hormel Quick Meal	1 pc.	3	5	2
	cheeseburger, bacon	Hormel Quick Meal	1 pc.	3	4	7
	cheeseburger, chili	Hormel Quick Meal	1 pc.	3	4	8
	fajita	Hot Pockets	1 pc.	2	4	6
	hamburger	Hormel Quick Meal	1 pc.	3	4	5
	steak, biscuit	Hormel Quick Meal	1 pc.	2	4	5
	steak, mushroom	Hormel Quick Meal	1 pc.	2	4	8
Bowtie entree, frozen	and chicken	Mrs. Paterson's Aussie Pie	1 pc.	3	3	2
	mushroom Marsala	Lean Cuisine Cafe Classics	1 pkg.	3	3	3
		Weight Watchers	1 pkg.	2	3	3
Broccoli pocket	and cheddar, frozen	Ken & Robert's Veggie Pockets	1 pc.	1	4	3
Broccoli pot pie	w/cheddar, frozen	Amy's	7.5 oz.	2	5	7

Food	Brand	Amount			
Broccoli-cheese in pastry	Pepperidge Farm	1 pc.	1	2	5
Burrito, frozen					
bean, black	Amy's	1 pc. or pkg.	1	6	3
bean and cheese	Old El Paso	1 pc. or pkg.	2	5	3
bean and cheese	Tina's	1 pc. or pkg.	2	5	3
bean and rice	Amy's	1 pc. or pkg.	1	4	2
bean, rice, and cheese	Amy's	1 pc. or pkg.	1	4	3
beef	Hormel Quick meal	1 pc. or pkg.	2	4	4
beef	Tina's Red Hot	1 pc. or pkg.	2	5	5
beef, nacho	Patio Britos	6 oz.	2	5	6
beef and bean	Patio Britos	6 oz.	2	5	6
beef and bean, hot	Old El Paso	1 pc. or pkg.	2	5	3
beef and bean, medium	Old El Paso	1 pc. or pkg.	2	5	3
beef and bean, mild	Old El Paso	1 pc. or pkg.	2	5	3
beef and bean, steak	Don Miguel	1 pc. or pkg.	1	5	3
cheese	Hormel Quick Meal	1 pc. or pkg.	1	6	2
cheese, nacho	Patio Britos	1 pc. or pkg.	2	4	4
chicken	Don Miguel	1 pc. or pkg.	2	5	3
chicken, and cheese, spicy	Patio Britos	1 pc. or pkg.	2	5	5
chicken son queso	Healthy Choice	1 pc. or pkg.	1	5	2
chili, red	Hormel Quick Meal	1 pc. or pkg.	2	4	4
pizza, cheese	Old El Paso	1 pc. or pkg.	2	4	3
pizza, pepperoni	Old El Paso	1 pc. or pkg.	2	3	3
pizza, sausage	Old El Paso	1 pc. or pkg.	2	3	3
black bean	Amy's	1 pkg.	1	4	2
Burrito, breakfast, frozen					
egg, scrambled	Swanson Great Starts Original	1 pkg.	2	3	3
egg, scrambled, w/bacon	Swanson Great Starts	1 pkg.	2	3	4
ham and cheese	Swanson Great Starts	1 pkg.	1	3	2
hot and spicy	Swanson Great Starts	1 pkg.	2	3	2
pizza, w/cheese, pepperoni	Swanson Great Starts	1 pkg.	3	3	3
sausage	Swanson Great Starts	1 pkg.	4	4	4
Burrito dinner, frozen					
beef	Chi-Chi's Burro	15 oz.	4	7	6
chicken	Chi-Chi's Burro	15 oz.	4	7	5
Cabbage, stuffed	frozen, w/potato — Lean Cuisine	9 1/2 oz.	2	2	2
Calzone, refrigerated	cheese — Stefano's	6-oz. pc.	3	4	9

PREPARED MEAL ITEM	SPECIFICATIONS	BRAND NAME	SERVING SIZE	PROTEIN BLOCKS	CARBOHYDRATE BLOCKS	FAT BLOCKS
	pepperoni	Stefano's	6-oz. pc.	3	5	9
	spinach	Stefano's	6-oz. pc.	3	5	6
Cannelloni dinner	frozen, w/potato	Amy's	10 oz.	2	3	4
Cannelloni entree	frozen, cheese	Lean Cuisine	9 1/8 oz.	3	3	2
Cheese Sandwich	frozen, grilled	Swanson Fun Feast	1 pkg.	4	6	7
Chicken dinner, frozen	barbeque, mesquite	The Budget Gourmet Light and Healthy	1 pkg.	3	3	2
	barbeque, mesquite	Healthy Choice	1 pkg.	3	5	1
	boneless	Swanson Hungry Man	1 pkg.	6	8	9
	breaded, country	Healthy Choice	1 pkg.	3	0	2
	broccoli Alfredo	Healthy Choice	1 pkg.	3	5	3
	Cantonese	Healthy Choice	1 pkg.	3	3	0
	Dijon	Healthy Choice	1 pkg.	3	4	1
	fried	Banquet Extra Helping	1 pkg.	5	7	13
	fried, country, w/gravy	Marie Callender's	1 pkg.	4	7	9
	fried, dark	Swanson	1 pkg.	6	5	9
	fried, dark	Swanson Budget	1 pkg.	5	5	7
	fried, dark	Swanson Hungry Man	1 pkg.	9	7	14
	fried, Southern	Banquet Extra Helping	1 pkg.	5	6	12
	fried, white	Banquet Extra Helping	1 pkg.	6	7	14
	fried, white	Swanson	1 pkg.	6	5	9
	fried, white, mostly	Swanson Hungry Man	1 pkg.	9	8	13
	glazed, Southwestern	Healthy Choice	1 pkg.	3	5	1
	grilled, patties	Swanson Hungry Man	1 pkg.	4	6	6
	grilled, white in garlic sauce	Swanson	1 pkg.	1	3	2
	herb, country	Healthy Choice	1 pkg.	3	4	1
	herbed	The Budget Gourmet Light and Healthy	1 pkg.	4	3	3
	honey mustard	The Budget Gourmet Light and Healthy	1 pkg.	3	4	2
	nuggets	Swanson	1 pkg.	4	5	6
	parmigiana	Banquet Extra Helping	1 pkg.	3	6	11
	parmigiana	The Budget Gourmet Light & Healthy	1 pkg.	3	3	3

parmigiana	Healthy Choice	1 pkg.	3	5	1
parmigiana	Marie Callender's	1 pkg.	4	6	9
parmigiana	Swanson	1 pkg.	4	4	6
parmigiana	Swanson Budget	1 pkg.	4	3	6
pasta and	Swanson Budget	1 pkg.	2	3	4
picante	Healthy Choice	1 pkg.	3	3	1
roasted, herb	The Budget Gourmet Light and Healthy	1 pkg.	2	3	2
roasted, herb	Swanson	1 pkg.	1	4	2
roasted, herb, mashed potatoes	Marie Callender's	1 pkg.	6	3	14
sweet and sour	Healthy Choice	1 pkg.	3	4	2
tenders platter	Swanson	1 pkg.	3	4	4
teriyaki	The Budget Gourmet Light and Healthy	1 pkg.	3	4	2
Chicken entree, canned					
teriyaki	Healthy Choice	1 pkg.	3	4	1
a la king	Swanson Main Dish	1 cup	5	2	7
a la king	Top Shelf	10 oz.	3	5	4
breast glazed	Top Shelf	10 oz.	3	2	2
and broccoli	Healthy Choice Hearty Handfuls	6.1 oz.	2	5	2
cacciatore	Top Shelf	10 oz.	3	3	1
chow mein	La Choy Bi-Pack	1 cup	1	0	1
chow mein	La Choy Entree	1 cup	1	2	1
and dumplings	Dinty Moore Cup	7 1/2 oz.	2	2	2
and dumplings	Swanson Main Dish	1 cup	3	2	4
fista	Top Shelf	10 oz.	4	5	5
w/mashed potatoes	Dinty Moore American Classics	10 oz.	3	3	1
and noodles	Dinty Moore American Classics	10 oz.	3	3	3
Oriental, w/noodles	La Choy	1 cup	2	1	2
and pasta	Chef Boyardee Bowl	7 1/2 oz.	2	2	0
spicy	La Choy Szechwan Bi-Pack	1 cup	1	1	1
stew	Dinty Moore	1 cup	2	2	4
stew	Dinty Moore Cup	7 1/2 oz.	1	2	3
stew	Swanson Main Dish	1 cup	3	3	1
sweet and sour	La Choy Bi-Pack	1 cup	1	2	1
teriyaki	La Choy Bi-Pack	1 cup	1	1	1

PREPARED MEALS

PREPARED MEAL ITEM	SPECIFICATIONS	BRAND NAME	SERVING SIZE	PROTEIN BLOCKS	CARBOHYDRATE BLOCKS	FAT BLOCKS
Chicken entree, freeze-dried	a la king and noodles	Mountain House	1 cup	3	3	3
	honey lime, w/rice	Mountain House	1 cup	1	5	1
	noodles and	Mountain House	1 cup	2	3	1
	Polynesian w/rice	Mountain House	1 cup	1	4	1
	rice and	Mountain House	1 cup	1	5	3
	stew	Mountain House	1 cup	2	2	3
	teriyaki, w/rice	Mountain House	1 cup	1	4	1
Chicken entree, frozen see also Chicken entree, refrigerated	a la king	Banquet Toppers	4.5-oz. bag	1	1	1
	a la king	Stouffer's	1 pkg.	2	4	3
	Alfredo	Stouffer's Lunch Express	1 pkg.	3	3	6
	au gratin	The Budget Gourmet Light and Healthy	1 pkg.	3	3	3
	baked and gravy, whipped potato	Stouffer's Homestyle	1 pkg.	3	2	4
	baked, whipped potato	Lean Cuisine	1 pkg.	3	3	2
	barbeque, glazed	Weight Watchers	1 pkg.	3	3	1
	barbeque, honey, w/potato, vegetables	Tyson	1 pkg.	3	5	5
	barbeque style	Banquet	1 pkg.	3	4	4
	barbeque w/potato, vegetables	Tyson BBQ	1 pkg.	4	5	3
	biryani	Curry Classics	1 pkg.	2	6	4
	blackened	Tyson	1 pkg.	3	4	1
	breaded cutlet, pasta marinara	Celentano	1 pkg.	2	3	6
	breast breaded	Tyson	2 pcs.	2	2	3
	breast breaded, southern	Tyson Breast Fillets	2 pcs.	2	1	2
	breast, in wine sauce	Lean Cuisine Café Classics	1 pkg.	2	2	2
	breast tenders	Banquet	3 pcs.	2	2	5
	breast tenders	Tyson	5 pcs.	2	2	5
	breast tenders, Southern	Banquet	3 pcs.	2	1	5
	w/broccoli and cheese	Tyson	1 pkg.	3	2	4

Item	Brand	Amount			
cacciatore	Healthy Choice	1 pkg.	3	3	1
Calypso	Lean Cuisine Café Classics	1 pkg.	2	4	2
carbonara	Lean Cuisine Café Classics	1 pkg.	3	3	3
chow mein	Banquet	1 pkg.	1	3	2
chow mein	Chun King	1 pkg.	2	5	5
chow mein	Lean Cuisine	1 pkg.	2	3	2
chow mein	Smart Ones	1 pkg.	2	3	1
chunks, breaded	Stouffer's Lunch Express		2	4	1
chunks, breaded	Country Skillet	5 pcs., 3.3 oz.	2	2	6
chunks, breaded	Tyson Breast Chunks	6 pcs., 3 oz.	2	1	5
chunks, breaded	Tyson Chick'n Chunks	6 pcs., 3 oz.	2	1	7
chunks, breaded, and cheddar	Banquet	4 pcs., 2.9 oz.	2	1	6
chunks, breaded, Southern	Banquet	5 pcs., 3.1 oz.	2	2	6
chunks, breaded, Southern	Country Skillet	5 pcs., 3.3 oz.	2	2	5
chunks, breaded, Southern	Tyson Chick'n Chunks	6 pcs., 3 oz.	1	1	6
Cordon Bleu	Weight Watchers	1 pkg.	2	3	2
creamed	Stouffer's	1 pkg.	2	1	7
creamy and broccoli	Stouffer's	1 pkg.	3	3	5
crouquettes	Goya	3 pcs.	2	3	4
drumlets	Swanson Fun Feast	1 pkg.	5	5	8
and dumplings	Banquet Family Size	1 cup	2	2	5
and dumplings	Banquet Home Style	1 pkg.	2	4	3
enchilada, see "Enchilada Entree"					
escalloped, and noodles	Stouffer's	1 pkg.	0	0	0
fajita, see "Fajita entree"					
fettuccine	The Budget Gourmet	1 pkg.	3	3	6
fettuccine	Lean Cuisine	1 pkg.	3	3	2
fettuccine	Stouffer's Homestyle	1 pkg.	4	3	5
fettuccine	Weight Watchers	1 pkg.	3	4	2
fettuccine	Healthy Choice	1 pkg.	3	4	2
w/broccoli and cheese	Lean Cuisine Lunch Express	1 pkg.	2	4	3
fiesta	Lean Cuisine	1 pkg.	3	4	2
fiesta	Smart Ones	1 pkg.	3	4	3
Francais	Tyson	1 pkg.	2	2	3
Francesca	Healthy Choice	1 pkg.	4	5	2

PREPARED MEALS

PREPARED MEAL ITEM	SPECIFICATIONS	BRAND NAME	SERVING SIZE	PROTEIN BLOCKS	CARBOHYDRATE BLOCKS	FAT BLOCKS
	French recipe	The Budget Gourmet Light and Healthy	1 pkg.	2	2	3
	fricassee, w/rice	Goya	1 pkg.	6	13	7
	fried	Banquet Meal	1 pkg.	3	3	9
	fried	Kid Cuisine High Flying	1 pkg.	3	5	6
	fried	Morton	1 pkg.	3	3	8
	fried	Swanson Fun Feast Frasslin'	1 pkg.	7	5	10
	fried, Southern	Banquet Meal	1 pkg.	3	4	10
	fried, whipped potato	Stouffer's Homestyle	1 pkg.	3	3	5
	fried, whipped potato	Swanson	1 pkg.	5	4	7
	fried, white meat	Banquet Meal	1 pkg.	3	3	9
	fried, pieces	Banquet Original	3 oz.	2	1	6
	fried, pieces	Country Skillet	3 oz.	2	1	6
	fried, breast	Banquet Original	5.5-oz. pc.	3	2	9
	fried, country	Banquet	3 oz.	2	1	6
	fried, drums and thighs	Banquet	3 oz.	2	1	6
	fried, honey BBQ, skinless	Banquet	3 oz.	4	1	4
	fried, hot 'n spicy	Banquet	3 oz.	2	1	6
	fried, skinless	Banquet	3 oz.	3	1	4
	fried, Southern	Banquet	3 oz.	2	1	6
	fried, wing, hot and spicy	Banquet	4 oz., 4 pcs.	2	0	5
	fried rice	Tyson Kit	1 cup	2	4	1
	garlic	Healthy Choice Hearty Handfuls	6.1 oz.	3	5	2
	garlic, milano	Healthy Choice	1 pkg.	3	3	1
	ginger, Hunan	Healthy Choice	1 pkg.	3	6	1
	glazed, country	Healthy Choice	1 pkg.	2	3	1
	glazed, w/rice, broccoli, carrots	Tyson	1 pkg.	2	3	2
	glazed, w/vegetable rice	Lean Cuisine	1 pkg.	3	2	2
	grilled, angel hair pasta	Stouffer's Lunch Express	1 pkg.	3	4	4
	grilled, w/corn, beans	Tyson	1 pkg.	3	2	1
	grilled, Italian, w/linguine	Tyson	1 pkg.	3	2	2
	grilled, salsa	Lean Cuisine Café Classics	1 pkg.	2	3	2
	grilled, gumbo	Goya Asopao de Pollo	1 pkg.	2	2	1

herb, w/radiatore, vegetables	Tyson	1 pkg.	3	5	2
honey mustard	Lean Cuisine Café Classics	1 pkg.	2	4	2
honey mustard	Healthy Choice	1 pkg.	3	4	1
honey mustard	Smart Ones	1 pkg.	2	3	2
honey mustard, w/gemelli	Tyson	1 pkg.	3	5	2
imperial	Healthy Choice	1 pkg.	2	3	1
Italian, w/fettuccine	Lean Cuisine	1 pkg.	3	3	2
Kiev	Tyson	1 pkg.	3	4	8
w/linguine	Stouffer's Lunch Express	1 pkg.	2	3	4
lo mein	Banquet	1 pkg.	3	4	2
mandarin	The Budget Gourmet Light & Healthy	1 pkg.	2	4	2
mandarin	Lean Cuisine Lunch Express	1 pkg.	2	4	2
mandarin	Healthy Choice	1 pkg.	3	4	1
marinara, w/pasta	Tyson	1 pkg.	4	6	3
Marsala	The Budget Gourmet	1 pkg.	3	3	2
Marsala	Smart Ones	1 pkg.	1	2	1
Marsala, w/potato, carrots	Tyson	1 pkg.	2	2	2
Marsala and vegetables	Healthy Choice	1 pkg.	3	3	0
Mediterranean	Lean Cuisine Café Classics	1 pkg.	3	3	1
mesquite	Tyson	1 pkg.	3	4	2
Mexican, and rice	Stouffer's Lunch Express	1 pkg.	2	4	3
Mirabella	Smart Ones	1 pkg.	2	2	1
Monterey	Stouffer's Homestyle	1 pkg.	3	3	3
and mushroom	Healthy Choice Hearty Handfuls	6.1 oz.	3	3	7
w/mushroom sauce	Tyson	1 pkg.	2	5	1
nibbles	Swanson	1 pkg.	3	3	1
and noodles	The Budget Gourmet	1 pkg.	4	3	7
and noodles	Stouffer's Homestyle	1 pkg.	3	3	8
noodle casserole	Swanson	1 pkg.	3	2	4
noodle casserole, w/vegetables	Swanson	1 pkg.	3	3	3
nuggets	Banquet	6 pcs., 3 oz.	2	1	5
nuggets	Banquet	6 pcs., 4.5 oz.	2	3	6
nuggets	Banquet, Homestyle	6.75 oz.	3	3	7
nuggets	Country Skillet	10 pcs., 3.3 oz.	2	2	6
nuggets	Kid Cuisine Cosmic	1 pkg.	3	5	5
nuggets	Morton	1 pkg.	2	3	6

PREPARED MEALS

PREPARED MEAL ITEM	SPECIFICATIONS	BRAND NAME	SERVING SIZE	PROTEIN BLOCKS	CARBOHYDRATE BLOCKS	FAT BLOCKS
	nuggets, mozzarella	Banquet	6 pcs., 2.9 oz.	2	2	5
	nuggets, Southern	Banquet	6 pcs., 4.5 oz.	2	2	7
	a l'orange	Lean Cuisine	1 pkg.	3	4	1
	orange glazed	The Budget Gourmet Light and Healthy	1 pkg.	2	6	1
	Oriental	Banquet	1 pkg.	2	3	3
	Oriental	The Budget Gourmet Light & Healthy	1 pkg.	3	4	2
	Oriental	Lean Cuisine	1 pkg.	3	3	2
	Oriental	Stouffer's Lunch Express	1 pkg.	2	6	4
	Parmesan	Lean Cuisine Café Classics	1 pkg.	3	2	2
	parmigiana	Banquet	4.7-oz. pc.	2	3	5
	parmigiana	Banquet Family Size	4.7-oz. pc.	2	3	4
	parmigiana	Stouffer's Homestyle	1 pkg.	4	3	3
	parmigiana	Tyson	1 pkg.	2	3	4
	parmigiana	Weight Watchers	1 pkg.	3	4	2
	parmigiana, Italian style	Banquet	4.6-oz. pc.	2	2	5
	patties, breaded	Banquet	1 pkg.	2	3	7
	patties, breaded	Banquet	2.3-oz. pc.	1	1	4
	patties, breaded	Country Skillet	2 1/2 oz. pc.	1	1	4
	patties, breaded	Morton	1 pkg.	2	2	5
	patties, breaded	Tyson Thick'n Crispy	2 1/2 oz. pc.	1	1	5
	patties, breaded, strips	Swanson	1 pkg.	4	3	6
	patties, breaded, breast	Tyson	2 1/2 oz. pc.	1	1	4
	patties, breaded, breast, Southern	Tyson	2 1/2 oz. pc.	2	1	4
	patties, breaded, w/cheddar	Tyson Chick'n with Cheddar	1 pc.	2	1	5
	patties, breaded, Southern	Tyson Chick'n Chunks	6 pcs., 3 oz.	1	1	6
	patties, breaded, Southern	Banquet	2.3-oz. pc.	1	1	3
	patties, breaded, Southern	Country Skillet	3.3-oz. pc.	1	1	4
	in peanut sauce	Lean Cuisine	1 pkg.	3	3	2
	penne pollo	Weight Watchers	1 pkg.	3	4	2
	piccata	Lean Cuisine Café Classics	1 pkg.	2	5	2

Description	Brand	Serving			
piccata, lemon herb	Smart Ones	1 pkg.	1	3	1
piccata, w/potato, broccoli	Tyson	1 pkg.	2	2	2
pie or pot pie	Banquet	1 pkg.	1	4	6
pie or pot pie	Banquet Family Size	1 pkg.	2	4	10
pie or pot pie	Empire Kosher	1 pkg.	3	3	7
pie or pot pie	Lean Cuisine	1 pkg.	3	4	3
pie or pot pie	Marie Callender's	10-oz. pie	2	6	15
pie or pot pie	Marie Callender's	1 cup, 8 1/2 oz.	2	5	10
pie or pot pie	Stouffer's	10 oz.	3	4	12
pie or pot pie	Stouffer's	1/2 of 16-oz. pkg.	2	4	12
pie or pot pie	Swanson	1 pkg.	5	5	7
pie or pot pie	Swanson Deluxe	1 pkg.	5	5	7
pie or pot pie	Swanson Hungry Man	1 pkg.	8	7	12
pie or pot pie	Tyson Meat Lovers	9-oz. pie	2	5	13
pie or pot pie	Tyson Meat Lovers	1 cup, 8.4 oz.	2	5	12
pie or pot pie au gratin	Marie Callender's	10-oz. pie	3	5	6
pie or pot pie au gratin	Marie Callender's	1 cup, 8 1/2 oz.	3	4	18
pie or pot pie and broccoli	Marie Callender's	10-oz. pie	3	9	16
pie or pot pie and broccoli	Marie Callender's	1 cup, 8 1/2 oz.	3	7	16
pie or pot pie, broccoli and cheese	Tyson	9-oz. pie	3	5	12
pie or pot pie, broccoli and cheese	Tyson	1 cup, 8.4 oz.	2	5	11
pie or pot pie, and vegetables	Tyson	9-oz. pie	2	5	12
pie or pot pie, and vegetables	Tyson	1 cup, 8.4 oz.	2	5	12
primavera, w/pasta	Banquet	1 pkg.	2	4	4
primavera, w/pasta	Tyson	1 pkg.	4	5	3
and rice, stir-fry casserole	Swanson	1 pkg.	1	5	1
w/rice	Goya Arroz con Pollo	1 pkg.	7	8	9
roast, glazed	Weight Watchers	1 pkg.	3	3	2
roasted, herb	Lean Cuisine Café Classics	1 pkg.	3	2	2
roasted, w/linguini; broccoli	Tyson	1 pkg.	3	2	2
sesame	Healthy Choice	1 pkg.	2	4	1
sesame, Shanghai	Healthy Choice	1 pkg.	3	4	2
stir-fry	Tyson Kit	1 cup	1	3	1

PREPARED MEALS

PREPARED MEAL ITEM	SPECIFICATIONS	BRAND NAME	SERVING SIZE	PROTEIN BLOCKS	CARBOHYDRATE BLOCKS	FAT BLOCKS
	supreme, w/potato, green beans	Tyson	1 pkg.	2	2	3
	sweet and sour	The Budget Gourmet	1 pkg.	3	6	2
	tikka	Curry Classics Makhanwala	1 pkg.	4	1	11
	and vegetables	Lean Cuisine	1 pkg.	3	3	2
	w/vegetables, garden	Stouffer's Lunch Express	1 pkg.	2	5	4
	walnut, crunchy	Chun King	1 pkg.	3	6	6
	wings, barbeque	Tyson	4 pcs.	3	0	5
	wings, teriyaki	Tyson	4 pcs.	3	0	4
Chicken entree, mix	stir-fry	Tyson	1 cup, prepared	1	2	1
Chicken entree, refrigerated see also "Chicken, refrigerated or frozen"	cutlet, breaded	Perdue	3 1/2-oz. pc.	1	2	4
	Italian	Perdue Short Cuts	3 oz.	3	0	1
	lemon pepper	Perdue Short Cuts	3 oz.	3	0	1
	mesquite	Perdue Short Cuts	3 oz.	3	0	1
	nuggets, breaded	Perdue	5 pcs., 3 oz.	1	1	4
	nuggets, breaded and cheese	Perdue	5 pcs., 3 oz.	2	1	5
	oven roasted	Perdue Short Cuts	3 oz.	3	0	1
	oven roasted, dark meat	Perdue	3 oz.	2	0	4
	oven roasted, white meat	Perdue	3 oz.	3	0	2
	tenderloins, breaded	Perdue	3 oz.	3	1	2
	wings, barbeque	Perdue	3 oz.	2	0	4
	wings, hot and spicy	Perdue	3 oz.	2	0	4
Chicken sandwich, frozen		Hormel Quick Meal	1 pc.	2	5	4
	broccoli and cheddar	Croissant Pockets	1 pc.	2	4	4
	and cheddar w/broccoli	Hot Pockets	1 pc.	2	4	4
	fajita	Lean Pockets	1 pc.	2	4	3
	glazed, supreme	Lean Pockets	1 pc.	1	4	2
	grilled	Hormel Quick Meal	1 pc.	3	4	3
	Parmesan	Lean Pockets	1 pc.	2	4	3

Chili, canned see also "Chili base"

Item	Brand	Serving			
pastry	Mrs. Paterson's Aussie Pie	1 pc.	2	5	8
w/beans	Chi-Chi's San Antonio	1 cup	3	2	6
w/beans	Gebhardt	1 cup	2	2	5
w/beans	Hormel	1 cup	3	2	6
w/beans	Hormel	7 1/2 oz. can	2	2	4
w/beans	Hormel Micro cup	1 cont.	2	2	4
w/beans	Hormel Micro cup	10.5-oz. cont.	3	3	6
w/beans	Just Rite	1 cup	3	3	8
w/beans	Libby's	1 cup	2	2	9
w/beans	Libby's Diner	7 3/4 oz.	3	3	7
w/beans	Nalley Real Hearty	1 cup	3	2	5
w/beans	Nalley Thick	1 cup	3	2	3
w/beans	Old El Paso	1 cup	3	1	2
w/beans	Van Camp's	1 cup	3	2	7
w/beans	Wolf	1 cup	3	2	6
w/beans, beef and hot dogs	Nalley Chili Dog	1 cup	3	2	4
w/beans cheddar	Nalley	1 cup	3	2	4
w/beans chunky	Hormel	1 cup	2	2	5
w/beans hot	Hormel	1 cup	3	2	6
w/beans hot	Hormel/Hormel Micro Cup	7 1/2 oz.	2	2	4
w/beans jalapeno	Wolf	1 cup	3	2	6
w/beans jalapeno, hot	Nalley	1 cup	3	2	3
w/out beans	Hormel	1 cup	3	1	10
w/out beans	Hormel	7 1/2 oz. can	3	1	10
w/out beans	Hormel Micro Cup	1 cont.	3	1	6
w/out beans	Libby's	1 cup	3	2	12
w/out beans	Nalley Big Chunk	1 cup	4	1	5
w/out beans	Wolf	1 cup	3	2	10
w/out beans, hot	Hormel	1 cup	3	1	10
w/out beans, jalapeno	Wolf	1 cup	3	2	10
w/out beans, onion	Nalley Walla Walla	1 cup	3	2	5
turkey w/beans	Hormel	1 cup	3	2	1
turkey w/out beans	Hormel	1 cup	3	2	1
vegetarian	Hormel	1 cup	2	3	0
vegetarian	Natural Touch	1 cup	3	1	4

PREPARED MEALS

PREPARED MEAL ITEM	SPECIFICATIONS	BRAND NAME	SERVING SIZE	PROTEIN BLOCKS	CARBOHYDRATE BLOCKS	FAT BLOCKS
	vegetarian	Worthington	1 cup	3	1	5
	vegetarian, all varieties except burrito flavor	Health Valley Nonfat	1/2 cup	1	1	0
	vegetarian, burrito flavor	Health Valley	1/2 cup	1	1	0
	w/macaroni	Hormel Chili Mac	7.5-oz. can	2	2	3
	w/macaroni	Hormel Chili Mac Micro Cup	1 cont.	2	2	3
Chili freeze-dried	w/beef, beans	Mountain House	1 cup	2	2	1
	w/beef, macaroni	Mountain House	1 cup	2	3	2
Chili frozen	w/beans	Stouffer's Entree	1 pkg.	2	2	3
	w/cornbread	Marie Callender's Dinner	1 pkg.	2	4	4
	three bean	Lean Cuisine Entree	1 pkg.	1	3	2
	vegetarian	Tabachnik Side Dish	1 pkg.	2	2	2
Chimichanga, frozen	beef	Old El Paso	4.5-oz. pc.	1	4	7
	beefsteak and bean	Don Miguel	7 oz.	2	6	4
	chicken	Don Miguel	7 oz.	2	5	4
	chicken	Old El Paso	4.5-oz. pc.	2	4	5
Chimichanga dinner, frozen	beef	Chi-Chi's	15 oz.	4	7	9
	chicken	Chi-Chi's	15 oz.	3	7	8
Chimichanga entree	frozen	Banquet	9.5 oz.	2	5	3
Egg breakfast, freeze-dried	w/bacon	Mountain House	1/2 cup	2	1	3
	w/bacon, precooked	Mountain House	1/2 cup	1	1	2
	omelet, cheese	Mountain House	1/2 cup	2	1	4
Egg breakfast, frozen see also specific listings	omelet, ham-cheese	Weight Watchers	1 pkg.	2	3	2
	patty, egg, w/Canadian bacon	Swanson Great Starts	1 pkg.	1	3	2
	patty, egg, w/pork and turkey	Swanson Great Starts	1 pkg.	2	3	3
	scrambled	Swanson Great Starts Egg Product	1 pkg.	3	2	4
	scrambled	Swanson Great Starts Low Fat	1 pkg.	3	2	4
	scrambled and bacon	Swanson Great Starts	1 pkg.	4	2	6
	scrambled w/homefries	Swanson Great Starts	1 pkg.	3	1	4

Food	Description	Brand	Amount	P	C	F
Egg breakfast sandwich, frozen	scrambled and sausage	Swanson Great Starts	1 pkg.	6	2	9
	w/cheese	Swanson Great Starts	1 pkg.	4	4	6
	muffin	Weight Watchers	1 pkg.	2	3	2
	muffin w/bacon and cheese	Swanson Great Starts	1 pkg.	3	3	5
	muffin w/Canadian bacon and cheese	Hormel Quick Meal	1 pkg.	2	3	3
	muffin w/sausage and cheese	Hormel Quick Meal	1 pkg.	2	3	8
	omelet	Weight Watchers Classic	1 pkg.	2	3	2
Eggplant entree, frozen	cutlets	Celentano	5 oz.	1	2	8
	parmigiana	Celentano	10-oz. pkg.	2	1	9
	parmigiana	Celentano 14 oz.	1/2 pkg.	2	1	7
	parmigiana	Celentano Value Pack	1 cup, 8 oz	1	1	8
	parmigiana	Mrs. Paul's	1/2 cup	3	2	5
	rollettes	Celentano	10 oz.	1	2	7
	rollettes	Celentano Great Choice	10 oz.	2	4	5
Enchilada, canned	beef	Gebhardt	2 pcs.	2	2	6
Enchilada, dinner, frozen	beef	Amy's	1 pkg.	1	4	3
	beef	Chi-Chi's Baja	1 pkg.	4	8	6
	beef	Healthy Choice, Rio Grande	1 pkg.	2	0	3
	beef	Patio	1 pkg.	2	5	3
	beef	Patio Chili 'n Beans Large	2 pcs.	2	3	2
	beef, chili sauce w/	Swanson	1 pkg.	4	6	6
	beef and cheese	Banquet Family	1 pc.	1	2	5
	cheese	Patio Chili 'n Beans	2 pcs.	2	3	2
	chicken	Patio	1 pkg.	2	5	3
	chicken	Chi-Chi's Suprema	1 pkg.	3	7	8
	chicken	Healthy Choice Suprema	1 pkg.	2	6	3
Enchilada entree, frozen	beef	Patio	1 pkg.	2	5	3
	beef	Banquet	1 pkg.	1	5	4
	beef and tamale, chili gravy w/	Patio Family	2 pcs.	1	3	2
	black bean	Morton	1 pkg.	1	4	2
	black bean	Amy's Family	4.38 oz.	1	2	1
	black bean and vegetable	Amy's Family	4.75 oz.	1	2	1
	cheese	Amy's	1 pkg.	2	2	3

PREPARED MEALS

PREPARED MEAL ITEM	SPECIFICATIONS	BRAND NAME	SERVING SIZE	PROTEIN BLOCKS	CARBOHYDRATE BLOCKS	FAT BLOCKS
	cheese	Amy's Family	4.38 oz.	1	1	3
	cheese	Banquet	1 pkg.	2	5	2
	cheese	Patio Family	2 pcs.	1	2	1
	cheese and rice	Stouffer's	1 pkg.	2	5	5
	chicken	Banquet	1 pkg.	2	5	3
	chicken, nacho grande	Weight Watchers	1 pkg.	2	4	3
	chicken and rice	Stouffer's	1 pkg.	2	5	5
	chicken Suiza	Healthy Choice	1 pkg.	2	4	1
	chicken Suiza	Weight Watchers	1 pkg.	2	3	3
	chicken Suiza, w/rice	Lean Cuisine	1 pkg.	2	5	2
Fajita, canned	beef	Nalley Superba	1 cup	2	2	2
	chicken	Nalley Superba	1 cup	2	2	2
Fajita entree, frozen	beef	Tyson Kit	3.6-oz. fajita	1	2	1
	chicken	Healthy Choice Fiesta	7 oz.	3	3	1
	chicken	Tyson Kit	3.6-oz. fajita	1	2	1
Fettuccine entree, frozen	Alfredo	Banquet	1 pkg.	2	4	6
	Alfredo	Healthy Choice	1 pkg.	2	4	2
	Alfredo	Lean Cuisine	1 pkg.	2	4	2
	Alfredo	Marie Callender's	1 cup	1	3	7
	Alfredo	Stouffer's	1 pkg.	2	4	13
	Alfredo, w/broccoli	Weight Watchers	1 pkg.	1	3	2
	Alfredo w/four cheeses	The Budget Gourmet	1 pkg.	3	5	8
	w/broccoli and chicken	Marie Callender's	1 cup	3	3	9
	primavera	Lean Cuisine	1 pkg.	2	3	3
	primavera	Marie Callender's	1 cup	1	3	3
	primavera	Stouffer's Lunch Express	1 pkg.	2	3	6
	battered portions w/chips	Swanson	1 pkg.	4	6	7
Fish dinner, frozen see also specific fish listings						
Fish entree, frozen see also specific fish listings	breaded sticks	Swanson Budget	1 pkg.	2	5	4
		Van de Kamp's Fish'n Fries	6.5 oz.	2	4	6

	Brand	Amount			
baked, w/ shells	Lean Cuisine	9 oz.	3	3	3
cakes	Mrs. Paul's	2 pcs.	2	2	3
and chips	Swanson	1 pkg.	3	4	4
fillets, battered	Gorton's	2 pcs.	1	2	6
fillets, battered	Mrs. Paul's	1 pc.	2	1	4
fillets, battered	Mrs. Paul's Crunchy	2 pcs.	3	2	4
fillets, battered	Van de Camp's	1 pc.	1	1	5
fillets, battered, lemon pepper	Gorton's	2 pcs.	1	2	6
fillets, breaded	Gorton's Crunchy	2 pcs.	3	2	4
fillets, breaded	Mrs. Paul's	2 pcs.	1	2	1
fillets, breaded	Mrs. Paul's Healthy Treasures	1 pc.	2	2	6
fillets, breaded	Van de Kamp's	2 pcs.	2	2	1
fillets, breaded	Van de Kamp's Crisp and Healthy	2 pcs.	1	2	5
fillets, breaded, garlic and herb	Gorton's Crunchy	2 pcs.	1	2	5
fillets, breaded, hot and spicy	Gorton's Crunchy	2 pcs.	2	2	7
fillets, breaded, potato	Gorton's	2 pcs.	2	0	5
fillets, breaded, Southern fried	Gorton's Crunchy	2 pcs.	3	0	2
fillets, grilled, Italian herb	Gorton's	1 pc.	2	2	2
fillets, grilled, lemon pepper	Gorton's	1 pc.	1	1	2
fillets, in sauce	Mrs. Paul's Kitchen	1 pc.	2	2	2
fillets, in sauce, lemon pepper	Healthy Choice	10.7 oz.	2	4	2
grilled, w/vegetables	Lean Cuisine Café Classics	8 7/8 oz.	3	1	7
w/macaroni and cheese	Stouffer's Homestyle	9 oz.	3	4	5
w/macaroni and cheese	Swanson	1 pkg.	2	2	6
nuggets	Van de Kamp's	8 pcs.	1	1	3
portions, battered	Gorton's	1 pc.	4	2	6
portions, battered	Mrs. Paul's	2 pcs.	2	3	7
portions, battered	Van de Kamp's	2 pcs.	2	2	3
portions, breaded	Mrs. Paul's	2 pcs.	2	3	7
portions, breaded	Van de Kamp's	3 pcs.	2	3	3
shapes, breaded	Mrs. Paul's Sea Pals	5 pcs.	2	4	4
sticks	Kid Cuisine Funtastic	1 pkg.	3	6	5
sticks	Swanson Fun Feast Frenzied	1 pkg.	1	5	7
sticks, battered	Gorton's	5 pcs.	3	2	4
sticks, battered	Mrs. Paul's	6 pcs.	3	1	5
sticks, battered	Mrs. Paul's Crispy Crunchy	6 pcs.	2	2	5

PREPARED MEALS

PREPARED MEAL ITEM	SPECIFICATIONS	BRAND NAME	SERVING SIZE	PROTEIN BLOCKS	CARBOHYDRATE BLOCKS	FAT BLOCKS
	sticks, breaded	Gorton's Crunchy	6 pcs.	2	2	5
	sticks, breaded	Mrs. Paul's	6 pcs.	2	2	4
	sticks, breaded	Mrs. Paul's Crispy Crunchy	5 pcs.	2	2	5
	sticks, breaded	Gorton's Value Pack	6 pcs.	1	2	4
	sticks, breaded	Van de Kamp's	6 pcs.	2	3	6
	sticks, breaded	Van de Kamp's Snack/Value Pack	6 pcs.	2	2	5
	sticks, breaded	Van de Kamp's Crisp and Healthy	6 pcs.	2	3	1
	sticks, breaded, mini	Mrs. Paul's	12 pcs.	2	2	4
	sticks, breaded, mini	Van de Kamps	13 pcs.	2	2	5
	sticks, breaded, potato	Gorton's	6 pcs.	1	2	5
Fish sandwich	fillet, frozen	Hormel Quick Meal	1 pc.	2	5	5
	fillet, frozen, w/cheese	Mrs. Paul's	1 pc.	3	4	5
Flounder entree, fillets, frozen	battered	Mrs. Paul's Crunchy	2 pcs.	3	2	5
	breaded	Mrs. Paul's Premium	1 pc.	3	2	4
	breaded	Van de Kamp's Light	1 pkg.	2	2	4
Frankfurter sandwich, frozen		Hormel Quick Meal Jumbo Dog	1 pc.	2	3	7
	bagel wrapped	Boar's Head Bagel Dog	1 pc.	2	0	9
	bagel wrapped	Hebrew National Bagel Dog	1 pc.	2	5	6
	on bun	Swanson Fun Feast	1 pc.	3	5	4
	w/cheese	Hormel Quick Meal Cheesey Dog	1 pc.	1	3	6
	chili w/cheese	Hormel Quick Meal	1 pc.	2	3	7
	corn dog	Hormel/Hormel Quick Meal	1 pc.	1	3	4
	corn dog, mini	Hormel Quick Meal	1 pc.	1	2	5
French toast, frozen		Aunt Jemima	2 pcs.	1	4	2
	cinnamon swirl	Downyflake	2 pcs.	1	5	2
	cinnamon swirl	Aunt Jemima	2 pcs.	1	4	2
	cinnamon swirl	Downyflake	2 pcs.	1	5	2
French toast breakfast, frozen	cinnamon swirl	Swanson Great Starts	2 pcs.	6	4	9
	w/sausage	Swanson Great Starts	2 pcs.	6	3	9
	sticks, mini	Swanson Kids Breakfast	2 pcs.	3	4	5

Food	Description	Brand	Serving			
Haddock entree, frozen	battered	Mrs. Paul's Crunchy	2 pcs.	3	3	4
	battered	Van de Kamp's	2 pcs.	2	2	5
	breaded	Mrs. Paul's	1 pc.	2	2	4
	breaded	Van de Kamp's	2 pcs.	2	2	6
	breaded	Van de Kamp's Light	1 pc.	2	2	3
Halibut entree	frozen, battered	Van de Kamp's	3 pcs.	2	3	7
Ham and asparagus	frozen, bake	Stouffer's	9 1/2 oz.	2	3	12
Ham and asparagus au gratin	frozen	The Budget Gourmet Light & Healthy	8.7 oz.	2	3	4
Ham and cheese sandwich	frozen	Croissant Pockets	1 pc.	2	4	6
	frozen	Hormel Quick Meal	1 pc.	3	5	3
	frozen	Hot Pockets	1 pc.	2	4	5
Herring salad		Vita	1/4 cup	1	2	1
Lamb curry entree	frozen	Curry Classics	10 oz.	5	1	10
Lasagna entree, canned		Hormel	7 1/2-oz. can	1	3	5
		Hormel Micro Cup	7 1/2 oz.	1	3	5
		Libby's Diner	7 3/4 oz.	1	2	2
		Nalley	1 cup	2	3	2
	and beef	Nalley	7 1/2-oz. can	1	2	2
	cheese, three	Hormel Micro Cup	10 1/2 oz.	2	3	6
	Italian	Nalley	7 1/2-oz. can	2	2	2
Lasagna entree, freeze dried		Top Shelf	10 oz.	3	3	5
		Mountain House	1 cup	2	2	3
Lasagna entree, frozen		Celentano	1 pkg.	3	5	5
		Celentano	1/2 of 14-oz. pkg.	2	3	3
	cheese	Celentano 25 oz.	1 cup	3	2	6
	cheese casserole	Celentano Great Choice	1 pkg.	3	4	1
	cheese, w/chicken scaloppini	Celentano Value Pack	1 cup	3	4	4
	cheese, four	Healthy Choice Roma	1 pkg.	4	6	2
		Lean Cuisine Classic	1 pkg.	3	4	2
		Lean Cuisine Lunch Express	1 pkg.	2	4	2
		Lean Cuisine Café Classics	1 pkg.	3	3	3
		Stouffer's	1 pkg.	3	4	6

PREPARED MEALS

PREPARED MEAL ITEM	SPECIFICATIONS	BRAND NAME	SERVING SIZE	PROTEIN BLOCKS	CARBOHYDRATE BLOCKS	FAT BLOCKS
	cheese, Italian	Weight Watchers	1 pkg.	3	4	3
	cheese, three	The Budget Gourmet	1 pkg.	3	4	5
	extra cheese	Marie Callender's	1 cup	2	3	5
	Florentine	Smart Ones	1 pkg.	1	3	1
	garden	Weight Watchers	1 pkg.	2	3	2
	w/meat sauce	Banquet	1 pkg.	2	4	3
	w/meat sauce	Banquet Bake at Home	8-oz. cup	2	3	2
	w/meat sauce	Banquet Family	1 cup	2	0	3
	w/meat sauce	The Budget Gourmet Light and Healthy	1 pkg.	2	3	2
	w/meat sauce	Lean Cuisine	1 pkg.	3	3	3
	w/meat sauce	Marie Callender's	7 oz.	2	3	6
	w/meat sauce	Stouffer's	1 pkg.	4	3	4
	w/meat sauce	Stouffer's	1/3 of 21-oz. pkg.	3	2	3
	w/meat sauce	Stouffer's Lunch Express	1 pkg.	3	4	3
	w/meat sauce	Swanson	1 pkg.	3	4	5
	w/meat sauce	Weight Watchers	1 pkg.	2	4	2
	w/meat sauce, casserole	Swanson	1 pkg.	2	4	3
	primavera	Celentano Great Choice	1 pkg.	2	3	2
	primavera	Celentano Selects	1 pkg.	2	3	1
	sausage, Italian	The Budget Gourmet	1 pkg.	3	4	7
	vegetable	Amy's Family	7 oz.	1	3	3
	vegetable	Banquet	1 pkg.	2	4	2
	vegetable	The Budget Gourmet Light & Healthy	1 pkg.	2	3	3
	vegetable	Lean Cuisine	1 pkg.	2	4	2
	vegetable	Stouffer's	1 pkg.	3	4	8
	vegetable	Stouffer's	1/12 of 96-oz. pkg.	2	3	6
	vegetable w/cheese	Amy's	1 pkg.	2	4	3
	vegetable, cheesy	Swanson	1 pkg.	3	4	4
	vegetable, tofu	Amy's	1 pkg.	3	4	3

Food	Description	Brand	Serving	Protein	Carbohydrate	Fat
Linguine entree, frozen	w/shrimp and clams	The Budget Gourmet Light & Healthy	1 pkg.	2	4	3
Lunch combinations	w/shrimp and clams, marinara	The Budget Gourmet	1 pkg.	2	4	4
	w/tomato sauce and sausage	The Budget Gourmet	1 pkg.	2	4	5
	bologna/American	Lunchables	1 pkg.	2	2	12
	bologna/wild cherry	Lunchables	1 pkg.	2	7	9
	chicken/turkey deluxe	Lunchables	1 pkg.	3	3	8
	ham/cheddar	Lunchables	1 pkg.	3	2	7
	ham/Swiss	Lunchables	1 pkg.	3	2	7
	ham/fruit punch	Lunchables	1 pkg.	2	6	7
	ham/fruit punch, low fat	Lunchables	1 pkg.	2	6	3
	ham/Surfer Cooler	Lunchables	1 pkg.	3	6	3
	pizza, mozzarella, cheddar	Lunchables	1 pkg.	3	3	5
	pizza, mozzarella, fruit punch	Lunchables	1 pkg.	3	7	6
	pizza/pepperoni, mozzarella	Lunchables	1 pkg.	2	3	5
	pizza/pepperoni, orange	Lunchables	1 pkg.	3	7	6
	salami/American	Lunchables	1 pkg.	3	2	10
	turkey/cheddar	Lunchables	1 pkg.	3	2	7
	turkey/ham	Lunchables	1 pkg.	3	3	7
	turkey/Monterey Jack	Lunchables	1 pkg.	3	2	7
	turkey/Pacific Cooler	Lunchables	1 pkg.	2	6	7
	turkey/Pacific Cooler, low fat	Lunchables	1 pkg.	2	6	3
	turkey/Surfer Cooler	Lunchables	1 pkg.	2	7	5
Macaroni dinner	and cheese, frozen	Swanson Budget	1 pkg.	2	4	4
Macaroni entree, canned	and beef	Kid's Kitchen Beefy	7 1/2 oz.	2	2	2
	and beef	Kid's Kitchen Cheezy Mac & Beef	7 1/2 oz.	2	4	2
	and beef	Libby's Diner	7 3/4 oz.	1	3	3
	and cheese	Chef Boyardee Bowl	7 1/2 oz.	1	3	0
	and cheese	Franco-American	1 cup	2	3	2
	and cheese	Hormel Micro Cup	7 1/2 oz.	2	3	3
	and cheese	Libby's Diner	7 3/4 oz.	2	3	4
	and cheese	Kid's Kitchen	7 1/2 oz.	2	3	7
Macaroni entree, frozen	and beef	Banquet Bake at Home	8-oz. cup	2	3	4
	and beef	Kid Cuisine Riproaring	1 pkg.	2	6	5
	and beef	Lean Cuisine	1 pkg.	2	4	3

PREPARED MEALS

PREPARED MEAL ITEM	SPECIFICATIONS	BRAND NAME	SERVING SIZE	PROTEIN BLOCKS	CARBOHYDRATE BLOCKS	FAT BLOCKS
	and beef	Marie Callender's	1 pkg.	2	4	4
	and beef	Nalley	1 pkg.	1	2	5
	and beef	Stouffer's	1 pkg.	3	4	7
	and beef	Weight Watchers	1 pkg.	2	2	2
	and beef, casserole	Healthy Choice	1 pkg.	2	3	3
	and beef, casserole	Swanson	1 pkg.	1	4	2
	broccoli	Swanson Mac & More	1 pkg.	2	3	3
	and cheese	Amy's	1 pkg.	3	6	3
	and cheese	Banquet	1 pkg.	2	5	4
	and cheese	Banquet Bake at Home	8 oz.	2	4	3
	and cheese	Banquet Family	1 cup	1	3	2
	and cheese	The Budget Gourmet Homestyle	1 pkg.	2	4	7
	and cheese	The Budget Gourmet Side Dish	6 oz.	2	3	4
	and cheese	Healthy Choice	1 pkg.	2	4	1
	and cheese	Kid Cuisine Magical	1 pkg.	1	7	4
	and cheese	Lean Cuisine	1 pkg.	2	4	2
	and cheese	Marie Callender's	1 pkg.	3	5	6
	and cheese	Morton	1 pkg.	1	4	1
	and cheese	Morton 16/28 oz.	1 cup	1	4	1
	and cheese	Stouffer's	1/2 of 12-oz. pkg.	2	3	6
	and cheese	Stouffer's	1/5 of 40-oz. pkg.	2	3	5
	and cheese	Swanson Entree	1 pkg.	2	4	3
	and cheese	Swanson Entree	1 cup	2	4	3
	and cheese	Swanson Mac & More Classic	1 pkg.	2	3	3
	and cheese	Tabatchnik Side Dish	1 pkg.	2	3	4
	and cheese	Weight Watchers	1 pkg.	2	4	2
	and cheese bake casserole, 3 cheese	Swanson	1 pkg.	3	6	5
	and cheese, and broccoli	Lean Cuisine Lunch Express	1 pkg.	2	3	2
	and cheese, w/cheddar and Parmesan	The Budget Gourmet Light & Healthy	1 pkg.	1	5	3

Food	Brand	Serving			
and cheese, cheddar, white	Swanson Mac & More	1 pkg.	2	3	2
and cheese, pie	Banquet	1 pkg.	1	4	1
and cheese, salsa	Swanson Mac & More	1 pkg.	3	3	2
Italiano	Swanson Mac & More	1 pkg.	5	4	1
soy cheeze	Amy's	1 pkg.	7	4	3
Manicotti entree, frozen — cheese	Celentano	1 pkg.	5	2	2
cheese	Celentano	1/2 of 14-oz. pkg.	1	4	2
cheese	Celentano Great Choice	1 pkg.	5	2	2
cheese	Celentano Value Pack	2 pcs., 8 oz.	5	3	3
cheese	Stouffer's	1 pkg.	2	3	2
cheese	Weight Watchers	1 pkg.	7	4	3
cheese, w/meat sauce	The Budget Gourmet	1 pkg.	3	4	2
cheese, three cheese	Healthy Choice	1 pkg.	2	3	2
Florentine	Celentano	1 pkg.	2	4	2
Florentine	Celentano Great Choice	1 pkg.	2	4	2
Meat loaf dinner, frozen	Banquet	1 pkg.	13	4	4
	Healthy Choice	1 pkg.	3	4	2
	Marie Callender's	1 pkg.	10	4	3
	Swanson	1 pkg.	5	4	4
	Swanson Budget	1 pkg.	6	3	4
	Swanson Hungry Man	1 pkg.	9	7	6
Meat loaf entree, frozen	Banquet Homestyle	1 pkg.	6	2	2
w/whipped potato	Lean Cuisine	1 pkg.	8	2	3
	Stouffer's Homestyle	1 pkg.	4	2	3
tomato sauce, w/	Morton	1 pkg.	5	1	1
w/sauce and vegetables	Swanson	1 pkg.	11	2	3
Meatball entree, frozen — kofta curry	Deep	1 pkg.	3	4	3
Swedish	The Budget Gourmet	1 pkg.	8	4	3
Swedish	Healthy Choice	1 pkg.	3	3	3
Swedish	Stouffer's	1 pkg.	6	3	2
Swedish	Weight Watchers	1 pkg.	3	3	3
Swedish, w/broccoli	Stouffer's Lunch Express	1 pkg.	11	4	3
Swedish, w/pasta	Lean Cuisine	1 pkg.	5	2	2
Swedish, w/pasta	Stouffer's Lunch Express	1 pkg.			
Meatball stew, canned	Dinty Moore	1 cup			

PREPARED MEAL ITEM	SPECIFICATIONS	BRAND NAME	SERVING SIZE	PROTEIN BLOCKS	CARBOHYDRATE BLOCKS	FAT BLOCKS
Mexican dinner, frozen see also specific listing		Dinty Moore Cup	7.5 oz.	2	2	5
		Patio	1 pkg.	2	5	5
	style	Patio Fiesta	1 pkg.	2	4	3
	style	Patio Ranchera	1 pkg.	2	5	5
	style	Banquet	1 pkg.	4	9	11
	style	Swanson Budget	1 pkg.	4	5	5
	style	Swanson Hungry Man	1 pkg.	8	8	12
	style, combination	Swanson	1 pkg.	4	5	6
		Banquet	1 pkg.	2	5	4
Mexican entree, frozen, see also specific listings	combination	Banquet	1 pkg.	2	5	4
Noodle entree, canned	w/beef	Hunt's Homestyle	1 cup	1	2	1
	w/beef	La Choy Bi-Pack	1 cup	2	2	0
	w/chicken	Dinty Moore	7 1/2 oz.	1	2	3
	w/chicken	Hormel Micro Cup	7 1/2 oz.	1	2	3
	w/chicken	Hormel Micro Cup	10 1/2 oz.	2	3	4
	w/chicken	La Choy Bi-Pack	1 cup	2	2	1
	w/chicken	Nalley Dinner	1 cup	1	2	2
	w/chicken	Nalley Dinner	7 1/2 oz.	1	2	2
	w/chicken, cacciatore or regular	Hunt's Homestyle	1 cup	2	2	1
	w/chicken, w/mushrooms	Hunt's Homestyle	1 cup	1	3	2
	w/franks	Van Camp's Noodle Weenee	1 can	1	4	3
	rings	Kid's Kitchen	7.5 oz.	2	2	2
	sweet and sour, w/chicken	La Choy Entree	1 cup	1	4	1
	w/vegetables	La Choy Entree	1 cup	1	3	0
	w/vegetables and beef	La Choy Entree	1 cup	1	3	1
	w/vegetables and chicken	La Choy Entree	1 cup	1	3	1
Noodle entree, frozen	and beef	Banquet Family	1 pkg.	2	2	2
	and chicken	Banquet Bake at Home	1 pkg.	1	2	3
	and chicken, escalloped	Marie Callender's	6 1/2 oz.	1	2	5

Food	Brand	Amount	P	C	F
escalloped, and turkey	The Budget Gourmet	1 pkg.	3	5	7
kung pao, and vegetables	Weight Watchers	1 pkg.	1	3	3
Romanoff	Stouffer's	1 pkg.	3	5	8
	Swanson Kids Breakfast Blast Mini	1 pkg.	2	6	3
Pancake breakfast, frozen					
w/bacon	Swanson Great Starts	1 pkg.	4	5	7
w/sausage	Swanson Great Starts	1 pkg.	5	5	8
silver dollar, eggs and	Swanson Great Starts	1 pkg.	3	2	5
silver dollar, and sausage	Swanson Great Starts	1 pkg.	4	3	6
Alfredo	Green Giant Pasta Accents	2 cups	1	2	3
Pasta dishes, frozen, see also "Pasta entree, frozen"					
Alfredo, w/broccoli	The Budget Gourmet Side Dish	5.8 oz.	1	2	4
cheddar, creamy	Green Giant Pasta Accents	2 1/3 cups	1	4	3
cheddar, white	Green Giant Pasta Accents	1 3/4 cups	1	4	4
garden herb	Green Giant Pasta Accents	2 cups	1	3	2
garlic	Green Giant Pasta Accents	2 cups	1	3	3
Florentine	Green Giant Pasta Accents	2 cups	2	4	3
primavera	Green Giant Pasta Accents	2 1/4 cups	2	4	4
spirals, and chicken	Libby's Diner	7 3/4 oz.	1	1	1
Pasta entree, canned, see also specific listings					
twists	Franco-American	1 cup	1	4	2
primavera	Mountain House	1 cup	1	3	2
Pasta entree, freeze-dried					
Roma	Alpine Aire	1 1/2 cups	3	5	0
cheddar bake w/	Lean Cuisine	1 pkg.	2	3	2
Pasta entree, frozen, see also "Pasta dishes, frozen" and specific pasta listings					
cheddar and broccoli	Banquet	1 pkg.	2	5	4
and chicken marinara	Lean Cuisine Lunch Express	1 pkg.	2	4	2
marinara twist	Lean Cuisine	1 pkg.	1	4	1
primavera, w/chicken	Marie Callender's	1 cup	2	2	6
rings	Swanson Fun Feast Razzlin'	1 pkg.	3	6	4
sausage and peppers	Banquet	1 pkg.	2	4	4

PREPARED MEALS

Zone Food Blocks for Prepared Meals 379

PREPARED MEAL ITEM	SPECIFICATIONS	BRAND NAME	SERVING SIZE	PROTEIN BLOCKS	CARBOHYDRATE BLOCKS	FAT BLOCKS
	and spinach Romano	Weight Watchers	1 pkg.	2	3	3
	w/tomato basil sauce	Weight Watchers	1 pkg.	2	3	3
	and tuna casserole	Lean Cuisine Lunch Express	1 pkg.	3	4	2
	and turkey Dijon	Lean Cuisine Lunch Express	1 pkg.	2	3	2
	vegetable Italiano	Healthy Choice	1 pkg.	1	5	0
	wheels and cheese	Swanson Fun Feast	1 pkg.	2	6	4
	wide ribbon w/ricotta	The Budget Gourmet	1 pkg.	2	6	2
Penne entree, canned	in meat sauce	Franco-American	1 cup	1	6	0
Penne entree, frozen	w/sausage	The Budget Gourmet Light & Healthy	1 pkg.	2	7	1
Pepper "steak" entree, vegetarian	spicy and ricotta	Weight Watchers	1 pkg.	2	6	0
	w/sun-dried tomato	Weight Watchers	1 pkg.	2	6	1
	frozen	Hain	10 oz.	4	4	2
Pepperoni bagel sandwich	frozen	Hormel Quick Meal	1 pc.	2	4	5
Pierogi, frozen or refrigerated	potato cheese	Empire Kosher	4 oz.	2	4	1
Pizza, frozen	potato onion	Empire Kosher	4 oz.	1	4	0
	potato onion	Giorgio	3 pcs.	1	4	1
	artichoke heart	Wolfgang Puck	1 pie	2	3	6
	Canadian bacon	Tombstone Original 12"	1/4 pie	3	4	5
	Canadian bacon	Totino's Party	1 pie	2	3	5
	Canadian bacon	Jeno's Crisp 'n Tasty	1 pie	2	5	6
	Canadian bacon	Celentano Thick Crust	1/2 pie	3	6	4
	cheese	Celeste Large	1/4 pie	2	3	5
	cheese	Celeste for One	1 pie	3	6	8
	cheese	Empire Kosher 3 Pack	1 pie	1	2	3
	cheese	Empire Kosher 10 oz.	1/2 pie	3	4	4
	cheese	Jeno's Crisp 'n Tasty	1 pie	3	5	6
	cheese	Jeno's Microwave	1 pie	1	3	6
	cheese	Swanson Fun Feast	1 pie	2	6	3
	cheese	Tombstone For One 1/2 Less Fat	1 pie	3	5	3

cheese	Totino's Microwave	1 pie	1	3	4
cheese	Totino's Party	1/2 pie	2	3	5
cheese	Totino's Party Family Size	1/3 pie	2	4	5
cheese, extra	Marie Callender's	1/2 pie	2	3	8
cheese, extra	Tombstone Original 9"	1/2 pie	3	4	6
cheese, extra	Tombstone Original 12"	1/4 pie	3	4	6
cheese, extra	Tombstone For One	1 pie	4	4	10
cheese, extra	Weight Watchers	1 pie	3	5	4
cheese, three	Pappalo's Deep Dish	1/4 pie	3	5	4
cheese, three	Pappalo's Deep Dish for One	1 pie	4	6	7
cheese, three	Pappalo's For One	1 pie	4	5	7
cheese, three	Pappalo's 9"	1/2 pie	3	5	5
cheese, three	Pappalo's 12"	1/4 pie	3	5	4
cheese, three	Totino's Select	1/3 pie	2	3	5
cheese, three, Italian	Tombstone Thin crust	1/4 pie	3	3	7
cheese, four	Celeste for One	1 pie	3	3	10
cheese, four	Tombstone Special Order 12"	1/5 pie	4	4	6
cheese, four	Wolfgang Puck	1/2 pie	3	4	5
cheese, four, hot and zesty	Celeste For One	1 pie	3	5	9
cheese, four, zesty	Celeste Large	1/4 pie	2	3	5
cheese, two, w/Canadian bacon	Totino's Select	1/3 pie	2	3	5
cheese, two, w/pepperoni	Totino's Select	1/3 pie	2	3	7
cheese, two, w/sausage	Totino's Select	1/3 pie	2	3	6
chicken and broccoli	Marie Callender's	1/2 pie	3	4	5
combination	Jeno's Microwave	1 pie	2	3	6
combination	Jeno's Crisp 'n Tasty	1 pie	2	5	9
combination	Totino's Microwave	1 pie	2	3	6
combination	Totino's Party	1/2 pie	2	4	7
combination	Totino's Party Family	1/4 pie	2	3	5
combination	Weight Watchers	1 pie	3	5	4
deluxe	Celeste Large	1/4 pie	2	3	6
deluxe	Celeste for One	1 pie	3	5	10
deluxe	Marie Callender's	1/2 pie	2	3	8
deluxe	Tombstone Original 9"	1/3 pie	2	3	5
deluxe	Tombstone Original 12"	1/4 pie	2	3	5
hamburger	Jeno's Crisp 'n Tasty	1 pie	3	5	8

PREPARED MEAL ITEM	SPECIFICATIONS	BRAND NAME	SERVING SIZE	PROTEIN BLOCKS	CARBOHYDRATE BLOCKS	FAT BLOCKS
	hamburger	Tombstone Original 9"	1/3 pie	2	3	5
	hamburger	Tombstone Original 12"	1/5 pie	2	3	5
	hamburger	Totino's Party	1/2 pie	2	3	6
	Italiano, zesty	Totino's Party	1/2 pie	2	4	7
	w/meat	Celeste Suprema for One	1 pie	4	5	10
	w/meat	Celeste Suprema, Large	1/5 pie	2	3	5
	meat, five	Marie Callender's	1/2 pie	2	4	5
	meat, four	Tombstone Special Order 9"	1/3 pie	3	4	7
	meat, four	Tombstone Special Order 12"	1/6 pie	2	3	6
	meat, four, combo, Italian	Tombstone Thin Crust	1/4 pie	3	3	8
	meat, three	Jeno's Crisp 'n Tasty	1 pie	3	5	9
	meat, three	Totino's Party	1/2 pie	2	3	6
	Mexican style, supreme taco	Tombstone Thin Crust	1/4 pie	2	3	8
	Mexican style, zesty	Totino's Microwave	1 pie	1	3	5
	Mexican style, zesty	Totino's Party	1/2 pie	2	4	6
	pepperoni	Celeste Large	1/4 pie	2	3	7
	pepperoni	Celeste Pizza for One	1 pie	3	5	9
	pepperoni	Hormel Quick Meal	1 pie	3	5	5
	pepperoni	Jeno's Microwave	1 pie	1	3	5
	pepperoni	Jeno's Crisp 'n Tasty	1 pie	2	5	9
	pepperoni	Marie Callender's	1/2 pie	2	3	10
	pepperoni	Pappalo's Deep Dish	1/5 pie	2	3	5
	pepperoni	Pappalo's Deep Dish for One	1 pie	4	7	9
	pepperoni	Pappalo's for One	1 pie	4	5	9
	pepperoni	Pappalo's 9"	1/2 pie	3	4	6
	pepperoni	Pappalo's 12"	1/4 pie	3	4	6
	pepperoni	Tombstone Original 9"	1/3 pie	2	3	6
	pepperoni	Tombstone Original 12"	1/5 pie	2	3	6
	pepperoni	Tombstone for One	1 pie	4	4	12
	pepperoni	Tombstone for One 1/2 Less Fat	1 pie	4	5	4
	pepperoni	Tombstone Special Order 9"	1/3 pie	3	4	7
	pepperoni	Tombstone Special Order 12"	1/6 pie	2	3	6
	pepperoni	Totino's Microwave	1 pie	1	3	5

	Product	Serving			
pepperoni	Totino's Party	1/2 pie	2	3	7
pepperoni	Totino's Party Family	1/3 pie	2	4	7
pepperoni	Weight Watchers	1 pie	3	5	4
pepperoni, double cheese	Tombstone Double Top	1/6 pie	3	3	7
pepperoni, Italian	Tombstone Thin Crust	1/4 pie	3	3	9
sausage	Celeste for One	1 pie	3	5	9
sausage	Jeno's Microwave	1 pie	1	3	5
sausage	Jeno's Crisp 'n Tasty	1 pie	2	5	9
sausage	Pappalo's Deep Dish	1/5 pie	2	4	4
sausage	Pappalo's 9"	1/2 pie	3	5	6
sausage	Pappalo's 12"	1/4 pie	3	4	5
sausage	Tombstone Original 9"	1/3 pie	2	3	5
sausage	Tombstone Original 12"	1/5 pie	2	3	9
sausage	Totino's Microwave	1 pie	1	4	5
sausage	Totino's Party	1/2 pie	2	3	7
sausage	Totino's Party Family	1/4 pie	2	3	5
sausage	Tombstone Double Top	1/6 pie	3	4	6
sausage, double cheese	Tombstone For One	1 pie	4	4	11
sausage, Italian	Tombstone ThinCrust	1/4 pie	3	3	8
sausage, Italian	Tombstone Special Order 9"	1/3 pie	3	4	6
sausage, three	Tombstone Special Order 12"	1/6 pie	2	3	6
sausage, three	Tombstone Original 12"	1/5 pie	2	3	5
sausage/mushroom	Marie Callender's	1/2 pie	2	3	9
sausage/pepperoni	Pappalo's Deep Dish	1/5 pie	2	4	5
sausage/pepperoni	Pappalo's Deep Dish For One	1 pie	4	6	9
sausage/pepperoni	Pappalo's for One	1 pie	4	5	9
sausage/pepperoni	Pappalo's 9"	1/2 pie	3	5	6
sausage/pepperoni	Pappalo's 12"	1/4 pie	3	4	6
sausage/pepperoni	Tombstone Original 9"	1/3 pie	2	3	7
sausage/pepperoni	Tombstone Original 12"	1/5 pie	2	3	6
sausage/pepperoni	Tombstone For One	1 pie	4	4	12
sausage/pepperoni	Totino's Select	1/3 pie	2	3	6
sausage/pepperoni, double cheese	Tombstone Double Top	1/6 pie	3	3	7
supreme	Jeno's Crisp 'n Tasty	1 pie	2	5	9
supreme	Pappalo's Deep Dish	1/5 pie	3	4	5

PREPARED MEALS

PREPARED MEAL ITEM	SPECIFICATIONS	BRAND NAME	SERVING SIZE	PROTEIN BLOCKS	CARBOHYDRATE BLOCKS	FAT BLOCKS
	supreme	Pappalo's Deep Dish for One	1 pie	4	6	9
	supreme	Pappalo's for One	1 pie	4	5	9
	supreme	Pappalo's 9"	1/3 pie	2	3	4
	supreme	Pappalo's 12"	1/4 pie	3	4	5
	supreme	Tombstone Original 12"	1/5 pie	2	3	6
	supreme	Tombstone Light	1/5 pie	4	3	3
	supreme, Italian	Tombstone ThinCrust	1/4 pie	3	3	3
	supreme	Tombstone For One	1 pie	3	4	8
	supreme	Tombstone For One 1/2 Less Fat	1 pie	4	5	11
	supreme	Totino's Microwave	1 pie	1	3	4
	supreme	Totino's Party	1/2 pie	2	4	6
	supreme	Totino's Select	1/3 pie	2	3	7
	supreme, super	Tombstone Special Order 9"	1/3 pie	3	3	6
	supreme, super	Tombstone Special Order 12"	1/6 pie	2	3	7
	tomato and mozzarella	Marie Callender's	1/2 pie	2	4	6
	vegetable	Celeste for One	1 pie	3	5	5
	vegetable	Tombstone Light	1/5 pie	4	3	8
	vegetable	Tombstone For One 1/2 Less Fat	1 pie	4	5	2
	vegetable, primavera	Marie Callender's	1/2 pie	2	4	3
Pizza, bagel		Empire Kosher	2-oz. pc.	1	2	5
Pizza, croissant, frozen	cheese	Pepperidge Farm	1 pc.	2	4	2
	deluxe	Pepperidge Farm	1 pc.	2	4	7
	pepperoni	Pepperidge Farm	1 pc.	2	4	9
Pizza, English muffin		Empire Kosher	2-oz. pc.	1	2	8
Pizza, French bread, frozen	bacon cheddar	Stouffer's	1 pc.	2	4	2
	cheese	Healthy Choice	1 pc.	3	5	7
	cheese	Lean Cuisine	6 oz.	3	5	1
	cheese	Stouffer's	1 pc.	2	4	3
	cheese, double	Stouffer's	1 pc.	3	4	5
	cheeseburger	Stouffer's	1 pc.	3	3	6
	deluxe	Lean Cuisine	6 1/8 oz.	3	4	9
	deluxe	Stouffer's	1 pc.	3	4	2
						7

	Brand	Serving	P	C	F
pepperoni	Healthy Choice	1 pc.	3	5	3
pepperoni	Lean Cuisine	5 1/4 oz.	3	5	2
pepperoni	Stouffer's	1 pc.	3	4	7
pepperoni and mushroom	Stouffer's	1 pc.	2	4	7
sausage	Healthy Choice	1 pc.	3	5	1
sausage	Stouffer's	1 pc.	3	4	7
sausage and pepperoni	Stouffer's	1 pc.	3	5	8
supreme	Healthy Choice	1 pc.	3	5	2
vegetable deluxe	Stouffer's	1 pc.	3	4	6
Pizza, Italian bread, frozen white	Stouffer's	1 pc.	2	4	9
cheese, four	Celeste	1 pc.	2	3	4
chicken, zesty	Celeste	1 pc.	2	3	3
deluxe	Celeste	1 pc.	2	4	4
pepperoni	Celeste	1 pc.	2	4	4
Pizza nuggets **Pizza pocket, frozen** frozen	Hormel Quick Meal	5 pcs.	1	3	3
deluxe	Amy's	1 pc.	2	4	3
pepperoni	Lean Pockets	1 pc.	2	4	3
pepperoni	Croissant Pockets	1 pc.	2	4	5
pepperoni and sausage	Hot Pockets	1 pc.	2	4	6
sausage	Hot Pockets	1 pc.	2	4	5
vegetable	Hot Pockets	1 pc.	2	4	5
vegetable, pepperoni style	Ken & Robert's Veggie Pockets	1 pc.	1	4	3
Pizza Pops pepperoni	Amy's	1 pc.	2	3	2
sausage, Italian	Totino's	1 pc.	2	3	5
sausage/pepperoni	Totino's	1 pc.	2	3	5
supreme	Totino's	1 pc.	2	3	6
Pizza rolls, frozen cheese, three	Totino's	1 pc.	2	3	5
combination	Totino's	1 pc.	2	4	5
hamburger and cheese	Totino's	1 pc.	2	4	6
meat, three	Totino's	1 pc.	2	4	5
nacho and beef	Totino's	1 pc.	2	4	5
pepperoni and cheese	Totino's	1 pc.	2	4	5
sausage and cheese	Totino's	1 pc.	2	4	6
sausage and mushroom	Totino's	1 pc.	2	4	5

PREPARED MEALS

PREPARED MEAL ITEM	SPECIFICATIONS	BRAND NAME	SERVING SIZE	PROTEIN BLOCKS	CARBOHYDRATE BLOCKS	FAT BLOCKS
Pork dinner	spicy, Italian style	Totino's	1 pc.	2	4	6
	frozen, barbeque	Swanson Hungry Man	1 pkg.	8	8	13
Pork entree, canned	chow mein	La Choy Bi-Pack	1 cup	1	1	1
Pork entree, freeze-dried	sweet and sour, w/rice	Mountain House	1 cup	1	4	3
Pork entree, frozen	cutlet	Banquet	1 pc.	2	4	8
	ribs, barbeque sauce	Swanson Fun Feast	1 pie	5	5	8
	rib-shape patty, barbeque	Swanson	1 pie	5	5	7
	sweet and sour	Chun King	1 pie	2	9	2
Pork sandwich	frozen, barbequed	Hormel Quick Meal	1 pc.	2	4	5
Potato dishes, canned	au gratin and bacon	Hormel	7 1/2 oz.	1	2	5
	scalloped, and ham	Hormel	7 1/2 oz.	1	2	5
	scalloped, and ham	Nalley	7 1/2 oz.	1	3	2
	sliced, and beef	Dinty Moore	7 1/2 oz.	1	3	3
		Goya Rellenos de Papa	2 pcs.	2	3	3
		Goya Rellenos de Papa Cocktail	6 pcs.	1	3	3
Potato dishes, frozen	au gratin	Stouffer's Side Dish	4.6 oz.	1	2	2
	baked, butter flavor	Ore-Ida Twice Baked	5 oz.	1	2	3
	baked, cheddar	Ore-Ida Twice Baked	5 oz.	1	3	3
	baked, sour cream/chive	Ore-Ida Twice Baked	5 oz.	1	3	2
	baked, broccoli/cheese	The Budget Gourmet Light & Healthy	1 pkg.	2	4	3
	baked, broccoli/cheese	Ore-Ida Twice Baked	1 pkg.	1	3	1
	baked, broccoli/cheese	Weight Watchers	1 pkg.	2	3	2
	baked, broccoli/cheese, cheddar	Lean Cuisine Lunch Express	1 pkg.	2	3	2
	cheddar/cheddared	The Budget Gourmet Side Dish	5.5 oz.	1	2	3
	cheddar/cheddared	Lean Cuisine Deluxe	1 pkg.	2	3	2
	cheddar/cheddared, and broccoli	The Budget Gourmet Side Dish	5.25 oz.	1	2	3
	cheddar/cheddared, pocket	Ken & Robert's Veggie Pockets	1 pc.	1	4	3
	scalloped	Stouffer's Side Dish	4.6 oz.	1	3	2
	scalloped, and ham	Swanson	1 pkg.	3	3	4

Food	Description	Brand	Serving	P	C	F
Radiatore entree	three cheese	The Budget Gourmet Side Dish	6.1 oz.	1	2	4
Ravioli entree, canned	vegetarian, frozen	Hain Bolognese	10 oz.	2	5	1
	beef, tomato sauce	Franco-American	1 cup	1	4	2
	beef, tomato sauce	Hunt's Homestyle	1 cup	1	3	3
	beef, tomato sauce	Libby's	7 3/4 oz.	2	2	3
	beef, tomato sauce	Nalley	1 cup	2	4	3
	beef, tomato sauce	Progresso	1 cup	1	5	3
	beef, tomato sauce	Top Shelf	10 oz.	3	3	2
	beef, tomato sauce, w/meat	Chef Boyardee	1 cup	2	4	3
	beef, tomato sauce, w/meat	Franco-American	1 cup	2	4	3
	beef, tomato sauce, mini, w/meat	Franco-American	1 cup	2	4	3
	beef, tomato sauce, mini, w/meat	Chef Boyardee Bowl	7 1/2 oz.	1	3	1
	cheese, tomato sauce	Chef Boyardee	1 cup	1	4	0
	cheese, tomato sauce	Progresso	1 cup	1	4	1
	cheese, tomato sauce, w/cheese	Chef Boyardee Bowl	7 1/2 oz.	1	4	0
	cheese, tomato sauce, w/meat	Chef Boyardee Bowl	7 1/2 oz.	1	3	1
	mini	Kid's Kitchen	7 1/2 oz.	1	4	2
	tomato sauce	Hormel Micro Cup	1 pkg.	1	4	4
Ravioli entree, frozen, cheese		The Budget Gourmet Light & Healthy	1 pkg.	2	4	4
		Kid Cuisine Raptor	1 pkg.	1	6	2
		Swanson Fun Feast Roaring	1 pkg.	2	7	3
	cheese	Lean Cuisine	1 pkg.	2	3	2
	Florentine	Smart Ones	1 pkg.	2	4	1
	in marinara sauce	Marie Callender's	1 pkg.	2	5	5
	parmigiana	Healthy Choice	1 pkg.	2	4	1
	Chinese fried	La Choy	1 cup	1	6	0
Rice dishes, canned	Mexican	Old El Paso	1/2 cup	0	10	3
	Spanish	Old El Paso	1 cup	0	3	0
	Spanish	Van Camp's	1 cup	1	4	1
Rice dishes, freeze-dried	wild, pilaf, w/almonds	AlpineAire	1 1/3 cups	1	10	2
Rice dishes, frozen, see also Rice entree,	Oriental w/vegetables	The Budget Gourmet	5.75 oz.	1	3	4

PREPARED MEALS

PREPARED MEAL ITEM	SPECIFICATIONS	BRAND NAME	SERVING SIZE	PROTEIN BLOCKS	CARBOHYDRATE BLOCKS	FAT BLOCKS
frozen and specific listings						
Rice dishes, mix	pilaf, w/ green beans	The Budget Gourmet	5.62 oz.	1	3	4
	and beans, black	Carolina/Mahatma	2 oz. dry, approx. 1 cup prepared	1	4	1
	and beans, black	Goya	2 oz. dry, approx. 1 cup prepared	1	3	0
	and beans, black, mediterranean, pilaf	Near East	2 oz. dry, approx. 1 cup prepared	1	5	2
	and beans, black, savory	Good Harvest	1/3 cup	1	3	1
	and beans, black, spicy	Spice Island Quick	1 pkg.	1	3	0
	and beans, Cajun	Lipton Rice & Sauce	1/2 pkg.	1	5	0
	and beans, Cajun	Rice-A-Roni	1 cup, prepared	1	5	2
	and beans, pinto	Mahatma	2 oz. dry, approx. 1 cup prepared	1	4	0
	and beans, red	Carolina/Mahatma	2 oz. dry, approx. 1 cup prepared	1	4	0
	and beans, red	Goya	2 oz. dry, approx. 1 cup prepared	1	4	0
	and beans, red	Rice-A-Roni	1 cup, prepared	1	5	2
	and beans, red, pilaf	Near East	2 oz. dry, approx. 1 cup prepared	1	4	1
	and beans, red, spicy	Good Harvest	1/3 cup	1	3	0
	and beans, red, spicy	Spice Island Quick Meal	1 pkg.	1	3	1
	and beans, Spanish	Fantastic Only A Pinch Cup	2.2 oz.	1	5	1
	and beans, tomato herb, pilaf	Near East	2 oz. dry, approx. 1 cup prepared	1	5	2
	and beans, vegetables, garden, pilaf	Near East	2 oz. dry, approx. 1 cup prepared	1	5	2
	beef/beef flavor	Country Inn	2 oz. dry, approx. 1 cup prepared	1	5	1
	beef/beef flavor	Golden Saute	1/3 pkg.	1	5	1

Food	Brand	Serving	Protein	Carbohydrate	Fat
beef/beef flavor	Lipton Rice & Sauce	1/2 pkg.	1	5	0
beef/beef flavor	Rice-A-Roni	1 cup, prepared	1	5	3
beef/beef flavor	Rice-A-Roni Less Salt	1 cup, prepared	1	6	2
beef/beef flavor	Success	2 oz. dry, approx. 1 cup prepared	1	5	0
beef/beef flavor, broccoli	Lipton Rice & Sauce	1/2 pkg.	1	5	0
beef/beef flavor, and mushroom	Rice-A-Roni	1 cup, prepared	1	5	2
beef/beef flavor, pilaf	Near East	2 oz. dry, approx. 1 cup prepared	1	5	2
broccoli, Alfredo	Lipton Rice & Sauce	1/2 pkg.	1	5	2
broccoli, cheese	Mahatma	2 oz. dry, approx. 1 cup prepared	1	4	1
broccoli, cheese	Rice-A-Roni Fast	1 cup, prepared	1	4	4
broccoli, cheese	Success	2 oz. dry, approx. 1 cup prepared	1	4	2
broccoli au gratin	Country Inn	1 cup prepared	1	4	1
broccoli au gratin	Rice-A-Roni	1 cup, prepared	1	5	6
broccoli au gratin	Rice-A-Roni Less Salt	1 cup, prepared	1	5	4
broccoli au gratin	Savory Classics	1 cup, prepared	1	5	2
brown and wild	Success	2 oz. dry, approx. 1 cup prepared	1	4	0
brown and wild, herb	Arrowhead Quick	1/4 pkg.	1	3	0
Cajun	Lipton Rice & Sauce	2 oz. dry, approx. 1 cup prepared	1	5	0
cheddar, white, w/herbs	Rice-A-Roni	1 cup, prepared	1	5	5
cheddar, broccoli	Lipton Rice & Sauce	1/2 pkg.	1	5	1
cheese	Country Inn	2 oz. dry, approx. 1 cup prepared	1	4	1
chicken/chicken flavor	Country Inn	2 oz. dry, approx. 1 cup prepared	1	5	0
chicken/chicken flavor	Golden Saute	1/3 pkg.	1	5	2
chicken/chicken flavor	Lipton Rice & Sauce	1/2 pkg.	1	5	1
chicken/chicken flavor	Rice-A-Roni	1 cup, prepared	1	6	3
chicken/chicken flavor	Rice-A-Roni Less Salt	1 cup, prepared	1	6	2
chicken/chicken flavor	Rice-A-Roni Fast	1 cup, prepared	1	4	2

PREPARED MEAL ITEM	SPECIFICATIONS	BRAND NAME	SERVING SIZE	PROTEIN BLOCKS	CARBOHYDRATE BLOCKS	FAT BLOCKS
	chicken/chicken flavor	Savory Classics	1 cup, prepared	1	6	3
	chicken/chicken flavor	Success Classic	2 oz. dry, approx.	1	3	0
	chicken/chicken flavor, creamy	Lipton Rice & Sauce	1 cup prepared	1	5	2
	chicken/chicken flavor, pilaf	Eastern Traditions	1/2 pkg. 2 oz. dry, approx.	1	4	0
	chicken/chicken flavor, pilaf	Knorr	1 cup prepared 1/3 cup	1	5	0
	chicken/chicken flavor, pilaf	Lundberg Quick Country	2 oz. dry, approx.	1	5	1
	chicken/chicken flavor, pilaf	Spice Island Quick	1 pkg.	1	4	0
	chicken/chicken flavor, pilaf, w/wild rice, Mediterranean	Near East	2 oz. dry, approx.	1	5	1
	chicken and broccoli	Country Inn	1 cup prepared 2 oz. dry, approx.	1	5	1
	chicken and broccoli	Golden Saute	1 cup prepared 1/2 pkg.	1	5	2
	chicken and broccoli	Lipton Rice & Sauce	1/2 pkg.	1	5	1
	chicken and broccoli	Rice-A-Roni	1 cup, prepared	1	5	2
	chicken and mushrooms	Rice-A-Roni	1 cup, prepared	1	6	5
	chicken w/vegetables	Country Inn	2 oz. dry, approx. 1 cup prepared	1	5	1
	chicken w/vegetables	Rice-A-Roni	1 cup, prepared	1	6	2
	chicken and wild rice	Country Inn	2 oz. dry, approx. 1 cup prepared	1	4	0
	chicken and wild rice, almond	Savory Classics	1 cup, prepared	1	6	3
	chili	Lundberg One Step	2 oz. dry, approx. 1 cup prepared	1	4	0
	curry	Lundberg One Step	1 cup prepared	1	4	1
	curry, pilaf	Near East	2 oz. dry, approx. 1 cup prepared	1	5	1
	fried	Golden Saute	1/2 pkg.	1	5	0
	fried	Rice-A-Roni	1 cup, prepared	1	6	4

Food	Brand	Serving Size			
garlic basil	Lundberg One Step	2 oz. dry, approx. 1 cup prepared	1	4	0
gumbo	Mahatma	2 oz. dry, approx. 1 cup prepared	0	3	1
herb, savory	Golden Saute	1/3 pkg.	1	5	2
herb and butter	Golden Saute	1/3 pkg.	1	5	2
herb and butter	Lipton Rice & Sauce	1/2 pkg.	1	5	1
herb and butter	Rice-A-Roni	1 cup, prepared	1	6	3
jambalaya	Mahatma	2 oz. dry, approx. 1 cup prepared	1	5	0
long grain and wild	Lipton Rice & Sauce Original	1/2 pkg.	1	5	0
long grain and wild	Mahatma	2 oz. dry, approx. 1 cup prepared	1	4	0
long grain and wild	Rice-A-Roni	1 cup, prepared	1	5	2
long grain and wild	Uncle Ben's Fast	2 oz. dry, approx. 1 cup prepared	1	4	0
long grain and wild	Uncle Ben's Original	2 oz. dry, approx. 1 cup prepared	1	4	0
long grain and wild, butter and herb	Uncle Ben's	2 oz. dry, approx. 1 cup prepared	1	4	1
long grain and wild, chicken w/almonds	Rice-A-Roni	1 cup, prepared	1	5	3
long grain and wild, chicken and herbs	Uncle Ben's	2 oz. dry, approx. 1 cup prepared	1	4	1
long grain and wild, mushroom and herb	Lipton Rice & Sauce	1/2 pkg.	1	5	1
long grain and wild, pilaf	Near East	2 oz. dry, approx. 1 cup prepared	1	4	2
long grain and wild, pilaf	Rice-A-Roni	1 cup, prepared	1	5	2
long grain and wild, vegetable herb	Uncle Ben's	2 oz. dry, approx. 1 cup prepared	1	4	1
medley	Lipton Rice & Sauce	1/2 pkg.	1	5	1
Mexican	Goya	2 oz. dry, approx. 1 cup prepared	0	4	0
Mexican	Pritikin	2 oz. dry, approx. 1 cup prepared	1	4	1

PREPARED MEAL ITEM	SPECIFICATIONS	BRAND NAME	SERVING SIZE	PROTEIN BLOCKS	CARBOHYDRATE BLOCKS	FAT BLOCKS
	Mexican	Savory Classics Fiesta	1 cup, prepared	1	6	2
	mushroom	Lipton Rice & Sauce	1/2 pkg.	1	5	0
	mushroom, brown	Uncle Ben's	2 oz. dry, approx.	1	4	1
			1 cup prepared			
	onion mushroom	Golden Saute	1/3 pkg.	1	5	1
	Oriental	Golden Saute	1/3 pkg.	1	5	2
	Oriental	Lipton Rice & Sauce	1/2 pkg.	1	5	1
	Oriental	Pritkin	2 oz. dry, approx.	1	4	1
			1 cup prepared			
	Oriental	Rice-A-Roni	2 oz. dry, approx.	1	6	2
			1 cup prepared			
	Oriental	Rice-A-Roni Fast	1 cup, prepared	1	5	4
	Oriental	Savory Classics	1 cup, prepared	1	5	4
	Oriental, and vegetables	Spice Island Quick	1 pkg.	1	4	1
	pilaf, see also specific listings	Casbah	1 oz.	0	2	0
	pilaf	Country Inn	2 oz. dry, approx.	1	5	0
			1 cup prepared			
	pilaf	Eastern Traditions	2 oz. dry, approx.	1	5	0
			1 cup prepared			
	pilaf	Eastern Traditions Harvest	2 oz. dry, approx.	1	4	0
			1 cup prepared			
	pilaf	Knorr Original	1/3 cup	1	5	0
	pilaf	Lipton Rice & Sauce	1/2 pkg.	1	5	0
	pilaf	Mahatma	2 oz. dry, approx.	1	5	0
			1 cup prepared			
	pilaf	Near East	2 oz. dry, approx.	1	5	2
			1 cup prepared			
	pilaf	Rice-A-Roni	1 cup, prepared	1	6	3
	pilaf	Success	2 oz. dry, approx.	1	5	0
			1 cup prepared			
	pilaf, almond, toasted	Near East	2 oz. dry, approx.	1	4	2
			1 cup prepared			

Food	Brand	Serving	P	C	F
pilaf, brown rice	*Near East*	2 oz. dry, approx. / 1 cup prepared	1	4	2
pilaf, brown rice, w/miso	*Fantastic Foods*	2 oz. dry, approx. / 1 cup prepared	1	6	1
pilaf, garden	*Savory Classics*	1 cup, prepared	1	4	2
pilaf, garlic herb	*Lundberg Quick*	2 oz. dry, approx. / 1 cup prepared	1	5	1
pilaf, lemon herb, w/jasmine rice	*Knorr Original*	1/3 cup	1	6	1
pilaf, Mediterranean	*Good Harvest*	1/3 cup	1	3	1
pilaf, mushroom, savory	*Lundberg Quick*	2 oz. dry, approx. / 1 cup prepared	1	4	1
pilaf, nutted	*Casbah*	1 oz.	0	2	0
pilaf, three grain	*Fantastic Foods*	2 oz. dry, approx. / 1 cup prepared	1	5	1
pilaf, primavera	*Goya*	2 oz. dry, approx. / 1 cup prepared	1	4	0
risotto	*Rice-A-Roni*	1 cup, prepared	1	5	3
risotto, broccoli au gratin	*Knorr*	1/3 cup	1	6	1
risotto, chicken	*Lipton Rice & Sauce*	1/2 pkg.	1	5	1
risotto, garlic primavera	*Lundberg*	1/4 cup	1	3	0
risotto, Italian herb	*Lundberg*	1/4 cup	1	3	0
risotto, Milanese	*Knorr*	1/3 cup	1	7	0
risotto, mushroom	*Knorr*	1/3 cup	1	7	0
risotto, onion herb	*Knorr*	1/4 cup	1	7	0
risotto, Parmesan, creamy	*Lundberg*	1/3 cup	1	3	1
risotto, primavera	*Knorr*	1/4 cup	1	7	0
tomato basil	*Lundberg*	1/3 cup	1	3	0
tomato-wild mushroom	*Good Harvest*	1/3 cup	1	3	0
Spanish	*Country Inn*	2 oz. dry, approx. / 1 cup prepared	0	5	2
Spanish	*Golden Saute*	1/2 pkg.	1	5	0
Spanish	*Good Harvest*	1/3 cup	1	3	0
Spanish	*Lipton Rice & Sauce*	1/2 pkg.	1	5	0
Spanish	*Mahatma*	2 oz. dry, approx. / 1 cup prepared	1	4	0

PREPARED MEALS

PREPARED MEAL ITEM	SPECIFICATIONS	BRAND NAME	SERVING SIZE	PROTEIN BLOCKS	CARBOHYDRATE BLOCKS	FAT BLOCKS
	Spanish	Rice-A-Roni	1 cup, prepared	1	5	3
	Spanish	Success	2 oz. dry, approx. 1 cup prepared	1	5	0
	Spanish, brown	Arrowhead Mills Quick	1/4 cup	1	3	0
	Spanish, brown rice pilaf	Fantastic Foods	2 oz. dry, approx. 1 cup prepared	1	6	1
	Spanish, pilaf	Casbah	1 oz.	0	2	0
	Spanish, pilaf	Knorr	1/3 cup	1	5	0
	Spanish, pilaf	Near East	2 oz. dry, approx. 1 cup prepared	1	5	2
	Spanish, pilaf, brown	Lundberg Quick Fiesta	2 oz. dry, approx. 1 cup prepared	1	4	1
	Stroganoff	Rice-A-Roni	1 cup, prepared	1	5	5
	vegetable, country	Spice Island Quick	1 pkg.	1	4	4
	vegetable, herb	Arrowhead Mills	1/4 pkg.	1	3	0
	wild and bean	Good Harvest	1/3 cup	1	3	1
	wild and vegetables	Spice Islands Quick	1 pkg.	0	4	0
	yellow	Goya	2 oz. dry, approx. 1 cup prepared	1	4	0
	yellow, saffron	Carolina/Mahatma	2 oz. dry, approx. 1 cup prepared	1	5	0
	and beans	Weight Watchers	1 pkg.	2	3	3
Rice entree, frozen, see also Rice dishes, frozen	and broccoli	Green Giant	1 pkg.	1	1	4
	and chicken, stir-fry	Lean Cuisine	1 pkg.	2	4	3
	fried, w/chicken	Chun King	1 pkg.	1	4	2
	fried, w/pork	Lean Cuisine	1 pkg.	2	5	2
	Mexican, w/chicken	Weight Watchers	1 pkg.	1	4	3
	pilaf Florentine	Weight Watchers	1 pkg.	1	5	2
	risotto, w/cheese and mushrooms	Weight Watchers	1 pkg.	2	4	3
	and vegetables	Green Giant Medley	1 pkg.	1	1	1

Food	Brand	Serving			
and vegetables, Hunan style	Weight Watchers	1 pkg.	2	3	1
and vegetables, Oriental	Green Giant International	1 pkg.	0	4	1
and vegetables, pilaf	Green Giant	1 pkg.	1	1	1
and vegetables, white and wild	Green Giant	1 pkg.	2	1	1
and vegetables, paella	Weight Watchers	1 pkg.	2	5	1
and vegetables, Peking style	Weight Watchers	1 pkg.	2	5	1
Rigatoni, canned — Italian garden sauce	Hunt's Homestyle	1 cup	2	3	1
Rigatoni entree, frozen — cream sauce, w/broccoli, chicken	Lean Cuisine	9 oz.	1	2	1
	The Budget Gourmet Light & Healthy	10.8 oz.	2	0	2
parmigiana	Marie Callender's	7.5 oz.	5	3	2
parmigiana	Marie Callender's Multi Serve	8 oz.	11	1	2
Shells, pasta, stuffed, frozen, w/out sauce — parmigiana	Celentano	4 shells	5	3	2
Shells, pasta, stuffed, entree	Celentano Value Pack	3 shells	4	2	2
	Celentano	1 pkg.	7	3	3
	Celentano	1/2 of 14-oz. pkg.	5	2	2
broccoli	Celentano Great Choice	1 pkg.	1	4	2
Florentine	Celentano Value Pack	3 shells, 8 oz.	5	4	2
marinara	Celentano Great Choice	1 pkg.	1	3	2
	Celentcno	1 pkg.	2	3	2
Shrimp dinner — frozen, Mariner	Healthy Choice	11 oz	4	6	4
	The Budget Gourmet Light & Healthy	1 cup	2	4	2
Shrimp entree, canned — chow mein	La Choy Bi-Pack	6 pcs.	0	1	0
Shrimp entree, frozen — beer batter	Gorton's	6 pcs.	1	2	5
breaded	Gorton's	1 pkg.	1	2	4
breaded	Mrs. Paul's	7 pcs.	4	3	5
breaded	Van de Kamp's	7 pcs.	2	3	3
breaded, butterfly	Van de Kamp's	1 cup	2	3	3
breaded, w/pasta	Marie Callender's	6 pcs.	2	3	5
breaded, scampi	Gorton's	1 pkg.	1	2	4
marinara	Healthy Choice	1 pkg.	1	4	0
marinara	Smart Ones	1 pkg.	1	4	1

PREPARED MEAL ITEM	SPECIFICATIONS	BRAND NAME	SERVING SIZE	PROTEIN BLOCKS	CARBOHYDRATE BLOCKS	FAT BLOCKS
	popcorn, breaded	Gorton's	1 cup	1	2	5
	popcorn, breaded	Van de Kamp's	4 oz.	2	3	4
	popcorn, breaded, garlic and herb	Gorton's	3.5 oz.	2	3	4
Sloppy Joe entree	and vegetables	Healthy Choice	12.5 oz.	2	5	1
	frozen	Swanson Fun Feast	1 pkg.	2	4	3
Soup, canned, ready-to-serve	bean	Grandma Brown's	1 cup	1	2	1
	bean, black	Goya	1 cup	1	3	1
	bean, black	Progresso	1 cup	1	2	1
	bean, black, w/bacon	Old El Paso	1 cup	1	2	0
	bean, black and vegetables	Health Valley	1 cup	1	1	0
	bean, salsa	Campbell's Home Cookin'	1 cup	0	3	2
	bean w/bacon and ham	Campbell's Microwave	1 cup	1	2	2
	bean and ham	Campbell's Chunky	1 cup	0	2	1
	bean and ham	Campbell's Chunky	10.75 oz.	2	3	3
	bean and ham	Campbell's Chunky Ham 'n Bean	10.75 oz.	0	3	3
	bean and ham	Campbell's Home Cookin'	1 cup	0	3	1
	bean and ham	Campbell's Home Cookin'	10.75 oz.	1	3	1
	bean and ham	Campbell's Home Cookin'	1 cup	0	3	1
	bean and ham	Healthy Choice	1 cup	1	3	1
	bean and ham	Progresso	1 cup	1	2	1
	beans and rice, creole	Campbell's Chunky	1 cup	2	3	3
	beans and rice, creole	Campbell's Chunky	10.75 oz.	2	3	3
	beef, barley	Progresso	1 cup	1	1	1
	beef, barley	Progresso Hearty Classics	1 cup	0	2	0
	beef, broth	Swanson	1 cup	1	0	0
	beef, chunky	Campbell's Microwave	1 cup	0	0	2
	beef, hearty	Old El Paso	1 cup	1	2	2
	beef, minestrone	Progresso	1 cup	1	2	1
	beef, noodle	Progresso	1 cup	1	1	1
	beef, pasta	Campbell's Chunky	1 cup	1	2	1
	beef, pasta	Campbell's Chunky	10.75 oz.	1	2	1
	beef, potato	Healthy Choice	1 cup	1	1	1

Food	Brand	Serving			
beef Stroganoff	Campbell's Chunky	1 cup	3	3	5
beef vegetable	Progresso Healthy Classics	1 cup	1	2	1
beef vegetable, country	Campbell's Chunky	1 cup	1	2	2
beef vegetable, country	Campbell's Chunky	10.75 oz.	1	2	2
beef vegetable and rotini	Progresso Pasta Soup	1 cup	1	1	1
borscht	Gold's	1 cup	0	2	0
broccoli, carotene	Health Valley	1 cup	1	1	0
broccoli, cream of	Progresso Healthy Classics	1 cup	0	1	1
broccoli and shells	Progresso Pasta Soup	1 cup	0	1	0
broccoli cheese	Campbell's Chunky	1 cup	2	1	4
chicken	Campbell's Chunky Old Fashioned	1 cup	1	2	2
chicken	Campbell's Chunky Old Fashioned	10.75 oz.	1	1	2
chicken	Progresso Chickarina	1 cup	1	2	1
chicken barley	Progresso	1 cup	1	1	1
chicken, hearty	Healthy Choice	1 cup	1	1	1
chicken, hearty	Progresso	10.75 oz.	1	1	1
chicken, minestrone	Progresso	1 cup	3	1	6
chicken, cream of	Campbell's Home Cookin'	1 cup	3	2	7
chicken, cream of	Campbell's Home Cookin'	10.75 oz.	1		3
chicken, cream of	Progresso	1 cup	1	2	1
chicken, cream of, w/mushrooms	Healthy Choice	1 cup	1	2	1
chicken, cream of, w/vegetables	Healthy Choice	1 cup	1	2	1
chicken broth	Campbell's Low Sodium	10.75 oz.	0	0	0
chicken broth	Campbell's Healthy Request	1 cup	0	0	0
chicken broth	College Inn	1 cup	0	0	0
chicken broth	College Inn Less Sodium	1 cup	0	0	1
chicken broth	Pritikin	1 cup	0	0	0
chicken broth	Progresso	1 cup	0	0	0
chicken broth	Swanson	1 cup	0	0	1
chicken broth	Swanson Natural Goodness	1 cup	0	0	0
chicken chowder, corn	Campbell's Healthy Request	1 cup	2	2	4
chicken chowder, mushroom	Campbell's Chunky	1 cup	1	1	1
chicken noodle	Campbell's Chunky Classic	1 cup	2	2	1
chicken noodle	Campbell's Chunky Classic	10.75 oz.	2	2	1
chicken noodle	Campbell's Home Cookin'	1 cup	1	1	1

PREPARED MEAL ITEM	SPECIFICATIONS	BRAND NAME	SERVING SIZE	PROTEIN BLOCKS	CARBOHYDRATE BLOCKS	FAT BLOCKS
	chicken noodle	Campbell's Home Cookin'	10.75 oz.	1	1	1
	chicken noodle	Campbell's Low Sodium	10.75 oz.	1	2	2
	chicken noodle	Campbell's Microwave	1 container	1	1	1
	chicken noodle	Healthy Choice Old Fashioned	1 cup	1	2	1
	chicken noodle	Progresso	1 cup	1	1	1
	chicken noodle	Progresso	10.75 oz.	1	1	1
	chicken noodle	Progresso Healthy Classics	1 cup	1	1	1
	chicken noodle	Weight Watchers	10.75 oz.	1	2	2
	chicken noodle, chunky	Campbell's Microwave	1 container	1	2	2
	chicken noodle, creamy	Campbell's Chunky	1 cup	3	1	6
	chicken noodle, creamy	Campbell's Chunky	10.75 oz.	3	1	7
	chicken noodle, hearty	Campbell's Healthy Request	1 cup	1	3	1
	chicken noodle, hearty	Old El Paso	1 cup	1	1	1
	chicken noodle, w/mushrooms	Campbell's Chunky	1 cup	1	2	1
	chicken pasta	Healthy Choice	1 cup	1	2	1
	chicken pasta	Pritikin	1 cup	1	2	0
	chicken pasta, penne, spicy	Progresso Pasta Soup	1 cup	1	2	1
	chicken rice	Campbell's Chunky	1 cup	1	2	1
	chicken rice	Campbell's Home Cookin'	1 cup	0	2	1
	chicken rice	Campbell's Home Cookin'	10.75 oz.	0	2	1
	chicken rice	Campbell's Microwave	1 cup	0	2	1
	chicken rice	Campbell's Healthy Request	1 cup	1	2	1
	chicken rice	Old El Paso	1 cup	1	2	1
	chicken rice	Pritikin	1 cup	1	1	0
	chicken rice	Weight Watchers	10.75 oz.	1	1	1
	chicken rice, w/rice	Campbell's Microwave	1 cup	1	1	1
	chicken rice, w/rice	Healthy Choice	1 cup	1	2	1
	chicken rice, w/vegetables	Progresso	1 cup	1	1	1
	chicken rice, w/vegetables	Progresso	10.75 oz.	1	2	1
	chicken rice, w/vegetables	Progresso Healthy Classics	1 cup	1	1	1
	chicken rice, wild rice	Progresso	1 cup	1	1	1
	chicken and rotini	Progresso Pasta Soup	1 cup	1	1	1
	chicken vegetable	Campbell's Chunky	1 cup	0	1	0

chicken vegetable	Campbell's Home Cookin'	1 cup	1	2	1
chicken vegetable	Campbell's Home Cookin'	10.75 oz.	1	2	1
chicken vegetable	Old El Paso	1 cup	1	1	1
chicken vegetable	Progresso Homestyle	1 cup	0	1	1
chicken vegetable, hearty	Campbell's Healthy Request	1 cup	1	2	1
chicken vegetable, nuggets	Campbell's Chunky	1 cup	1	2	2
chicken vegetable, nuggets	Campbell's Chunky	10.75 oz.	1	2	2
chicken vegetable and penne	Progresso Pasta Soup	1 cup	1	1	1
chili beef w/beans	Campbell's Chunky	1 cup	1	3	2
chili beef w/beans	Campbell's Chunky	10.75 oz.	1	3	2
chili beef w/beans	Campbell's Microwave	1 container	1	3	2
chili beef w/beans	Healthy Choice	1 cup	1	3	0
clam chowder, Manhattan	Campbell's Chunky	1 cup	1	2	1
clam chowder, Manhattan	Campbell's Chunky	10.75 oz.	1	2	1
clam chowder, Manhattan	Progresso	1 cup	1	1	1
clam chowder, New England	Campbell's Chunky	1 cup	2	2	5
clam chowder, New England	Campbell's Chunky	10.75 oz.	3	3	6
clam chowder, New England	Campbell's Home Cookin'	1 cup	3	1	5
clam chowder, New England	Campbell's Microwave	1 container	2	1	5
clam chowder, New England	Campbell's Healthy Request	1 cup	1	1	1
clam chowder, New England	Healthy Choice	1 cup	1	2	0
clam chowder, New England	Progresso	1 cup	1	2	3
clam chowder, New England	Progresso Healthy Classics	1 cup	1	2	1
clam chowder, New England, chunky	Campbell's Microwave	1 container	3	3	6
clam rotini chowder	Progresso Pasta Soup	1 cup	1	2	3
corn, country, and vegetable	Health Valley	1 cup	1	1	0
corn chowder	Campbell's Chunky	1 cup	2	2	5
corn chowder	Campbell's Chunky	10.75 oz.	3	2	6
corn chowder	Progresso	1 cup	1	2	3
corn chowder, chicken	Healthy Choice	1 cup	1	3	1
egg flower	Rice Road	1 cup	0	2	1
escarole, in chicken broth	Progresso	1 cup	0	0	0
garlic pasta	Progresso Healthy Classics	1 cup	0	2	0
hot and sour	Rice Road	1 cup	0	1	1

PREPARED MEALS

PREPARED MEAL ITEM	SPECIFICATIONS	BRAND NAME	SERVING SIZE	PROTEIN BLOCKS	CARBOHYDRATE BLOCKS	FAT BLOCKS
	Italian, carotene	Health Valley Fat Free	1 cup	1	1	0
	lentil	Healthy Choice	1 cup	1	3	0
	lentil	Pritikin	1 cup	1	2	0
	lentil	Progresso	1 cup	1	2	1
	lentil	Progresso	10.75 oz.	1	2	1
	lentil	Progresso Healthy Classics	1 cup	1	2	1
	lentil and carrots	Health Valley Fat Free	1 cup	1	1	0
	lentil, hearty	Campbell's Home Cookin'	1 cup	0	2	0
	lentil, hearty	Campbell's Home Cookin'	10.75 oz.	1	3	1
	lentil w/sausage	Progresso	1 cup	1	2	2
	lentil and shells	Progresso Pasta Soup	1 cup	1	2	1
	macaroni and bean	Progresso	1 cup	1	1	2
	meatballs and pasta pearls	Progresso Pasta Soup	1 cup	1	2	2
	minestrone	Campbell's Chunky	1 cup	1	2	2
	minestrone	Healthy Choice	1 cup	1	2	0
	minestrone	Pritikin	1 cup	1	2	0
	minestrone	Progresso	10.75 oz.	1	2	1
	minestrone	Progresso	1 cup	1	2	1
	minestrone	Progresso Healthy Classics	1 cup	1	2	1
	minestrone	Weight Watchers	10.75 oz.	1	2	1
	minestrone, hearty	Campbell's Healthy Request	1 cup	0	2	1
	minestrone, Italian	Health Valley	1 cup	0	1	0
	minestrone, shells	Progresso Pasta Soup	1 cup	1	2	2
	minestrone, Tuscany	Campbell's Home Cookin'	1 cup	1	2	2
	minestrone, Tuscany	Campbell's Home Cookin'	10.75 oz.	1	2	3
	minestrone, zesty	Progresso	1 cup	1	1	2
	mushroom, cream of	Campbell's Home Cookin'	1 cup	2	1	4
	mushroom, cream of	Campbell's Home Cookin'	1 cup	3	1	6
	mushroom, cream of	Campbell's Low Sodium	1 cup	2	2	5
	mushroom, cream of	Healthy Choice	1 cup	0	2	0
	mushroom, cream of	Progresso	1 cup	0	1	3
	mushroom rice	Campbell's Home Cookin'	1 cup	0	2	0
	Oriental broth	Swanson	1 cup	0	0	0

Item	Brand	Amount			
pasta Bolognese	Health Valley Healthy Pasta	1 cup	1	1	0
pasta, cacciatore	Health Valley Healthy Pasta	1 cup	1	2	0
pasta, Chinese	Rice Road	1 cup	0	1	1
pasta, fagioli	Health Valley Healthy Pasta	1 cup	1	1	0
primavera	Health Valley Healthy Pasta	1 cup	1	2	0
Romano	Health Valley Healthy Pasta	1 cup	1	4	0
pea, split	Campbell's Low Sodium	1 cup	1	3	1
pea, split	Grandma Brown's	1 cup	1	2	0
pea, split	Pritikin	1 cup	1	3	1
pea, split	Progresso Healthy Classics	1 cup	1	3	0
pea, split and carrots	Health Valley	1 cup	1	2	1
pea, split, green	Progresso	1 cup	1	3	1
pea, split, w/ham	Campbell's Chunky	10.75 oz.	0	3	1
pea, split, w/ham	Campbell's Chunky	1 cup	0	3	1
pea, split, w/ham	Campbell's Home Cookin'	10.75 oz.	0	3	1
pea, split, w/ham	Campbell's Home Cookin'	1 cup	1	3	1
pea, split, w/ham	Campbell's Healthy Request	1 cup	1	3	1
pea, split, w/ham	Healthy Choice	1 cup	1	3	1
pea, split, w/ham	Progresso	1 cup	1	2	0
penne, hearty, chicken broth	Progresso Pasta Soup	1 cup	0	1	0
penne, zesty	Campbell's Healthy Request	1 cup	0	2	1
pepper steak	Campbell's Chunky	1 cup	1	2	1
pepper steak	Campbell's Chunky	10.75 oz.	3	2	6
potato ham chowder	Campbell's Chunky	10.75 oz.	1	2	3
sirloin burger, chunky	Campbell's Microwave	1 cup	1	2	3
sirloin burger, w/vegetable	Campbell's Chunky	1 cup	1	2	2
steak and potato	Campbell's Chunky	1 cup	1	2	1
steak and potato	Campbell's Low Sodium	10.75 oz.	1	2	2
tomato	Campbell's Chunky	10.75 oz.	0	3	2
tomato	Progresso	1 cup	1	1	1
tomato	Progresso	1 cup	1	1	1
tomato, beef and rotini	Campbell's Home Cookin'	10.75 oz.	1	3	1
tomato, garden	Healthy Choice	1 cup	0	2	1
tomato, garden	Progresso	1 cup	1	1	0
tomato, hearty, rotini	Campbell's Home Cookin'	10.75 oz.	0	1	2
tomato, tortellini	Progresso Pasta Soup	1 cup		2	1
tomato, vegetable	Progresso Pasta Soup	1 cup		1	
	Campbell's Healthy Request	1 cup			

PREPARED MEALS

PREPARED MEAL ITEM	SPECIFICATIONS	BRAND NAME	SERVING SIZE	PROTEIN BLOCKS	CARBOHYDRATE BLOCKS	FAT BLOCKS
	tomato, vegetable	Health Valley	1 cup	1	1	0
	tomato, vegetable, garden	Progresso Healthy Classics	1 cup	0	2	0
	tortellini, in chicken broth	Progresso	1 cup	1	2	5
	tortellini, creamy	Progresso	1 cup	0	1	1
	turkey w/wild rice	Healthy Choice	1 cup	1	2	1
	turkey w/wild rice, vegetable	Campbell's Healthy Request	1 cup	0	2	1
	vegetable	Campbell's Chunky	1 cup	1	2	1
	vegetable	Campbell's Chunky	10.75 oz.	1	3	1
	vegetable	Campbell's Microwave	1 container	0	2	1
	vegetable	Campbell's Healthy Request	1 cup	0	2	0
	vegetable	Progresso	1 cup	0	1	1
	vegetable	Progresso Healthy Classics	1 cup	0	1	1
	vegetable	Weight Watchers	10.75 oz.	0	2	0
	vegetable, barley	Health Valley Fat Free	1 cup	1	2	0
	vegetable, carotene	Health Valley Fat Free	1 cup	0	1	0
	vegetable, country	Campbell's Home Cookin'	1 cup	0	2	0
	vegetable, country	Campbell's Home Cookin'	10.75 oz.	0	3	0
	vegetable, country	Healthy Choice	1 cup	0	2	0
	vegetable, 5 bean	Health Valley	1 cup	1	2	0
	vegetable, 14 garden	Health Valley Fat Free	1 cup	1	1	0
	vegetable, garden	Healthy Choice	1 cup	1	3	0
	vegetable, garden	Old El Paso	1 cup	1	2	1
	vegetable, harborside	Campbell's Home Cookin'	1 cup	0	2	1
	vegetable, hearty	Campbell's Healthy Request	1 cup	0	2	0
	vegetable, hearty	Pritikin	1 cup	0	2	0
	vegetable, hearty, w/pasta	Campbell's Chunky	1 cup	1	2	1
	vegetable, hearty, w/rotini	Progresso Pasta Soup	1 cup	0	2	0
	vegetable, Italian	Campbell's Home Cookin'	1 cup	1	1	1
	vegetable, Italian	Campbell's Home Cookin'	10.75 oz.	1	2	2
	vegetable, Mediterranean	Campbell's Chunky	1 cup	1	2	2
	vegetable, Southwestern	Campbell's Home Cookin'	1 cup	0	2	1
	vegetable, Southwestern	Campbell's Healthy Request	1 cup	0	3	0
	vegetable, vegetarian	Pritikin	1 cup	0	2	0

Food	Brand	Amount			
vegetable beef	Campbell's Chunky	1 cup	1	2	2
vegetable beef	Campbell's Chunky	10.75 oz.	1	2	2
vegetable beef	Campbell's Home Cookin'	1 cup	0	2	1
vegetable beef	Campbell's Home Cookin'	10.75 oz.	0	2	1
vegetable beef	Campbell's Low Sodium	10.75 oz.	1	2	2
vegetable beef	Campbell's Microwave	1 container	0	1	1
vegetable beef	Healthy Choice	1 cup	1	2	0
vegetable beef, hearty	Campbell's Healthy Request	1 cup	0	0	1
vegetable broth	Pritikin	1 cup	0	0	0
vegetable broth	Swanson	1 cup	0	0	0
asparagus, cream of	Campbell's	0.5 cup	1	1	2

Soup, canned, condensed

Food	Brand	Amount			
bean, w/bacon	Campbell's	0.5 cup	1	2	2
bean, w/bacon	Campbell's Healthy Request	0.5 cup	0	2	1
bean, black	Campbell's	0.5 cup	0	2	1
beef, broth, double rich	Campbell's	0.5 cup	0	0	0
beef, consomme	Campbell's	0.5 cup	0	0	0
beef, noodle	Campbell's	0.5 cup	0	1	0
beef, w/vegetables, barley	Campbell's	0.5 cup	1	1	1
broccoli, cream of	Campbell's	0.5 cup	0	1	1
broccoli, cream of	Campbell's Healthy Request	0.5 cup	1	1	2
broccoli, cheese	Campbell's	0.5 cup	1	1	1
celery, cream of	Campbell's	0.5 cup	1	1	3
celery, cream of	Campbell's Reduced Fat	0.5 cup	0	1	2
celery, cream of	Campbell's Healthy Request	0.5 cup	1	1	1
cheese, cheddar	Campbell's	0.5 cup	1	1	1
cheese, nacho	Campbell's	0.5 cup	0	1	3
chicken, alphabet, w/vegetables	Campbell's	0.5 cup	0	1	3
chicken broth	Campbell's	0.5 cup	1	0	1
chicken, cream of	Campbell's	0.5 cup	1	1	1
chicken, cream of	Campbell's Reduced Fat	0.5 cup	1	1	3
chicken, cream of	Campbell's Healthy Request	0.5 cup	0	1	1
chicken, cream of, and broccoli	Campbell's	0.5 cup	1	1	1
chicken, cream of, and broccoli	Campbell's Healthy Request	0.5 cup	0	1	3
chicken, dumplings	Campbell's	0.5 cup	1	1	1
chicken, gumbo	Campbell's	0.5 cup	0	1	1

PREPARED MEALS

PREPARED MEAL ITEM	SPECIFICATIONS	BRAND NAME	SERVING SIZE	PROTEIN BLOCKS	CARBOHYDRATE BLOCKS	FAT BLOCKS
	chicken mushroom, creamy	Campbell's	0.5 cup	1	1	3
	chicken noodle	Campbell's	0.5 cup	0	1	1
	chicken noodle	Campbell's Healthy Request	0.5 cup	0	1	1
	chicken noodle, creamy	Campbell's	0.5 cup	1	1	2
	chicken noodle	Campbell's Homestyle	0.5 cup	0	1	1
	chicken noodle O's	Campbell's	0.5 cup	1	1	1
	chicken w/rice	Campbell's	0.5 cup	0	1	1
	chicken w/rice	Campbell's Healthy Request	0.5 cup	0	1	1
	chicken and stars	Campbell's	0.5 cup	0	1	1
	chicken, vegetable	Campbell's	0.5 cup	0	1	1
	chicken, vegetable	Campbell's Healthy Request	0.5 cup	0	1	1
	chicken, vegetable, Southwestern	Campbell's	0.5 cup	0	2	0
	chicken, wild rice	Campbell's	0.5 cup	0	0	0
	chicken wonton	Campbell's	0.5 cup	0	2	2
	chili beef w/beans	Campbell's	0.5 cup	1	1	2
	clam chowder, Manhattan	Campbell's	0.5 cup	0	2	0
	clam chowder, New England	Campbell's	0.5 cup	0	2	1
	clam chowder, New England	Doxsee	0.5 cup	0	2	1
	corn, golden	Campbell's	0.5 cup	1	2	1
	minestrone	Campbell's	0.5 cup	0	1	1
	minestrone	Campbell's Healthy Request	0.5 cup	0	2	0
	mushroom, beefy	Campbell's	0.5 cup	1	0	1
	mushroom, cream of	Campbell's Reduced Fat	0.5 cup	1	1	2
	mushroom, cream of	Campbell's Healthy Request	0.5 cup	0	1	1
	mushroom, golden	Campbell's	0.5 cup	1	1	1
	noodle, curly, chicken broth	Campbell's	0.5 cup	0	1	1
	noodle, double, chicken broth	Campbell's	0.5 cup	0	1	1
	noodle and ground beef	Campbell's	0.5 cup	1	1	1
	onion, creamy	Campbell's	0.5 cup	1	1	2
	onion, French, w/beef stock	Campbell's	0.5 cup	0	1	1
	oyster stew	Campbell's	0.5 cup	1	1	2
	pea, green	Campbell's	0.5 cup	1	3	1

Food	Brand	Serving			
pea, split, w/ham and bacon	Campbell's	0.5 cup	1	3	1
pepper, cream of, Mexican	Campbell's	0.5 cup	1	1	2
pepperpot	Campbell's	0.5 cup	1	1	2
potato, cream of	Campbell's	0.5 cup	1	1	1
Scotch broth	Campbell's	0.5 cup	1	1	1
shrimp, cream of	Campbell's	0.5 cup	1	2	2
tomato	Campbell's	0.5 cup	0	2	1
tomato	Campbell's Healthy Request	0.5 cup	0	2	1
tomato, bisque	Campbell's	0.5 cup	0	2	1
tomato, cream of	Campbell's Homestyle	0.5 cup	0	2	1
tomato, fiesta	Campbell's	0.5 cup	0	2	0
tomato, Italian, w/basil, oregano	Campbell's	0.5 cup	0	2	0
tomato, rice	Campbell's Old Fashioned	0.5 cup	0	2	1
turkey noodle	Campbell's	0.5 cup	0	1	1
turkey, vegetable	Campbell's	0.5 cup	0	1	1
vegetable	Campbell's	0.5 cup	0	1	1
vegetable	Campbell's Homestyle	0.5 cup	0	1	1
vegetable	Campbell's Old Fashioned	0.5 cup	0	1	1
vegetable	Campbell's Healthy Request	0.5 cup	0	2	0
vegetable beef	Campbell's	0.5 cup	0	1	1
vegetable beef	Campbell's Healthy Request	0.5 cup	0	1	1
vegetable, California style	Campbell's	0.5 cup	0	2	0
vegetable, hearty	Campbell's Healthy Request	0.5 cup	0	2	0
vegetable, hearty, w/pasta	Campbell's	0.5 cup	0	1	0
vegetable, vegetarian	Campbell's	0.5 cup	0	1	0
Soup, canned, semi-condensed, undiluted					
bacon, lettuce, tomato w/chicken broth	Pepperidge Farm	0.7 cup	1	1	2
black bean w/sherry	Pepperidge Farm	0.7 cup	0	2	1
broccoli, cream of	Pepperidge Farm	0.7 cup	0	1	2
chicken curry	Pepperidge Farm	0.7 cup	1	2	3
chicken w/rice	Pepperidge Farm	0.7 cup	1	1	1
chicken w/rice, w/bacon and ham	Campbell's	0.7 cup	1	2	1
clam chowder, Manhattan	Pepperidge Farm	0.7 cup	0	1	1

PREPARED MEALS

PREPARED MEAL ITEM	SPECIFICATIONS	BRAND NAME	SERVING SIZE	PROTEIN BLOCKS	CARBOHYDRATE BLOCKS	FAT BLOCKS
	clam chowder, New England	Pepperidge Farm	0.7 cup	1	1	3
	consomme, Madrilene	Pepperidge Farm	0.7 cup	0	1	0
	corn chowder	Pepperidge Farm	0.7 cup	0	1	3
	crab	Pepperidge Farm	0.7 cup	0	1	1
	gazpacho	Pepperidge Farm	0.7 cup	0	1	1
	hunter's, w/turkey, beef	Pepperidge Farm	0.7 cup	1	1	2
	lobster bisque	Pepperidge Farm	0.7 cup	2	1	4
	minestrone	Pepperidge Farm	0.7 cup	1	1	1
	mushroom, shiitake	Pepperidge Farm	0.7 cup	1	1	1
	onion, French	Pepperidge Farm	0.7 cup	0	1	0
	oyster stew	Pepperidge Farm	0.7 cup	2	1	3
	pea, green, w/ham	Pepperidge Farm	0.7 cup	1	3	2
	vichyssoise	Pepperidge Farm	0.7 cup	1	1	3
	watercress	Pepperidge Farm	0.7 cup	1	1	1
Soup, frozen	barley mushroom	Tabatchnik	1 cup	0	1	0
	barley mushroom, no salt	Tabatchnik	1 cup	0	1	0
	bean, Yankee	Tabatchnik	1 cup	1	2	1
	broccoli, cream of	Tabatchnik	1 cup	0	1	1
	cabbage	Tabatchnik	1 cup	0	1	0
	cheddar vegetable, Wisconsin	Tabatchnik	1 cup	0	1	3
	chicken w/noodles and dumplings	Tabatchnik	1 cup	0	1	1
	chicken w/noodles and vegetables	Tabatchnik	1 cup	0	1	0
	corn chowder	Tabatchnik	1 cup	0	2	2
	lentil, Tuscany	Tabatchnik	1 cup	1	2	0
	minestrone	Tabatchnik	1 cup	1	2	0
	pea	Tabatchnik	1 cup	1	2	1
	pea, no salt	Tabatchnik	1 cup	1	2	1
	potato, New England	Tabatchnik	1 cup	0	2	2
	potato, old-fashioned	Tabatchnik	1 cup	0	2	0
	spinach, cream of	Tabatchnik	1 cup	0	1	1
	vegetable	Tabatchnik	1 cup	1	2	0

Food	Brand / Product	Serving			
vegetable, no salt	Tabatchnik	1 cup	1	2	0
barley, vegetable, hearty	Fantastic Cup	1 pkg.	1	3	0
bean	Bean Cuisine Bouillabaisse	1 serving	1	1	0
bean, black	Bean Cuisine Island	1 serving	1	2	0
bean, black	Knorr Cup	1 pkg.	1	3	0
bean, black	Smart Soup	1 pkg.	1	2	1
bean, black, hearty	Fantastic Jumpin' Cup	1 pkg.	1	3	0
bean, black, Santa Fe	Campbell's Soupsations	1 pkg.	0	5	1
bean, black, spicy, w/couscous	Health Valley	0.3 cup	1	3	0
bean, black, zesty, w/rice	Health Valley	0.3 cup	1	2	0
bean, 5, hearty	Fantastic Cup	1 pkg.	1	4	0
bean, navy	Knorr Cup	1 pkg.	1	2	0
bean, white	Bean Cuisine Provencale	1 serving	1	1	0
bean and ham	Hormel Micro Cup	1 pkg.	1	2	1
beef vegetable	Hormel Micro Cup	1 pkg.	1	1	0
broccoli-cheese, cheddar, creamy	Fantastic Cup	1 pkg.	1	2	1
broccoli-cheese, creamy	Cup-a-Soup	1 pkg.	0	1	1
broccoli-cheese, w/ham	Hormel Micro Cup	1 pkg.	0	1	4
broccoli-cheese, and rice	Uncle Ben's Hearty	1 pkg.	1	3	1
chicken, cream of	Campbell's Instant	1 pkg.	0	2	1
chicken, hearty, supreme	Cup-a-Soup	1 pkg.	0	1	1
chicken noodle	Cup-a-Soup	1 pkg.	0	1	1
chicken noodle, hearty	Cup-a-Soup	1 pkg.	0	1	1
chicken noodle	Hormel Micro Cup	1 pkg.	1	1	0
chicken, rice	Hormel Micro Cup	1 pkg.	1	1	0
chicken, vegetable	Smart Soup	1 pkg.	2	2	1
chili, hearty	Fantastic Cha-Cha Cup	1 pkg.	1	3	1
clam chowder, New England	Hormel Micro Cup	1 pkg.	0	3	1
corn chowder	Knorr Cup	1 pkg.	0	2	0
corn chowder	Smart Soup	1 pkg.	1	3	2
corn chowder and potato, creamy	Fantastic Cup	1 pkg.	0	2	1
corn chowder w/tomatoes	Health Valley	0.5 cup	0	2	0
couscous	Casbah Moroccan Stew Cup	1 pkg.	1	4	0

PREPARED MEAL ITEM	SPECIFICATIONS	BRAND NAME	SERVING SIZE	PROTEIN BLOCKS	CARBOHYDRATE BLOCKS	FAT BLOCKS
	couscous, w/lentil, hearty	Fantastic Cup	1 pkg.	1	4	0
	gumbo, New Orleans	Campbell's Soupsations	1 pkg.	0	4	1
	lentil	Smart Soup	1 pkg.	0	3	0
	lentil, hearty	Campbell's Soup/Recipe	1 pkg.	0	4	1
	lentil, hearty	Campbell's Soupsations	1 pkg.	2	4	5
	lentil, hearty	Fantastic Country Cup	1 pkg.	1	3	0
	lentil, hearty	Knorr Cup	1 pkg.	1	4	0
	lentil, w/couscous	Health Valley	0.3 cup	0	3	0
	minestrone	Smart Soup	1 pkg.	0	2	0
	minestrone, hearty	Fantastic Cup	1 pkg.	1	3	0
	minestrone, hearty	Knorr Cup	1 pkg.	0	3	0
	mushroom, cream of	Cup-a-Soup	1 pkg.	0	1	1
	mushroom, creamy	Fantastic Cup	1 pkg.	1	2	0
	noodle	Nissin Top Ramen Damae	1 pkg.	0	3	3
	noodle	Nissin Top Ramen Oriental	1 pkg.	0	3	3
	noodle, chicken free	Fantastic Cup	1 pkg.	1	2	0
	noodle, Oriental	Campbell's Ramen Low Fat	1 pkg.	0	5	1
	noodle, ring noodle	Cup-a-Soup	1 pkg.	0	1	0
	noodle, beef	Campbell's Instant	1 pkg.	0	2	1
	noodle, beef	Campbell's Ramen Fried Cup	1 pkg.	2	4	4
	noodle, beef	Campbell's Ramen Low Fat	1 pkg.	0	5	1
	noodle, beef	Nissin Cup Noodles	1 pkg.	1	3	4
	noodle, beef	Nissin Top Ramen	1 pkg.	0	3	3
	noodle, beef	Nissin Top Ramen Low Fat	1 pkg.	0	3	0
	noodle, beef, onion	Nissin Cup Noodles	1 pkg.	1	4	4
	noodle, beef, spicy	Nissin Top Ramen	1 pkg.	0	3	3
	noodle, chicken	Campbell's Ramen	1 pkg.	2	4	4
	noodle, chicken	Campbell's Ramen Low Fat	1 pkg.	0	5	0
	noodle, chicken	Campbell's/Sanwa Ramen	1 pkg.	2	4	4
	noodle, chicken	Knorr Cup	1 pkg.	0	2	1
	noodle, chicken	Nissin Cup Noodles	1 pkg.	1	3	4
	noodle, chicken	Nissin Top Ramen	1 pkg.	0	3	3
	noodle, chicken	Nissin Top Ramen Low Fat	1 pkg.	0	3	0

Food	Brand	Amount	Protein	Carbohydrate	Fat
noodle, chicken, broth	Campbell's Instant	1 pkg.	1	2	0
noodle, chicken, curry	Sanwa Ramen Pride	1 pkg.	5	4	2
noodle, chicken, mushroom	Nissin Cup Noodles	1 pkg.	4	4	1
noodle, chicken, mushroom	Nissin Top Ramen	1 pkg.	3	3	0
noodle, chicken, sesame	Nissin Top Ramen	1 pkg.	3	3	0
noodle, chicken, spicy	Nissin Cup Noodles	1 pkg.	4	4	1
noodle, crab	Nissin Cup Noodles	1 pkg.	4	4	1
noodle, lobster	Nissin Cup Noodles	1 pkg.	2	5	0
noodle, pork	Campbell's Ramen Low Fat	1 pkg.	1	4	1
noodle, pork	Nissin Cup Noodles	1 pkg.	4	3	0
noodle, pork	Nissin Top Ramen	1 pkg.	3	4	2
noodle, shrimp	Campbell's Ramen	1 pkg.	5	5	0
noodle, shrimp	Campbell's Ramen Low Fat	1 pkg.	0	0	1
noodle, shrimp	Nissin Cup Noodles	1 pkg.	4	4	0
noodle, shrimp	Nissin Top Ramen	1 pkg.	3	3	2
noodle, shrimp	Sanwa Ramen Pride	1 pkg.	5	4	1
noodle, shrimp, picante	Nissin Cup Noodles	1 pkg.	4	4	2
noodle, shrimp, Thai	Sanwa Ramen Pride	1 pkg.	4	4	2
noodle, vegetable, beef	Sanwa Ramen Pride	1 pkg.	4	4	1
noodle, vegetable, curry	Fantastic Cup	1 pkg.	0	3	0
noodle, vegetable, egg, in broth	Campbell's Soupsations	1 pkg.	1	3	1
noodle, vegetable, garden	Nissin Cup Noodles	1 pkg.	4	3	0
noodle, vegetable, hearty	Campbell's Instant	1 pkg.	1	3	2
noodle, vegetable, miso	Fantastic Cup	1 pkg.	0	3	1
noodle, vegetable, tomato	Campbell's/Sanwa Ramen Pride	1 pkg.	5	4	1
noodle, vegetable, tomato	Fantastic Cup	1 pkg.	0	3	1
noodle, vegetable, tomato	Health Valley Fat Free	0.5 cup	0	2	1
pasta, Italiano	Health Valley Pasta Cup Fat Free	0.5 cup			
pasta, marinara, Parmesan, or Mediterranean					
pasta and bean	Casbah Pasta Fasul	1 pkg.	1	1	1
pasta and bean	Bean Cuisine Ultima	1 serving	1	2	1
pea, green	Cup-a-Soup	1 pkg.	0	2	0
pea, split	Bean Cuisine Thick as Fog	1 serving	1	2	1
pea, split	Knorr Cup	1 pkg.	1	3	1
pea, split	Smart Soup	1 pkg.	1	3	1
pea, split, hearty	Fantastic Cup	1 pkg.	1	3	1

PREPARED MEALS

PREPARED MEAL ITEM	SPECIFICATIONS	BRAND NAME	SERVING SIZE	PROTEIN BLOCKS	CARBOHYDRATE BLOCKS	FAT BLOCKS
	potato cheese, w/ham	Hormel Micro Cup	1 pkg.	0	2	4
	potato leek	Knorr Cup	1 pkg.	0	3	0
	potato leek	Smart Soup	1 pkg.	1	2	0
	rice	Casbah Thai Yum	1 pkg.	0	3	0
	rice and beans	Casbah La Fiesta	1 pkg.	1	3	0
	rice and beans, black	Uncle Ben's Hearty	1 pkg.	1	2	1
	rice and beans, Cajun	Casbah Jambalaya	1 pkg.	0	3	0
	rice and beans, Cajun	Fantastic Cup	1 pkg.	1	5	1
	rice and beans, Caribbean	Fantastic Cup	1 pkg.	1	4	1
	rice and beans, curry, Bombay	Fantastic Cup	1 pkg.	1	4	1
	rice and beans, Mexican	Campbell's Soupsations	1 pkg.	0	4	1
	rice and beans, Northern Italian	Fantastic Cup	1 pkg.	1	5	0
	rice and beans, red	Smart Soup	1 pkg.	1	3	1
	rice and beans, Szechuan	Fantastic Cup	1 pkg.	1	4	1
	rice and beans, Tex-Mex	Fantastic Cup	1 pkg.	1	5	1
	tomato	Cup-a-Soup	1 pkg.	0	2	0
	tomato, basil	Uncle Ben's Hearty	1 pkg.	0	2	1
	tomato, rice Parmesano	Fantastic Cup	1 pkg.	1	4	1
	tomato, vegetable	Campbell's Soupsations	1 pkg.	0	3	1
	vegetable, barley, hearty	Fantastic Cup	1 pkg.	0	3	0
	vegetable, chicken flavor	Cup-a-Soup	1 pkg.	1	1	0
	vegetable, chicken flavor	Knorr Cup	1 pkg.	0	2	0
	vegetable, chicken flavor, creamy	Cup-a-Soup	1 pkg.	0	1	1
Spaghetti dinner	and meatballs, frozen	Swanson	1 pkg.	3	3	4
Spaghetti dishes, mix	w/meat sauce	Kraft Dinner	5.5 oz.	2	5	4
	mild	Kraft American Dinner	2 oz.	1	4	1
	tangy	Kraft Italian Dinner	2 oz.	1	4	1
Spaghetti entree, canned		Franco-American Garfield Pizzos	1 cup	0	4	1
	w/beef	Franco-American Garfield Pizzos	1 cup	2	3	4
	w/franks	Franco-American SpaghettiO's	1 cup	2	3	4
	w/franks	Van Camp's Weenee	1 can	1	4	3

Category	Food	Brand	Serving Size			
	w/franks, rings	Kid's Kitchen	7 1/2 oz.	1	4	2
	w/meatballs	Campbell's Superiore/Franco-American	1 cup	2	3	3
	w/meatballs	Franco-American SpaghettiO's	1 cup	2	3	4
	w/meatballs	Hormel Micro Cup	7 1/2 oz.	1	3	2
	w/meatballs	Libby's Diner	7 3/4 oz.	0	3	2
	w/meatballs	Top Shelf	10 oz.	2	3	4
	w/meatballs, mini meatballs	Kid's Kitchen	7 1/2 oz.	2	3	3
	w/meatballs, rings	Kid's Kitchen	7 1/2 oz.	2	4	3
	rings	Kid's Kitchen	7 1/2 oz.	1	4	2
	tomato-cheese sauce	Franco-American	1 cup	0	4	1
	tomato-cheese sauce	Franco-American SpaghettiO's	1 cup	0	4	1
Spaghetti entree, freeze-dried	w/meat, sauce	Mountain House	1 cup	2	3	2
Spaghetti entree, frozen	Bolognese	Banquet	1 pkg.	2	4	5
	Bolognese	Healthy Choice	1 pkg.	2	4	1
	marinara	Marie Callender's	1 pkg.	2	4	3
	w/meat sauce	The Budget Gourmet Light & Healthy	1 pkg.	2	5	2
	w/meat sauce	Lean Cuisine	1 pkg.	2	5	2
	w/meat sauce	Morton	1 pkg.	1	3	1
	w/meat sauce	Stouffer's Lunch Express	1 pkg.	2	4	3
	w/meat sauce	Weight Watchers	1 pkg.	2	4	2
	w/meatballs	Lean Cuisine	1 pkg.	2	4	2
	w/meatballs	Stouffer's	1 pkg.	3	5	5
Spinach dishes, frozen	au gratin	The Budget Gourmet Side Dish	5.5 oz.	1	1	4
	creamed	Green Giant	1/2 cup	1	1	1
	creamed	Seabrook	1/2 cup	1	1	2
	creamed	Stouffer's Side Dish	1/2 of 9-oz. pkg.	1	1	4
	creamed	Tabatchnick	7.5 oz.	0	1	1
	feta pocket	Amy's	1 pc.	1	3	2
	Indian	Deep Palak Paneer	5 oz.	1	0	6
	souffle	Stouffer's Side Dish	4 oz.	1	0	3
Stir-fry entree, frozen	lo-mein	Green Giant Create a Meal!	2 1/3 cups, as packaged	1	3	0

PREPARED MEAL ITEM	SPECIFICATIONS	BRAND NAME	SERVING SIZE	PROTEIN BLOCKS	CARBOHYDRATE BLOCKS	FAT BLOCKS
	lo-mein	Green Giant Create a Meal!	1 1/4 cups, prepared	5	3	2
	sweet and sour	Green Giant Create a Meal!	2 3/4 cups, as packaged	0	3	0
	sweet and sour	Green Giant Create a Meal!	1 1/4 cups, prepared	4	3	2
	Szechuan	Green Giant Create a Meal!	2 3/4 cups, as packaged	1	2	2
	Szechuan	Green Giant Create a Meal!	1 1/4 cups, prepared	4	2	5
	teriyaki	Green Giant Create a Meal!	2 3/4 cups, as packaged	1	2	0
	teriyaki	Green Giant Create a Meal!	1 1/4 cups, prepared	4	2	2
	teriyaki	Lean Cuisine Lunch Express	9 oz.	2	4	2
	vegetable almond	Green Giant Create a Meal!	2 3/4 cups, as packaged	1	2	2
	vegetable almond	Green Giant Create a Meal!	1 1/3 cups, prepared	5	2	4
Tamale, canned	beef	Gebhardt	2 pcs.	1	2	7
	beef, hot-spicy or regular	Gebhardt Jumbo	2 pcs.	1	2	8
	beef, jumbo	Just Rite	3 pcs.	1	2	6
	chicken	Nalley	3 pcs.	1	3	6
		Old El Paso	3 pcs.	1	3	6
		Van Camp's	2 pcs.	1	2	4
		Hormel	7 1/2 oz. can	1	2	7
		Hormel	3 pcs.	2	2	7
		Hormel	2 pcs.	1	2	7
		Hormel	3 pcs.	1	3	3
Tamale, frozen	Mexican, frozen	Goya	1 pc.	1	3	6
Tamale pie		Amy's	8 oz.	1	3	1
Tortellini dishes	cheese, frozen	The Budget Gourmet Side Dish	6.25 oz.	1	3	3
Tortellini entree, canned	cheese	Chef Boyardee	1 cup	1	5	0

Food	Description	Brand	Amount			
	cheese	Franco-American	1 cup	1	5	1
	meat	Chef Boyardee	1 cup	1	5	1
	meat	Franco-American	1 cup	2	4	3
	ground beef	Chef Boyardee	7 1/2 oz.	1	4	1
Tuna casserole, frozen, noodle		Stouffer's	1 pkg.	3	4	3
Turkey dinner, frozen	breast	Swanson	1 pkg.	2	4	4
	breast, w/pasta	Weight Watchers	1 pkg.	2	4	2
	breast, stuffed	Healthy Choice	1 pkg.	3	4	1
		Swanson	1 pkg.	2	3	2
		The Budget Gourmet Light & Healthy	1 pkg.	3	2	2
	mostly white meat	Swanson	1 pkg.	1	4	2
	mostly white meat	Swanson Hungry Man	1 pkg.	3	6	5
	and gravy, w/dressing	Banquet	1 pkg.	5	6	7
	and gravy, w/dressing	Marie Callender's	1 pkg.	5	5	6
Turkey entree, canned	gravy and dressing	Dinty Moore American Classics	10 oz.	3	3	3
	gravy and dressing	Libby's Diner	7 oz.	2	2	2
	stew	Dinty Moore	1 cup	1	2	1
	stew	Dinty Moore Cup	7.5 oz.	2	2	3
Turkey entree, freeze-dried	tetrazzini	Mountain House	1 cup	3	2	2
Turkey entree, frozen	breast, stuffed	Lean Cuisine Homestyle	1 pkg.	3	3	2
	fettuccine alla crema	Weight Watchers	1 pkg.	2	2	2
	glazed	Healthy Choice	1 pkg.	4	5	1
	glazed	The Budget Gourmet Light & Healthy	1 pkg.	2	4	1
	and gravy, w/dressing	Lean Cuisine Café Classics	1 pkg.	2	3	2
	gravy and	Banquet Homestyle	1 pkg.	2	3	3
	gravy and	Swanson	1 pkg.	1	3	2
	gravy and w/dressing	Banquet Family	2 slices	1	0	3
	medallions	Banquet Toppers	5-oz. bag	2	1	1
	pie or pot pie	Morton	1 pkg.	1	2	3
		Smart Ones	1 pkg.	1	3	1
		Banquet	1 pkg.	1	4	7

PREPARED MEAL ITEM	SPECIFICATIONS	BRAND NAME	SERVING SIZE	PROTEIN BLOCKS	CARBOHYDRATE BLOCKS	FAT BLOCKS
	pie or pot pie	Empire Kosher	1 pkg.	3	4	8
	pie or pot pie	Lean Cuisine	1 pkg.	3	3	3
	pie or pot pie	Marie Callender's	1 pkg.	2	6	15
	pie or pot pie	Stouffer's	1 pkg.	3	4	11
	pie or pot pie	Swanson	1 pkg.	5	5	8
	pie or pot pie	Swanson Hungry Man	1 pkg.	7	7	11
	pie or pot pie	Tyson	1 pkg.	2	5	11
	open face, w/potato	The Budget Gourmet	1 pkg.	2	3	5
	roast	Healthy Choice Country Inn	1 pkg.	4	3	1
	roast, breast, and stuffing	Lean Cuisine	1 pkg.	2	5	1
	roast, w/mushrooms	Healthy Choice Country	1 pkg.	3	3	1
	roast, and stuffing	Stouffer's Homestyle	1 pkg.	3	3	4
	tetrazzini	Stouffer's	1 pkg.	3	4	8
Turkey sandwich, frozen	w/broccoli	Mrs. Paterson's Aussie Pie	1 pc.	2	3	9
	w/broccoli and cheese	Lean Pockets	1 pc.	2	3	3
	and ham w/cheddar	Hot Pockets	1 pc.	2	4	4
	and ham w/cheddar	Lean Pockets	1 pc.	2	3	2
Veal dinner, parmigiana, frozen		Swanson	1 pkg.	4	4	6
Veal entree, parmigiana, frozen		Swanson Hungry Man	1 pkg.	5	7	8
		Banquet	9 oz.	2	3	5
Vegetable dinner, frozen		Morton	8.75 oz.	1	3	4
	w/spaghetti	Swanson	1 pkg.	3	3	4
	patties	Stouffer's Homestyle	11 7/8 oz.	3	4	6
		Banquet Family	1 patty	1	2	5
	loaf	Amy's Country	1 pkg.	2	6	4
		Amy's	1 pkg.	1	4	2
	curry	Patak's	1/2 cup	1	2	3
Vegetable entree, frozen	Chinese, and chicken	The Budget Gourmet Light & Healthy	1 pkg.	0	4	3
	country, and beef	Lean Cuisine	1 pkg.	2	3	1

Food		Brand	Serving			
	Italian, and chicken	The Budget Gourmet Light & Healthy	1 pkg.	1	5	2
	pilaf, Indian	Deep	1 cup	1	5	1
	pot pie	Amy's	1 pkg.	1	4	6
	pot pie	Amy's Nondairy	1 pkg.	1	5	3
	pot pie, w/beef	Morton	1 pkg.	1	4	6
	pot pie, w/cheese	Banquet	1 pkg.	1	5	6
	pot pie, w/chicken	Morton	1 pkg.	1	3	6
	pot pie, w/turkey	Morton	1 pkg.	1	3	6
	Shepherd's pie, nondairy	Amy's	1 pkg.	1	2	1
Vegetable entree mix	stew	Knorr	1 pkg.	1	3	1
Vegetable pocket, frozen, see also specific listings	Bar-B-Q	Ken & Robert's Veggie Pockets	1 pc.	1	4	3
	Greek	Ken & Robert's Veggie Pockets	1 pc.	1	4	3
	Indian	Ken & Robert's Veggie Pockets	1 pc.	1	4	3
	Oriental	Ken & Robert's Veggie Pockets	1 pc.	1	4	3
	pot pie	Amy's	1 pc.	1	4	2
	pot pie	Ken & Robert's Veggie Pockets	1 pc.	1	4	3
	Santa Fe	Ken & Robert's Veggie Pockets	1 pc.	1	4	3
	Tex-Mex	Ken & Robert's Veggie Pockets	1 pc.	1	4	3
Vegetarian entree, see also specific listings	canned	Loma Linda Swiss Stake	1 pc.	1	0	2
	canned	Worthington Numete	3/8" slice	1	0	3
	canned	Worthington Protose	3/8" slice	2	0	2
	canned, choplet	Worthington	2 pcs.	2	0	1
	canned, cuts, dinner	Loma Linda Swiss Stake	2 pcs.	2	0	1
	canned, cutlet	Worthington	1 pc.	2	0	0
	canned, cutlet, multigrain	Worthington 20 oz.	2 pcs.	2	0	1
	canned, cutlet, multigrain	Worthington 50 oz.	1 pc.	2	0	1
	frozen	Worthington FriPats	1 patty	2	0	2
	frozen	Worthington Stakelets	1 pc.	2	0	3
	frozen, croquettes	Worthington Golden	4 pcs.	2	1	3
	frozen, dinner entree	Natural Touch	3-oz. patty	3	0	5
	frozen, nuggets, w/rice	Hain Hawaiian	10 oz.	2	5	2

PREPARED MEAL ITEM	SPECIFICATIONS	BRAND NAME	SERVING SIZE	PROTEIN BLOCKS	CARBOHYDRATE BLOCKS	FAT BLOCKS
	frozen, roast, dinner	Worthington	3/4" slice	2	0	4
	mix, dry, loaf, dinner	Loma Linda	1/3 cup	2	0	1
	mix, dry, patty	Loma Linda	1/3 cup	2	0	0
Waffle breakfast	frozen	Swanson Kids Breakfast Blast	1 pkg.	4	4	6
Ziti dishes, frozen	marinara sauce	The Budget Gourmet Side Dish	6.25 oz.	1	3	3

PART IV

Zone Food Blocks for Fast Foods

More than 50 percent of all meals are now eaten outside the home, and the majority of those come from fast-food restaurants. As you can see in this section, most meals are both carbohydrate-rich and overloaded with fat—a deadly combination. The excess carbohydrate will rapidly increase insulin levels which then drives the excess fat into storage in your adipose tissue. But by using the Zone Food Blocks, you can go into any fast-food outlet and, by picking and choosing (and discarding most of the excess carbohydrates), make a reasonably good Zone meal.

FAST FOOD RESTAURANT FOOD ITEM	SPECIFICATIONS	PROTEIN BLOCKS	CARBOHYDRATE BLOCKS	FAT BLOCKS
ARBY'S				
Breakfasts				
bacon	2 strips	1	0	2
biscuit, plain		1	4	5
blueberry muffin		0	4	3
cinnamon-nut danish		1	7	4
croissant, plain		1	3	4
egg portion		0	0	3
French Toastix	6 sticks	1	5	7
ham		1	0	0
sausage		1	0	5
Swiss cheese	1/2 oz.	1	0	1
table syrup		0	3	0
Lunch items				
chicken fingers	2 pieces	2	2	5
chicken sandwich	breaded fillet	4	5	9
	Cordon Blue	5	5	11
	grilled, deluxe	3	4	7
	grilled, BBQ	3	5	4
	roast, club	4	4	10

FAST FOOD RESTAURANT FOOD ITEM	SPECIFICATIONS	PROTEIN BLOCKS	CARBOHYDRATE BLOCKS	FAT BLOCKS
	roast, deluxe, light	3	3	2
	roast, deluxe, sesame seed bun	3	4	7
	roast, Santa Fe	4	4	7
sandwich, ham 'n cheese		3	4	5
sandwich, ham 'n cheese melt		3	4	4
sandwich, fish fillet		3	5	9
sandwich, roast beef	Arby's Melt w/cheddar	3	4	6
sandwich, roast beef	Arby's Q	3	5	6
sandwich, roast beef	Bac'n Cheddar deluxe	3	4	11
sandwich, roast beef	Beef'n Cheddar	4	4	9
sandwich, roast beef	deluxe, light	3	3	3
sandwich, roast beef	giant	5	4	9
sandwich, roast beef	junior	2	4	5
sandwich, roast beef	regular	3	3	6
sandwich, roast beef	super	4	5	9
sandwich, roast turkey deluxe	light	3	3	2
sandwich, sub roll	French dip	4	4	7
sandwich, sub roll	hot Ham'n Swiss	4	5	8
sandwich, sub roll	Italian sub	4	5	12
sandwich, sub roll	Philly Beef'n Swiss	6	5	16
sandwich, sub roll	roast beef sub	5	4	14
sandwich, sub roll	triple cheese melt	5	5	15
sandwich, sub roll	turkey sub	4	5	9
salads	garden	0	1	0
salads	roast chicken	3	1	1
salads	side salad	0	0	0
soups	Boston clam chowder	1	2	3
soups	broccoli, cream of	1	1	3
soups	cheese, Wisconsin	1	2	6
soups	chicken noodle	1	1	1
soups	chili, timberline	3	1	3
soups	potato w/bacon	1	2	2
soups	vegetable, lumberjack	0	1	1
potatoes, baked	plain 11.5 oz.	1	8	0
potatoes, baked	w/margarine and sour cream	1	9	8
potatoes, baked	Broccoli 'n Cheddar	2	9	7
potatoes, baked	deluxe	3	9	12
potato cakes	2 pcs.	0	2	4
fries	curly	1	4	5
fries	cheddar curly	1	4	6
fries	french	0	3	4
sauces/dressings	Arby's Sauce	0	0	0
sauces/dressings	barbecue sauce	0	1	0
sauces/dressings	beef stock au jus	0	0	0
sauces/dressings	blue cheese dressing	0	0	10
sauces/dressings	buttermilk ranch dressing, reduced calorie	0	1	0
sauces/dressings	cheddar dressing	0	0	1

FAST FOOD RESTAURANT FOOD ITEM	SPECIFICATIONS	PROTEIN BLOCKS	CARBOHYDRATE BLOCKS	FAT BLOCKS
sauces/dressings	honey French dressing	0	2	8
sauces/dressings	honey mayonnaise, reduced calorie	0	0	2
sauces/dressings	Horsey Sauce	0	0	2
sauces/dressings	Italian dressing, reduced calorie	0	0	0
sauces/dressings	Italian sub sauce	0	0	2
sauces/dressings	mayonnaise	0	0	4
sauces/dressings	mayonnaise, light	0	0	0
sauces/dressings	Parmesan sauce	0	0	2
sauces/dressings	red ranch dressing	0	1	2
sauces/dressings	tartar sauce	0	0	5
sauces/dressings	Thousand Island dressing	0	1	9
desserts and shakes				
apple turnover		1	5	5
cheesecake, plain		1	3	8
cherry turnover		1	5	4
chocolate chip cookie		0	2	2
Polar Swirl	Butterfinger	2	7	6
Polar Swirl	Heath	2	8	7
Polar Swirl	Oreo	2	7	7
Polar Swirl	Snickers	2	8	6
Polar Swirl	peanut butter cup	3	7	8
shake	chocolate	2	8	4
shake	jamocha	2	7	3
shake	vanilla	2	6	4

BURGER KING

Breakfasts				
biscuit	w/bacon, egg, cheese	3	4	10
biscuit	w/sausage	2	4	13
Croissan'wich	sausage, egg, cheese	3	3	15
French toast sticks		1	7	9
hash browns		0	3	4
Lunch items				
BK Big Fish		4	6	14
BK Broiler chicken		4	4	10
cheeseburger	regular	3	3	6
cheeseburger	double	6	3	12
cheeseburger	double w/bacon	6	3	13
chicken sandwich		4	6	14
Double Whopper	regular	7	5	19
Double Whopper	w/cheese	7	5	21
hamburger		3	3	18
Whopper		4	5	13
Whopper	w/cheese	5	5	15

FOOD ITEM	SPECIFICATIONS	PROTEIN BLOCKS	CARBOHYDRATE BLOCKS	FAT BLOCKS
Whopper Jr.		3	3	8
Whopper Jr.	w/cheese	3	3	9
Chicken Tenders	6 pcs.	2	1	4
dipping sauces 1 oz.	*A.M. Express*	0	2	0
dipping sauces 1 oz.	barbecue sauce	0	1	0
dipping sauces 1 oz.	*Bull's Eye*	0	1	0
dipping sauces 1 oz.	honey	0	3	0
dipping sauces 1 oz.	ranch	0	0	6
dipping sauces 1 oz.	sweet and sour	0	1	0
side dishes				
fries, medium		1	4	7
onion rings		1	4	5
salad, w/out dressing	chicken, broiled	3	0	3
salad, w/out dressing	garden	1	0	2
salad, w/out dressing	side	0	0	1
salad dressings 1/2 oz.				
	blue cheese	0	0	5
	French	0	1	3
	Italian, light	0	0	0
	ranch	0	0	6
	Thousand Island	0	1	4
desserts and shakes				
Dutch apple pie		0	4	5
shakes, medium	chocolate	1	6	2
shakes, medium	chocolate, w/syrup	1	9	2
shakes, medium	strawberry, w/syrup	1	9	2
shakes, medium	vanilla	1	6	2

CARL'S JR

Breakfast 1 serving				
bacon	2 strips	0	0	1
breakfast burrito		3	3	9
English muffin w/margarine		1	3	3
French toast dips	w/out syrup	1	4	8
quesadilla, breakfast		2	3	5
sausage	1 patty	1	0	6
scrambled eggs		2	0	4
Sunrise Sandwich		2	3	7
table syrup	1 oz.	0	2	0
chicken stars	6 pcs.	2	1	5
sauces	barbeque	0	1	0
	honey sauce	0	3	0
	mustard sauce	0	1	0
	salsa	0	0	0
	sweet 'n sour sauce	0	1	0

FAST FOOD RESTAURANT FOOD ITEM	SPECIFICATIONS	PROTEIN BLOCKS	CARBOHYDRATE BLOCKS	FAT BLOCKS
Lunch items				
Sandwiches	Big Burger	4	5	7
	Carl's Catch Fish Sandwich	2	5	10
	chicken bacon Swiss	4	6	12
	chicken, barbeque	4	3	2
	chicken club	5	4	10
	chicken, ranch	3	6	10
	chicken, Santa Fe double cheeseburger, 1/2 lb.	4	4	10
	double cheeseburger, 1/3 lb.	5	4	14
	Double Western Bacon Cheeseburger	8	3	19
	Famous Big Star hamburger	4	4	13
	hamburger	2	2	3
	Hot & Crispy sandwich	2	4	7
	Super Star hamburger	6	4	18
	Western Bacon Cheeseburger	5	6	12
"Great Stuff" potato	bacon and cheese	3	8	10
	broccoli and cheese	2	8	7
	potato, plain	1	7	0
	sour cream and chive	1	7	5
Entree Salads-to-Go	chicken	4	1	3
	garden	0	0	1
salad dressings 2 oz.	blue cheese	0	0	11
	French, fat free	0	2	0
	house	0	0	7
	Italian, fat free	0	0	0
	Thousand Island	0	1	8
side dishes	*CrossCut Fries,* large	1	6	11
	fries, regular	1	5	7
	hash brown nuggets	0	3	6
	onion rings	1	7	9
	zucchini	1	4	8
bakery products	blueberry muffin	1	5	5
	bran muffin	1	6	4
	cheese danish	1	5	7
	cheesecake, strawberry swirl	1	3	6
	chocolate cake	0	5	3
	chocolate chip cookie	0	5	6
	cinnamon roll	1	7	4
shake, small	chocolate	1	8	2
	strawberry	1	9	2
	vanilla	2	6	3

CHICK-FIL-A

chicken dishes	3.7 oz.	3	0	3
	chargrilled, 2.8 oz.	4	0	1
	Chick-fil-A Nuggets, 8 pack	4	1	5

FAST FOOD RESTAURANT FOOD ITEM	SPECIFICATIONS	PROTEIN BLOCKS	CARBOHYDRATE BLOCKS	FAT BLOCKS
	Chick-n-Strips, 4 pcs.	4	1	3
	Chick-n-Strips Salad	5	2	3
	salad, chargrilled garden	4	1	1
	salad plate	3	4	2
chicken sandwiches	regular	3	3	3
	chargrilled	4	4	1
	chargrilled, deluxe	4	4	1
	chargrilled club, w/out dressing	5	4	4
	Chick-n-Q	4	4	4
	deluxe	4	3	3
	salad, whole wheat	4	5	2
side dishes, small	carrot raisin salad	1	3	1
	chicken soup 1 cup	2	1	0
	coleslaw	1	1	2
	tossed salad	1	1	0
	Waffle fries, salted	0	5	3
	Waffle fries, unsalted	0	5	3
desserts	brownies, fudge nut	1	5	5
	cheesecake	2	1	7
	cheesecake, w/blueberry	2	1	8
	cheesecake, w/strawberry	2	1	8
	Icedream, small cone	2	2	1
	Icedream, small cup	2	6	3
	lemon pie	0	2	7

CHURCH'S CHICKEN

chicken, edible portion	breast 2.8 oz.	3	0	4
	leg 2 oz.	2	0	3
	Tender Strip 1.1 oz	1	0	1
	thigh 2.8 oz.	2	1	5
	wing 3.1 oz.	3	1	5
sides	biscuit	0	3	5
	Cajun rice	0	2	2
	coleslaw	1	1	2
	corn on cob	1	2	1
	fries	0	3	4
	okra	0	2	5
	potatoes and gravy	0	1	1
apple pie		0	4	4

DAIRY QUEEN/BRAZIER

DQ Homestyle
burgers

	cheeseburger	3	3	6
	double cheeseburger	5	3	10
	deluxe double cheeseburger	5	3	10

FAST FOOD RESTAURANT FOOD ITEM	SPECIFICATIONS	PROTEIN BLOCKS	CARBOHYDRATE BLOCKS	FAT BLOCKS
	cheeseburger w/bacon, double	6	3	12
	hamburger	2	3	4
	hamburger, deluxe, double	4	3	7
	Ultimate burger	6	3	14
Sandwiches				
	chicken fillet, breaded	3	4	7
	breaded w/cheese	4	4	8
	grilled	3	3	3
fish fillet		2	4	5
fish fillet w/cheese		3	4	7
hot dog	plain	1	2	5
	w/cheese	2	2	6
	w/chili	2	2	5
	w/chili and cheese	2	2	7
chicken strip basket	w/gravy	5	9	14
	w/BBQ sauce	5	9	12
side dishes				
fries	large	1	5	6
	regular	1	4	5
	small	0	3	3
onion rings	regular	1	3	4
desserts and shakes				
banana split		1	10	4
Blizzard	*Butterfinger*, regular	2	13	9
	Butterfinger, small	2	9	6
	chocolate chip cookie dough, regular	2	16	12
	chocolate chip cookie dough, small	2	11	8
	chocolate sandwich cookie, regular	2	11	8
	chocolate sandwich cookie, small	1	9	6
	Heath, regular	2	13	11
	Heath, small	1	9	7
	Reese's peanut butter cup, regular	3	11	1
	Reese's peanut butter cup, small	2	9	8
	strawberry, regular	2	10	5
	strawberry, small	1	7	4
Buster Bar		1	4	9
cone, chocolate	regular	1	6	4
	small	1	4	3
cone, chocolate-dipped	regular	1	7	8
	small	1	5	6
cone, vanilla	large	1	7	4
	regular	1	6	3
	small	1	4	2
DQ cake, undecorated	heart, 1/10 cake	1	4	3
	log, 1/8 cake	1	5	3

FAST FOOD RESTAURANT FOOD ITEM	SPECIFICATIONS	PROTEIN BLOCKS	CARBOHYDRATE BLOCKS	FAT BLOCKS
	round, 8", 1/8 cake	1	6	4
	round, 10", 1/12 cake	1	6	4
	sheet, 1/20 cake	1	6	4
DQ caramel & nut bar		1	4	4
DQ fudge bar		1	1	0
DQ Lemon Freez'r	1/2 cup	0	2	0
DQ sandwich		0	3	2
DQ Treatzza Pizza 1/8 pie	*Heath*	0	3	2
	M&M	0	3	2
	peanut butter fudge	1	3	3
	strawberry-banana	0	3	2
DQ vanilla orange bar		0	2	0
Dilly bar	chocolate	0	2	4
	chocolate mint	0	2	4
	toffee, w/*Heath*	0	3	4
Fudge Nut bar		1	4	8
malt, chocolate	regular	3	17	7
	small	2	12	5
Misty	cooler, strawberry	0	5	0
	slush, regular	0	8	0
	slush, small	0	6	0
Peanut Buster parfait		2	11	10
Queen's Choice Big Scoop	chocolate	1	3	5
	vanilla	1	3	5
shake, chocolate	regular	2	14	7
	small	2	10	5
soft-serve, *DQ*	chocolate, 1/2 cup	1	2	2
	vanilla, 1/2 cup	0	2	2
Starkiss		0	2	0
strawberry shortcake		1	8	5
sundae, chocolate	regular	1	8	3
	small	1	6	2
yogurt, *Breeze*	*Heath*, regular	2	14	6
	Heath, small	2	9	3
	strawberry, regular	2	11	3
	strawberry, small	1	7	0
yogurt, frozen	*DQ* Nonfat 1/2 cup	0	2	0
	regular cup	1	5	0
	cone	1	7	0
	strawberry sundae	1	7	0

DOMINO'S PIZZA

1/4 of 12" pie (2 slices) except as noted

deep dish				
	cheese	3	7	8
	ham	4	7	8
	pepperoni	4	7	10
	sausage and mushroom	4	7	9

FAST FOOD RESTAURANT FOOD ITEM	SPECIFICATIONS	PROTEIN BLOCKS	CARBOHYDRATE BLOCKS	FAT BLOCKS
	veggie	3	7	12
	X-tra cheese and pepperoni	4	7	11
hand tossed	cheese	2	5	3
	ham	2	5	3
	pepperoni	3	5	5
	sausage and mushroom	3	5	5
	veggie	2	5	3
	X-tra cheese and pepperoni	3	5	6
thin crust, 1/3 pie	cheese	2	4	5
	ham	3	4	6
	pepperoni	3	4	8
	sausage and mushroom	3	5	7
	veggie	2	4	6
	X-tra cheese and pepperoni	3	4	9

JACK-IN-THE-BOX

Breakfast

Breakfast Jack		3	3	4
Country Crock Spread	.2 oz.	0	0	1
croissant	sausage	3	4	16
	supreme	3	4	12
hash browns		0	1	4
jelly, grape	.5 oz.	0	1	0
pancake platter		2	6	4
pancake syrup	1 1/2 oz.	0	3	0
sandwich, breakfast	sourdough	3	3	7
	ultimate	5	4	12
scrambled egg pocket		4	3	7

sandwiches

beef, Monterey roast		4	4	10
cheeseburger	regular	2	4	5
	double	3	4	8
	ultimate	7	3	26
	bacon bacon	5	5	15
	Colossus	8	3	28
	The Outlaw Burger	4	6	13
chicken		3	4	6
chicken, Caesar		4	4	9
chicken, spicy crispy		3	6	9
chicken, supreme		4	5	12
chicken fajita pita		3	3	3
chicken fillet, grilled		4	4	6
The Really Big Chicken Sandwich		6	6	19
fish supreme		3	5	11
hamburger	regular	2	3	4
	quarter-pounder	4	4	9

FAST FOOD RESTAURANT FOOD ITEM	SPECIFICATIONS	PROTEIN BLOCKS	CARBOHYDRATE BLOCKS	FAT BLOCKS
	sourdough, grilled	5	4	14
Jumbo Jack		4	5	11
Jumbo Jack w/cheese		4	5	13
entrees				
chicken teriyaki bowl		4	12	1
taco		1	1	4
taco, super		2	2	6
salads				
chicken, garden		3	1	3
side		1	0	1
finger foods				
chicken strips	4 pcs.	4	2	4
chicken strips	6 pcs.	6	3	7
egg rolls	3 pcs.	0	6	8
egg rolls	5 pcs.	1	9	14
jalapenos, stuffed	7 pcs.	2	3	9
jalapenos, stuffed	10 pcs.	3	4	13
potato wedges w/bacon, cheddar		3	5	19
side dishes				
fries	small	0	3	4
	regular	1	5	6
	jumbo	1	5	6
	super scoop	1	8	10
	seasoned, curly	1	4	7
onion rings		1	4	8
sauces				
barbeque	1 oz.	0	1	0
buttermilk	.9 oz.	0	0	4
soy	.3 oz.	0	0	0
sweet and sour	1 oz.	0	1	0
tartar	1 oz.	0	0	5
dressings, 2 oz.	blue cheese	0	1	6
	buttermilk, house	0	1	10
	Italian, low calorie	0	0	1
	Thousand Island	0	1	8
condiments				
cheese 1 slice	American	0	0	1
	Swiss style	0	0	1
croutons	.4 oz.	0	1	1
guacamole	.9 oz.	0	0	1
hot sauce pkt.		0	0	0
ketchup pkt.		0	0	0
mayonnaise pkt.		0	0	6
mustard pkt.		0	0	0
mustard pkt., Chinese hot		0	0	0
salsa	1 oz.	0	0	0
sour cream	1.1 oz.	0	0	2

FAST FOOD RESTAURANT FOOD ITEM	SPECIFICATIONS	PROTEIN BLOCKS	CARBOHYDRATE BLOCKS	FAT BLOCKS
desserts				
apple turnover		0	5	6
cheesecake		1	3	6
cheesecake, chocolate chip cookie dough		1	5	6
shakes	chocolate	1	8	2
	strawberry	1	7	2
	vanilla	1	7	2
KFC				
Original Recipe	breast	5	1	7
	drumstick	2	0	2
	thigh	3	1	6
	wing, whole	2	1	3
Colonel's Rotisserie Gold	breast/wing	6	0	6
	breast/wing, w/out skin	5	0	2
	thigh/leg	4	0	8
	thigh/leg w/out skin	4	0	4
Extra Tasty Crispy	breast	4	3	9
	drumstick	2	1	4
	thigh	3	2	8
	wing/whole	1	1	4
Hot and Spicy	breast	5	2	12
	drumstick	2	1	4
	thigh	3	1	9
	wing, whole	1	1	5
	chicken pot pie	4	7	13
Crispy Strips	4 pcs.	4	1	7
Hot Wings	6 pcs.	4	2	11
Kentucky Nuggets	6 pcs.	2	2	6
sandwiches				
chicken		4	5	7
Colonel's chicken		3	4	9
BBQ chicken		2	3	3
sides/specials				
BBQ baked beans		1	2	1
beans, red, and rice		1	2	1
biscuit		0	2	4
coleslaw		0	1	2
corn-on-the-cob		1	2	4
corn bread		0	3	4
garden rice		0	2	0
macaroni & cheese		1	2	3
mashed potato w/gravy		0	2	2
Mean Greens		0	1	1
potato salad		0	2	4
potato wedges		0	2	3

FAST FOOD RESTAURANT

FOOD ITEM	SPECIFICATIONS	PROTEIN BLOCKS	CARBOHYDRATE BLOCKS	FAT BLOCKS
LITTLE CAESARS				
Baby Pan!Pan!	2 sqs.	5	7	8
Crazy Bread		0	2	1
Crazy Sauce	6 oz.	1	1	0
Pan!Pan!, 1 medium slice	cheese only	1	2	2
	pepperoni	2	2	3
Pizza!Pizza!, 1 medium slice	cheese only	2	3	2
	pepperoni	2	3	3
salads, individual	antipasto	2	1	4
	Caesar	1	1	2
	Greek	1	1	3
	tossed	1	2	1
dressings, 1.5 oz.	blue cheese	0	1	5
	Caesar	0	0	9
	French	0	1	5
	Greek	0	0	10
	Italian	0	0	7
	Italian, fat free	0	0	0
	ranch	0	1	7
	Thousand Island	0	1	6
sandwich, cold	ham and cheese	4	8	12
	Italian	4	8	12
	veggie	3	8	10
sandwich, hot	Cheeser	6	8	13
	Meatsa	8	8	19
	pepperoni	6	8	16
	supreme	6	8	15
	veggie	5	8	8
LONG JOHN SILVER'S				
clams	3 oz.	2	3	6
chicken	batter-dipped, 1 pc.	1	1	2
	Flavorbaked, 1 pc.	3	0	1
	popcorn, 3.3 oz.	2	2	5
fish	batter-dipped, 1 pc.	2	1	4
	Flavorbaked, 1 pc.	2	0	1
	popcorn, 3.6 oz.	2	3	5
shrimp	batter-dipped, 1 pc.	0	0	1
	popcorn, 3.3 oz.	2	3	5
sandwiches 1 pc.				
chicken, *Flavorbaked*		3	3	3
fish, batter-dipped, w/out sauce		2	4	4
fish, *Flavorbaked*		3	3	5
Ultimate Fish		3	5	7
sides, 1 serving				
cheese sticks	1.6 oz.	1	1	3
coleslaw		0	2	2

FAST FOOD RESTAURANT FOOD ITEM	SPECIFICATIONS	PROTEIN BLOCKS	CARBOHYDRATE BLOCKS	FAT BLOCKS
corn cobbette, 1 pc.	w/butter	0	2	3
	plain	0	2	0
fries	3 oz.	0	3	5
green beans		0	0	0
hushpuppy	1 pc.	0	1	1
potato	baked	1	5	0
rice pilaf		0	3	2
side salad		0	0	0
dressings				
French	fat free, 1 1/2 oz.	0	2	0
Italian	1 oz.	0	0	5
ranch	1 oz.	0	0	6
	fat free, 1 1/2 oz.	0	1	0
Thousand Island	1 oz.	0	1	3
sauces, condiments				
honey mustard	.4 oz.	0	1	0
malt vinegar	.3 oz.	0	0	0
margarine	.2 oz.	0	0	1
shrimp sauce	.4 oz.	0	0	0
sour cream	1 oz.	0	0	2
sweet 'n' sour	.4 oz.	0	1	0
tartar sauce	.4 oz.	0	1	1

MCDONALD'S

breakfast biscuit	plain	1	3	4
	bacon, egg, and cheese	2	4	8
	sausage	1	3	10
	sausage and egg	2	4	12
breakfast burrito		2	2	7
breakfast dishes	eggs, scrambled, 2	2	0	4
	hash browns	0	1	3
	hotcakes, plain	1	6	2
	hotcakes, w/syrup, margarine	1	11	5
	sausage	1	0	5
breakfast muffin	English	1	3	1
	Egg McMuffin	2	3	4
	Sausage McMuffin	2	3	8
	Sausage McMuffin w/egg	3	3	10
danish and muffin	apple bran muffin	1	4	0
	apple danish	1	6	.5
	cheese danish	1	5	7
	cinnamon raisin danish	1	6	7
	cinnamon roll	1	5	7
	raspberry danish	1	6	5
sandwiches				
Arch Deluxe		4	4	10
Arch Deluxe, w/bacon		5	4	11

FAST FOODS

FAST FOOD RESTAURANT FOOD ITEM	SPECIFICATIONS	PROTEIN BLOCKS	CARBOHYDRATE BLOCKS	FAT BLOCKS
Big Mac		4	5	9
cheeseburger		2	4	5
Filet-O-Fish		2	4	5
hamburger		2	4	3
McChicken		2	5	10
McGrilled Chicken Classic		3	3	1
Quarter Pounder		3	4	7
Quarter Pounder, w/cheese		4	4	7
Chicken McNuggets	4 pcs.	2	1	4
	6 pcs.	3	2	6
	9 pcs.	4	3	9
McNuggets sauce pkt.	barbeque	0	1	0
	honey	0	1	0
	honey mustard	0	0	2
	hot mustard	0	1	1
	sweet and sour	0	1	0
french fries	small	0	3	3
	large	1	6	7
	Super Size	1	7	9
salads	chicken, fajita	3	1	2
	garden	1	1	1
salad bacon bits	1 pkg.	0	0	0
salad croutons	1 pkg.	0	1	1
salad dressing, 1 pkg.	blue cheese	0	1	6
	ranch	0	1	7
	red French, reduced calorie	0	3	3
	Thousand Island	0	2	4
	vinaigrette, lite	0	1	1
desserts and shakes				
baked apple pie		0	4	4
McDonaldland Cookies	1 pkg.	1	4	3
shake, small	chocolate	2	7	2
	strawberry	2	7	2
	vanilla	2	7	2
sundae	hot fudge	1	6	2
sundae nuts	1/4 oz.	0	0	1
yogurt, frozen, lowfat	cone, vanilla	1	3	0
	hot caramel sundae	1	7	1
	strawberry sundae	1	6	0

PIZZA HUT

1 slice of medium pie, except as noted				
Bigfoot 1 slice	cheese	1	3	2
	pepperoni	1	3	2
	pepperoni, mushroom, and sausage	2	3	3
breadsticks	5 pcs.	3	14	5

FAST FOOD RESTAURANT FOOD ITEM	SPECIFICATIONS	PROTEIN BLOCKS	CARBOHYDRATE BLOCKS	FAT BLOCKS
hand-tossed	cheese	2	3	2
	beef	2	3	3
	ham	2	3	2
	Meat Lovers	2	3	4
	pepperoni	2	3	3
	Pepperoni Lovers	2	3	0
	pork topping	2	3	3
	sausage, Italian	2	3	4
	supreme	2	3	4
	supreme, super	2	3	4
	Veggie Lovers	2	3	2
pan pizza	cheese	2	3	4
	beef	2	3	4
	ham	2	3	7
	Meat Lovers	2	3	6
	pepperoni	2	3	4
	Pepperoni Lovers	2	3	6
	pork topping	2	3	5
	sausage, Italian	2	3	5
	supreme	2	3	5
	supreme, super	2	3	6
	Veggie Lovers	1	3	3
Personal Pan Pizza, 1 pie	pepperoni	4	7	9
	supreme	5	7	11
Thin 'N Crispy	cheese	2	2	3
	beef	2	2	4
	ham	1	2	2
	Meat Lovers	2	2	4
	pepperoni	2	2	3
	Pepperoni Lovers	2	2	5
	pork topping	2	2	4
	sausage, Italian	2	2	4
	supreme	2	2	4
	supreme, super	2	2	5
	Veggie Lovers	1	2	2

SIZZLER

hot entrees

hamburger on bun	w/lettuce, tomato	6	4	11
chicken breast	5 oz.	4	1	1
hibachi, w/pineapple		4	0	1
Santa Fe		4	0	1
Malibu chicken patty		3	1	6
salmon	8 oz.	5	0	4
shrimp, broiled	5 oz.	3	0	2
shrimp, fried	4 pcs.	3	4	1
shrimp, mini	4 oz.	2	3	0
shrimp scampi	5 oz.	4	0	1

FAST FOODS

FAST FOOD RESTAURANT FOOD ITEM	SPECIFICATIONS	PROTEIN BLOCKS	CARBOHYDRATE BLOCKS	FAT BLOCKS
steak, Dakota, ranch	6 oz.	4	0	7
	8 oz.	5	0	9
	9.5 oz.	7	0	11
swordfish	8 oz.	6	0	5
side dishes				
cheese toast		1	2	7
french fries	4 oz.	1	5	4
potato, baked, pulp		0	2	0
rice pilaf	6 oz.	1	5	2
sauces 1 1/2 oz.	buttery dipping	0	0	12
	cocktail sauce	0	1	0
	hibachi sauce	0	1	0
	Malibu sauce	0	0	10
	sour dressing	0	0	3
	tartar sauce	0	1	6
hot bar				
chicken wings	1 oz.	1	0	7
focaccia bread	2 pcs.	0	1	2
marinara sauce	1 oz.	0	0	0
meatballs	4	1	0	4
nacho sauce	2 oz.	1	0	3
pasta, fettuccine	2 oz.	0	2	0
pasta, spaghetti	2 oz.	0	2	0
potato skins	2 oz.	0	2	3
refried beans	1/4 cup	1	1	0
saltines	2 pcs.	0	0	0
taco filling	2 oz.	0	0	3
taco shells	1 pc.	0	1	1
soup, 4 oz.	broccoli, cheese	0	1	3
	chicken noodle soup	0	0	0
	clam chowder	0	1	2
	minestrone soup	0	1	0
	vegetable sirloin	1	1	1
salads, prepared, 2 oz.				
carrot and raisin		0	1	3
Chinese chicken		1	1	1
jicama, spicy		0	0	0
Mediterranean Minted Fruit		0	1	0
Mexican Fiesta		0	1	0
pasta, seafood, Louis		0	1	1
potato, old-fashioned		0	1	2
potato, red herb		0	1	3
seafood Louis		0	0	1
teriyaki beef		1	0	1
tuna pasta		1	1	3
dressings, 1 oz.				
blue cheese		0	0	4

FAST FOOD RESTAURANT FOOD ITEM	SPECIFICATIONS	PROTEIN BLOCKS	CARBOHYDRATE BLOCKS	FAT BLOCKS
guacamole		0	0	1
honey mustard		0	0	5
Italian, lite		0	0	0
Parmesan, Italian		0	0	3
ranch		0	0	4
ranch, lite		0	0	3
rice vinegar, Japanese		0	0	0
salsa		0	0	0
sour dressing		0	0	2
Thousand Island		0	0	5

WENDY'S

sandwiches

		PROTEIN	CARBOHYDRATE	FAT
bacon cheeseburger, Jr.		3	4	7
Big Bacon Classic		5	5	11
cheeseburger	Jr.	2	4	4
	Jr., Deluxe	3	4	5
	Kid's Meal	2	3	4
chicken	grilled	3	4	2
	breaded	4	5	6
	spicy	3	4	7
	club	5	5	8
hamburger	single, plain	4	3	5
	single, everything	4	4	7
	Jr.	2	4	3
	Kid's Meal	2	3	3

sandwich components

		PROTEIN	CARBOHYDRATE	FAT
American cheese		0	0	2
American cheese Jr.		0	0	1
bacon	1 slice	0	0	1
ketchup	1 tsp.	0	0	0
mayonnaise	1 1/2 tsp.	0	0	1
mustard	1/2 tsp.	0	0	0
onion	4 rings	0	0	0
pickles	4 slices	0	0	0
chicken nuggets	5 pcs.	2	1	5
nuggets sauce, 1 oz.	barbeque	0	1	0
	honey	0	1	0
	honey mustard	0	1	4
	spicy buffalo wing	0	0	1
	sweet and sour	0	1	0
chili	small, 8 oz.	2	2	2
	large, 12 oz.	3	3	3
	cheddar cheese, shredded, 2 Tbsp.	1	0	2
	saltine crackers, 2	0	0	0
baked potato	plain	1	7	0

FAST FOODS

FOOD ITEM	SPECIFICATIONS	PROTEIN BLOCKS	CARBOHYDRATE BLOCKS	FAT BLOCKS
	bacon and cheese	2	8	6
	broccoli and cheese	1	8	5
	cheese	2	8	8
	chili and cheese	3	8	8
	sour cream w/chive	1	7	2
fries	small	0	3	4
	medium	1	5	6
	Biggie	1	6	8
Salads-to-go, fresh, w/out dressing	deluxe garden	1	1	2
	grilled chicken	4	1	3
	side salad	1	0	1
	side salad, Caesar	1	1	2
	taco salad	4	5	10
	soft breadstick	1	3	1
dressing, 2 Tbsp.	blue cheese	0	0	6
	French	0	1	3
	French, fat free	0	1	0
	French, sweet red	0	1	3
	Italian, reduced fat/calorie	0	0	1
	Italian, Caesar	0	0	5
	ranch, *Hidden Valley*	0	0	3
	ranch, *Hidden Valley*, reduced fat/calorie	0	0	2
	Thousand Island	0	0	4
desserts	chocolate chip cookie	1	4	4
	Frosty, small	1	6	3
	Frosty, medium	2	8	4
	Frosty, large	2	10	6

APPENDIX

A. ZONE BLOCK HELP

The average female will need meals consisting of three blocks, and the average male will require meals containing four blocks. If you want even more precision, refer to *Mastering the Zone* or call this toll-free information line which will provide you with an analysis of your percent body fat, your lean body mass, and the number of Zone Food Blocks you need per day: 1-800-233-3426. The analysis only takes a few seconds over the phone, and all the information you need will be sent to you in a hard copy format.

Make sure you have the following information ready:

Females:

(1) Your barefoot height in inches.
(2) Your waist measurement in inches at your belly button.
(3) Your hip measurement in inches at the widest point.

Males:

(1) Your weight in pounds.
(2) Your waist measurement in inches at your belly button.
(3) Your wrist measurement in inches of your dominant hand just inside your wrist bone.

B. COMPUTER PROGRAMS BASED ON THE ZONE FOOD BLOCK METHOD

A very simple-to-use program called *Mastering the Zone* has been written by Dr. Rene Espy. This program will not only calculate your percent body fat and Zone Food Block requirements, but will also scale any of the meals found in *Mastering the Zone* and *Zone Perfect Meals in Minutes* to you (or your family's) unique block requirements and print out a shopping list for those food items. In addition, it will allow you to make your own Zone meals based on Zone Food Blocks. This program is available for both IBM-compatibles and Macintosh computers.

Another recommended computer program would be Zone Manager 2.0. Although similar in nature to *Mastering the Zone*, this program is based on grams, not Zone Food Blocks. This program is only available for IBM-compatible computers.

For more information on either of these programs, call 1-800-233-3426.